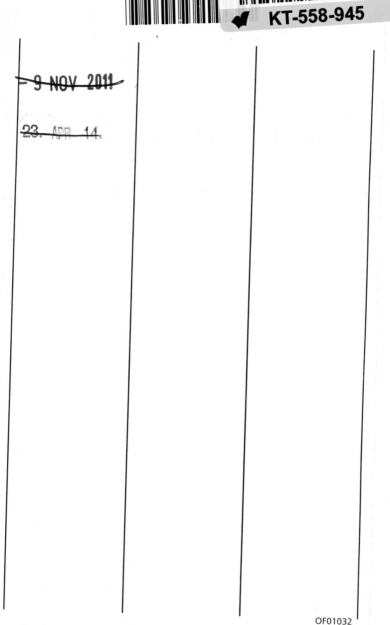

Books should be returned to the SDH Library on or before
the date stamped above unless a renewal has been arranged

Salisbury District Hospital Library

Telephone: Salisbury (01722) 336262 extn. 4430 / 33
Out of hours answer machine in operation

Contemporary Play Therapy

Theory, Research, and Practice

Edited by
CHARLES E. SCHAEFER
HEIDI GERARD KADUSON

THE GUILFORD PRESS
New York   London

©2006 The Guilford Press
A Division of Guilford Publications, Inc.
72 Spring Street, New York, NY 10012
www.guilford.com

Printed in the United States of America

This book is printed on acid-free paper.

Last digit is print number: 9 8 7 6 5 4 3 2

Library of Congress Cataloging-in-Publication Data

Contemporary play therapy: theory, research, and practice / edited by Charles
E. Schaefer, Heidi Gerard Kaduson.
    p. cm.
  Includes bibliographical references and index.
  ISBN-13: 978-1-59385-304-4 ISBN-10: 1-59385-304-1 (hardcover : alk. paper)
  ISBN-13: 978-1-59385-633-5 ISBN-10: 1-59385-633-4 (paperback : alk. paper)
  1. Play therapy. I. Schaefer, Charles E. II. Kaduson, Heidi.
  RJ505.P6C67 2006
  618.92′891653—dc22

               2006006359

To our children—
Karine, Eric, Jay, Nicole, and Kimberly—
for showing us the true meaning of play

About the Editors

Charles E. Schaefer, PhD, RPT-S, a nationally renowned child psychologist, is Professor of Psychology at Fairleigh Dickinson University in Teaneck, New Jersey. He is cofounder and director emeritus of the Association for Play Therapy, and founder and codirector of the Play Therapy Training Institute in Hightstown, New Jersey. He has written or edited more than 50 books on parenting, child psychology, and play therapy, including *The Therapeutic Use of Child's Play, Foundations of Play Therapy, Handbook of Play Therapy, Play Therapy with Adolescents,* and *Empirically Based Play Interventions for Children.* Dr. Schaefer maintains a private practice in child psychotherapy in Hackensack, New Jersey.

Heidi Gerard Kaduson, PhD, RPT-S, specializes in evaluation and intervention services for children with a variety of behavioral, emotional, and learning problems. She is past president of the Association for Play Therapy and codirector of the Play Therapy Training Institute. She has lectured internationally on play therapy, attention-deficit/hyperactivity disorder, and learning disabilities. Dr. Kaduson's publications include *The Playing Cure* and *101 Favorite Play Therapy Techniques* (Volumes I, II, and III). With Charles E. Schaefer, she is coeditor of *Short-Term Play Therapy for Children, Second Edition.* Dr. Kaduson maintains a private practice in child psychotherapy in Monroe Township, New Jersey.

Contributors

Jennifer Baggerly, PhD, LMHC-S, RPT-S, is Associate Professor
in the Counselor Education Program at the University of South Florida,
Tampa, Florida.

Helen E. Benedict, PhD, RPT-S, is Professor and Director of Clinical Training
in the Department of Psychology and Neuroscience at Baylor University,
Waco, Texas.

David Bond, LCSW, is a therapist at the Chadwick Center for Children
and Families, Children's Hospital and Health Center, San Diego, California.

Ann Cattanach PhD, MSc, RDth, is a child care consultant therapist in
Scotland. She is also a Teaching Fellow at the University of York,
United Kingdom.

Kristin Condon, PsyD, is Director of School Consultation Programming
and Director of Training, Shared Vision, Inc., Oak Brook, Illinois.

Erika Felix, PhD, is a researcher at the Center for School-Based Youth
Development, University of California, Santa Barbara, California.

Bess Sirmon Fjordbak, MS, CCC-SLP, is in the Department of Communication
Sciences and Disorders at the University of Georgia, Athens, Georgia.

Ulrike Franke, RPT-S, CTT-T, SLP, SLP-T, is Assistant Professor
in the Department of Special Education at the Educational College
in Heidelberg, Germany, and in private practice in Oftersheim, Germany.

Steve Harvey, PhD, ADTR, RDT, RPT-S, is a consultant psychologist
at the Taranaki District Health Board, New Plymouth, New Zealand.

Kathryn S. Jacobi, PsyD, is Chief Psychologist at the child development center
of one of Israel's central region HMOs. She also has a private practice
in Zichron Yaacov, Israel.

Mary Margaret Kelly, PhD, is Professor in the Department of Psychology at Millersville University, Millersville, Pennsylvania.

Myra M. Lawrence, PsyD, is Professor at the Illinois School of Professional Psychology, Argosy University/Chicago, and CEO and Clinical Director of Shared Vision, Inc., Oak Brook, Illinois.

Debra May, LLAM, Dip SW, MA Play Therapy, is in private practice, Grimsby, United Kingdom.

Emily Nicholson, PsyD, is a postdoctoral fellow at Shared Vision, Inc., Oak Brook, Illinois.

Byron E. Norton, EdD, is a psychologist with Family Psychological Services in Greeley, Colorado.

Carol C. Norton, EdD, is a psychologist with Family Psychological Services in Greeley, Colorado.

Hope C. Odenwalt, MS, is an adjunct professor in the Department of Psychology at Millersville University, Millersville, Pennsylvania. She provides crisis intervention services in Lancaster, Pennsylvania.

Dee C. Ray, PhD, LPC, NCC, RPT-S, is Assistant Professor and Director of the Child and Family Resource Clinic in the Counseling Program at the University of North Texas, Denton, Texas.

Roberto Robles, LCSW, works for Kaiser Permanente in Northern California and is a child development instructor at the University of California at Davis Extension, Davis, California.

Janine Shelby, PhD, RPT-S, is Director of the Child Trauma Clinic at Harbor–UCLA Medical Center, Los Angeles, California.

Herbert H. G. Wettig, Dipl-Psych, is principal and senior researcher at the Theraplay Institute in Leonberg, Germany.

Paul R. White, LCSW, is in private practice in Rockford, Illinois.

Preface

Play therapy is the oldest and most popular form of child therapy. Widely practiced across the world, it is expanding at an exponential rate. Most child mental health professionals are well aware of the fact that it is through play that children are best able to form therapeutic alliances, express themselves, relate to others, learn new knowledge and skills, boost their egos, master stress, and develop their sense of self.

Over the past decade, the practice of play therapy has witnessed a number of innovations and refinements of existing procedures. The goal of this volume is to present a state-of-the-art overview of the latest advances and developments in the field, including the three main pillars of play therapy: theory, research, and practice.

The reader will learn the latest advances in narrative, dynamic, experiential, and object relations play therapy from distinguished experts in each domain. An update on the status of the growing movement toward evidence-based play therapy is provided, together with descriptions of research on the effectiveness of specific play interventions, such as Theraplay and play therapy with homeless children. Also described are guidelines on using play therapy with sexually abused children, adolescent girls displaying relational aggression, and victims of natural disasters, as well as a discussion of culturally competent play therapy with Latino clients. In addition, practical strategies for the effective use of clay play and for promoting resiliency in children are detailed.

The new directions and applications in play therapy found in this book should be of interest to both beginning and experienced play therapists who wish to keep abreast of this evolving field.

CHARLES E. SCHAEFER
HEIDI G. KADUSON

Contents

PART III. APPLICATIONS

PART I

THEORY

CHAPTER 1

Object Relations Play Therapy

Applications to Attachment Problems and Relational Trauma

HELEN E. BENEDICT

Object relations play therapy is a relational approach to play therapy grounded in attachment-based object relations theory. This approach uses play therapy techniques to provide a developmentally appropriate intervention for young children who show emotional and behavioral problems. Object relations theories, including the attachment theory of John Bowlby (1988) as well as theoretical formulations of Donald Winnicott (1965, 1971a, 1971b) and Margaret Mahler, are interpersonal and relational models of human development and functioning (Mahler & Furer, 1968; Mahler, Pine, & Bergman, 1975). Thus, object relations play therapy focuses on the relationship between the therapist and child in a play setting to help the child with difficulties experienced in interpersonal relationships.

THEORETICAL BACKGROUND

Object relations theories are a loosely organized collection of models that share certain fundamental assumptions (Glickhauf-Hughes & Wells, 1997). While each model has proposed unique understandings, all the models are held together by three basic ideas. First, object relations theorists believe that interpersonal relationships are the central motivational force of human development. Research has provided considerable support for this assumption. For example, infants' sensory capacities, from the distance of optimal visual focus to the well-documented preference for attending to facial configurations, are specifically prepared to respond to human interactions (Sigelman & Rider, 2005). Similarly, recent work in neuroscience has shown that early brain development is experience-dependent, requiring attuned interactive events to develop fully (Schore, 2003).

The second assumption is that humans, through experiences relating to others, develop cognitive-affective structures about the self, the other, and the relationships between them, called object relations. These structures, or internal working models, develop slowly over the first 2–3 years of life and depend for their development on the actual interactions between the infant and others as well as the infant's perceptions of those interactions. Over time, the experiences and perceptions become encoded as cognitive-affective templates that serve to guide both the understanding of self and others and actual behavior in relationships (Bowlby, 1988).

The third assumption is that object relations start to develop at the beginning of life, initially through the relationship between the infant and the primary caregiver or attachment figure. The initial object relations develop a basic structure in the first few years of life following a pattern that is neurologically based and dependent on the nature of the infant's interpersonal experiences. These object relations influence the child's interpersonal relationships and are also influenced by ongoing relationships. In therapy, the therapist–child relationship becomes an arena where internal working models that are maladaptive can be altered into object relations that are more adaptive in the child's world.

Object relations theorists argue that the development of object relations over the first 3 years of life creates relatively enduring patterns of interpersonal relationships. These patterns emerge out of two important developmental processes: the development of attachment and the development of appropriate autonomy within that attachment relationship. Considerable research on the development of attachment has revealed wide individual differences in the security of attachment, ranging from secure attachment through insecure avoidant or resistant attachments and disorganized attachment to disorders of nonattachment (Hinshaw-Fuselier, Heller, Parton, Robinson, & Boris, 2004; Schuder & Lyons-Ruth, 2004; Zeanah & Boris, 2000). Similarly, the process of developing appropriate autonomy, as elaborated in Margaret Mahler's model of separation-individuation, shows variability in the infant's and toddler's ability to achieve what Mahler called "emotional object constancy"

(Mahler & Furer, 1968; Mahler et al., 1975). Thus, the enduring object relational patterns that emerge in the first 3 years can range from healthy, adaptive internal working models to maladaptive internal working models associated strongly with various types of developmental psychopathology in childhood and adulthood.

Psychotherapy, including play therapy, based on an object relations model proposes that change occurs when a "secure-base" relationship exists between the therapist and child. Within this relationship, the therapist, by failing to conform to the maladaptive expectations of the child's negative internal working models, challenges the child to amend those maladaptive object relations in healthy directions (Benedict, 2003; Benedict & Hastings, 2002).

CHARACTERISTICS OF OBJECT RELATIONS PLAY THERAPY

The core feature of object relations play therapy is clearly the relationship between the therapist and the child. Developing a secure-base relationship with the child is the first and most important task for the therapist (Lieberman & Van Horn, 2004). A secure-base relationship is one in which the child experiences attachment to the therapist coupled with a sense of safety in the relationship, freeing the child to explore his or her psychological world (Bowlby, 1988). This task presents a considerable challenge to the therapist because those children most likely to be helped by object relations play therapy are those who have experienced relational trauma early in life and have emerged from the first 3 years of development with attachment and/or relational problems. As such, they are typically slow to trust others, have primarily negative internal working models of the self and others, and often resist interpersonal connections because of the pain associated with previous relational traumas (Hinshaw-Fuselier et al., 2004; Schore, 2003; Schuder & Lyons-Ruth, 2004).

The process of building a secure-base relationship with the child can require both considerable time and diligent attention to the characteristics of the therapist and the setting. Foremost among the therapist characteristics needed for successful development of a secure-base relationship is attunement. Attunement, a term taken from the attachment research literature, is best defined as "interactive synchrony," in which the caregiver or therapist deliberately tunes her activities to the child's cues during interaction, engaging when the child signals readiness and allowing the child to disengage when he or she feels it is necessary (Schore, 2003). For the therapist, such attunement can be facilitated by adopting a child-responsive stance to therapy (Benedict, 2003). Instead of adopting either a directive or nondirective approach, the therapist chooses her activity level and degree of directiveness in response to cues from the child. Another important facet of attunement is assuring that all the therapist's responses and behaviors are matched to the child's developmental level.

Several other therapist characteristics and behaviors can be identified that facilitate the development of the therapist–child relationship. As is true of most therapy approaches, the therapist needs to be warm and accepting of the child. In addition, the therapist must be emotionally constant for the child. This entails maintaining predictability about her behaviors and reactions as well as providing a constant therapeutic environment. The latter can be achieved by limiting changes in the play materials, preserving traces of the child's play, and having a box (like a locker) where the child can leave personal things in the playroom knowing other children will not disturb his or her things.

To facilitate the development of a secure-base therapeutic relationship, it is essential the therapist ensure that the playroom is both psychologically and physically safe for the child (Benedict & Mongoven, 1997). Physical safety, while typically easy to maintain for most young children, is difficult to provide when the child has experienced relational trauma. Such children often have poor self-regulation and a negative sense of self, both of which can lead to dangerous and risky behaviors by the child (Schuder & Lyons-Ruth, 2004; Zeanah & Boris, 2000).

Psychological safety is both harder to define and more difficult to provide. All of the characteristics already described, including attunement, child-responsiveness, warmth and acceptance, developmental appropriateness, and constancy, contribute to the child's sense of safety. The therapist's ability to contain intense, poorly controlled, and negative affects such as rage, shame, and despair while maintaining acceptance of the child also contributes to the child's perceived psychological safety. Finally, allowing the child to control the interaction and activities (except where the child's or therapist's safety is threatened) also increases the child's sense of safety. One way to do this is to use an "invitational" approach when responding in an attuned fashion to the child's cues for the therapist to be directive (Gil, 1991). Invitations, in this context, are potential directives by the therapist that may serve to alter the direction of play or offer interpretations. They are invitational in nature because they are offered by the therapist in a tentative manner; there are no negative consequences should the child choose to decline or ignore the invitation.

Once the therapist–child relationship has been established, the second phase of therapy begins. During this phase, the goal of therapy is to modify the child's object relations or internal working models. This overarching goal is achieved in several ways, all of which involve challenging the existing maladaptive object relations. These challenges occur both through the relationship between the child and therapist and through the child's play.

Many challenges to the child's object relations occur within the therapist–child relationship. Once the therapist–child relationship is developed, the child feels attachment to the therapist and, thus, closely attends to the therapist's attitudes and behaviors. Where, in the past, the child often experienced trauma in relationships, in the therapy situation, the child is no longer traumatized. Each time the therapist fails to confirm the child's expectation of a negative interaction with a significant other, the negative internal working model is challenged. For example, a negative internal working model of the other would lead to expectations that others will hurt one. When the child experiences the therapist as accepting and attuned regardless of the child's behavior, the child's internal working model of the other becomes open to the idea that not all people are going to hurt one. Similarly, a negative object relation of the self, that the self is bad and unlovable, would begin to shift to the idea that maybe the self is actually lovable. Just as it required innumerable interactions to form the object relations in the first place, it requires many reiterations of such challenging interactions to shift the child's object relations.

Challenges to the child's object relations and healing of the memories and cognitions arising from relational trauma also occur through play. When a child has experienced relational trauma, he or she acquires distorted cognitions of causation and time, intense, negative affective reactions toward many people and things in his or her world, and traumatic affect-laden memories in addition to the maladaptive object relations described earlier. These distorted cognitions and affects and traumatic memories often must be resolved before the child can begin to heal the negative internal working models that have emerged out of the traumatic relationships. Sometimes, they interfere with developing a secure-base therapist–child relationship. Play, especially thematic play, is an important avenue to correcting distorted cognitive understandings and resolving both affective reactions and traumatic memories. Some of this work actually occurs during the initial relationship development phase of therapy, while much of it occurs in the second phase of therapy.

Thematic play is where the child imagines roles, relationships, and events and enacts these through playful use of objects, role play, and actions. For young children, thematic play serves as a communicative medium to convey their concerns, feelings, and ideas. Thus, for the child, play is a language that is far more fluent than words. In play therapy, it is often the therapist's understanding of and response to the child's play that facilitates therapeutic change. Extensive research (Benedict, 1997, 2004a; Benedict & Hastings, 2002; Benedict et al., 1996) has shown that children play a variety of easily recognizable themes, varying the characters and outcomes repeatedly to convey unique meanings, including aggressive themes (e.g., good guy–bad guy, aggressor–victim, and death play), family themes (e.g., separation, reunion, and nurturance), and safety themes (e.g., danger and rescue). An example of an aggressive theme would be for a child to make a dinosaur puppet attack a baby alligator and then have the daddy alligator bite the dinosaur. A nurturing theme could be a child making dinner and then feeding the therapist (who, on the child's instruction, was pretending to be a child). The therapist, by identifying the child's themes and their possible meanings, can begin to understand the child's psychological world. Using the child-responsive invitations described earlier, the therapist can communicate to the child within the metaphor and enable the child to use the play to gain resolution and new understanding of troubling feelings, cognitions, and memories.

Research identifying play themes has revealed that complete understanding of the child's play not only requires recognizing its themes, but also identifying the affects and interpersonal interactions presented through it (Benedict, 2004a; Benedict, Hastings, Ato, Carson, & Nash, 1998). These affects (e.g., sadness, anger, and jealousy) and interpersonal interactions (e.g., helping, sharing, protecting, and controlling) can also be reliably identified by sensitive therapists. Most important, the affects and interactions identified give a relatively direct view of the child's internal working models of self, other, and relationships between self and other. With this understanding, the therapist can use child-responsive invitations to challenge the distorted and negative object relations through play. Thus, thematic play is central to both the healing of traumatic experiences and challenging the child's object relations.

Object relations play therapy, a relational, developmental approach to young children, is most effective when used with children who have experienced relational trauma, especially when the trauma was experienced in the first 5 years of life. Relational trauma, as we see in the next section, typically leads to disturbed attachment relationships and negative or distorted object relations or ideas about the self, other, and relationships between self and other. Object relations play therapy directly addresses the primary therapeutic needs of relationally traumatized children. It addresses relationship issues and the child's internal working model and helps resolve specific trauma-related cognitions, affects, and memories.

APPLICATIONS TO ATTACHMENT
AND RELATIONAL TRAUMA

A growing body of research and clinical work has confirmed that relational traumas, such as abuse, family violence, and disrupted attachment, are tragically common in children's lives. Research has also confirmed that such experiences, especially in the first 3 years of life, have long-term consequences for the child and correlate with later development of significant psychopathology. It has long been recognized that attachment does not always develop in a secure manner (Ainsworth, Blehar, Waters, & Wall, 1978; Main & Solomon, 1986). Recent research has identified many of the factors, such as abuse or maltreatment, associated with insecure attachment or attachment failure (Cassidy & Shaver, 1999; Schore, 1994; Stern, 1985). It has become increasingly evident that any significant disruption of the attuned caregiving needed by the infant constitutes relational trauma. The typical outcome of relational trauma is some type of insecure attachment or failure to attach (Schuder & Lyons-Ruth, 2004).

There are many circumstances now recognized in which "good-enough mothering" (Winnicott, 1965) does not occur. These impeding circumstances to forming a secure attachment may take several forms. They include biologically based impediments coming from the infant, such as unrecognized hearing impairment, autism, or extreme prematurity, and the various forms of easily recognized "grossly pathological care," such as neglect or abuse (Cicchetti, Toth, & Lynch, 1995; American Psychiatric Association, 1994). The impediment can also occur in more subtle ways with caregivers unable to provide attuned care to the infant for a variety of reasons. Such caregivers might frighten, fail to soothe, or fail to attune to the infant (Hinshaw-Fuselier et al., 2004; Schuder & Lyons-Ruth, 2004).

Just as there are many contributing factors to the development of insecure attachment or the failure to attach, there are many symptomatic presentations of children who have experienced relational trauma (Hinshaw-Fuselier et al., 2004; Lieberman & Pawl, 1988; Zeanah & Boris, 2000; Zeanah, Mammen, & Lieberman, 1993; Zero to Three, 1994). Zeanah and his colleagues propose that relational trauma can best be understood and treated by examining three broad categories of attachment disorders.

First, they describe disorders of nonattachment, or reactive attachment disorders of infancy and early childhood (RAD; American Psychiatric Association, 1994). The second category has been labeled secure-base distortions and has four different presentations identified. The final category, according to Zeanah and his colleagues, is disrupted attachment, a category that has recently been described in more detail by Hinshaw-Fuselier and her colleagues (2004). Each of these presentations is described in more detail below.

Disorders of nonattachment, or RAD, has been recognized as a clinical disorder at least since the publication of DSM-III in 1980. Two subtypes of nonattachment have been identified in terms of the child's characteristic way of interacting with others. In the inhibited type, the child typically is withdrawn and resists interaction with others. In the disinhibited type, the child is indiscriminately social, seeks interaction with strangers, and shows no preferred attachment figure. Both subtypes have in common disturbances in seeking comfort, showing affect, exploring of the environment, and self-regulation. This is the most pathological type of attachment problem, and successful intervention is both extremely challenging and time-consuming. More and more, these children are being presented for treatment. Most of them have experienced extreme forms of relational trauma, including prolonged orphanage care with subsequent adoption, severe abuse and neglect, and/or repeated foster placements.

Secure-base distortions, the second broad category, occur when the child remains in the care of the original caregiver but has developed an insecure attachment with him or her. This insecure attachment can be primarily avoidant, resistant (or ambivalent), or disorganized, a distinction based on the interaction between the mother and child in the strange situation paradigm (Cicchetti et al., 1995). Zeanah's group proposed that there are four subtypes of secure-base distortions: self-endangerment; clinging/inhibited; hypercompliance/vigilance; and role reversal (Zeanah & Boris, 2000).

The first type of secure-base distortion is labeled self-endangerment. These children typically explore the environment freely but do not consistently maintain a "safe haven" with the caregiver. As a result, they often engage in reckless, dangerous, and provocative behavior and are especially likely to do so when in the presence of the primary caregiver. They also exhibit aggression, which can be self-directed or directed at the caregiver. In many ways, they and disinhibited nonattached children present similar challenges to the therapist; the similar treatment of these two groups is discussed later (Benedict, 2004b).

Secure-base distortions can also present as clinging and inhibited. These children refuse to separate from the caregiver and do not readily explore new settings. This distortion is most likely to be seen when in a new situation with the caregiver present. These children can appear quite ambivalent about the caregiver, alternating affectionate or clingy behavior with resistance to relational initiatives made by the caregiver. Often, their behavior becomes less clingy when the situation becomes familiar, but they remain inhibited and do not readily engage in activities or social relationships. These children experience a subtle relational trauma through difficult relationships with the caregiver. These relationships can include such patterns as overly restrictive parenting, emotional neglect, or parents who have a preoccupied adult attachment pattern (Siegel, 1999).

A third type of secure-base distortion, hypercompliance/vigilance, seems to be the presentation most likely when there is overt physical abuse, family violence, or other overt trauma (Kirkpatrick & Williams, 1997; Kolbo, Blakely, & Engelman, 1996; Levoy, Rivinus, Matzko, & McGuire, 1991; Prior, 1996; Wooley, 1998) . The symptoms seen in such children overlap with those of posttraumatic stress disorder (American Psychiatric Association, 1994). The children are inhibited in exploring the environment, emotionally constricted and watchful, hypervigilant, and hypercompliant. They seem more afraid of displeasing the caregiver than of separating from the caregiver. Thus, while much of their presenting behavior is similar to children in the clinging/inhibited type, other behaviors, including their play, are quite different (Benedict, 2004b).

The final subtype of secure-base distortion is called role reversal (Zeanah & Boris, 2000). Other clinicians tend to call these children "burdened" or "parentified" (Hall, 1996; Hastings, 2001; Jurkovic, 1997; Kaplan, 1997; Solomon, George, & DeJong, 1995). Children who show role reversal seem preoccupied with the well-being of the caregiver. Indeed, the relationship seems to be inverted, with the child assuming responsibility for the caregiver rather than the caregiver assuming responsibility for the child. Such children can be extremely controlling with the caregiver and, in therapy, with the therapist. They tend to show hyperindependence and will often ignore hurts and needs to avoid seeking or accepting help or comfort from others. These children are often living with caregivers who have significant psychopathology, especially personality disorders, dissociative disorders, or a combination of substance abuse problems with depression or personality problems. As with the other types of secure-base distortions, this type requires special adjustments on the part of the therapist for therapy to succeed.

The third category of attachment disorders is disrupted attachment. In their original formulation, Zeanah and Boris (2000) gave few details of the behaviors of this group. From my clinical work, it appeared that the behavior and clinical needs of these children varied with the type of attachment relationship they had had with the caregiver before the disruption (Benedict, 2004b). Boris was subsequently part of a working group that proposed a new category called disrupted attachment disorder, or DAD (Hinshaw-Fuselier et al., 2004). The group suggested that the attachment relationship before the disruption was important, distinguishing between secure and insecure attachments. However, it also felt that the disruption itself was sufficiently stressful to cause problems even when there was a previously secure attachment relationship with the departed caregiver. Thus, the group suggested that the disruption elicits one or more of the following behaviors: irritability, angry protest, searching for the missing caregiver, clinginess with the replacement caregiver, and/or anger or withdrawal at reminders of the lost caregiver. Accompanying symptoms may include lack of play, diminished appetite or hoarding, disrupted sleep patterns, flat or sad affect, emotional withdrawal, or lethargy. This syndrome requires treatment even with securely attached children. The difficulties are multiplied exponentially when the child and departed caregiver had an insecure relationship. This latter group of children often presents the greatest challenge to therapists. In addition, for all children with disrupted attachment, the discontinuity in the caregiving relationship further complicates clinical interventions including play therapy because of the unique issues presented by the new caregiver.

Clearly, relational trauma in young children is a complex phenomenon. Children can present with a wide variety of symptoms that can result from the interplay of multiple causal factors. Object relations play therapy, because it focuses on the child–therapist relationship and modifying the particular child's maladaptive internal working models of relationships, is ideally suited to make appropriate adjustments in treatment in light of these variations. In the following section, several cases are presented. Each case highlights one of the attachment disorder presentations described above. The dynamic issues presented by the child are characterized along with the specific treatment goals most suited to that attachment presentation. Then the actual play therapy techniques used to achieve those goals are outlined and the treatment of the child summarized. Because this chapter is focused on play therapy, most of the details of related work with the parents or caregivers have been omitted. For all cases, all identifying details have been altered to protect the confidentiality of the child and family, although the clinical issues and techniques specific to the attachment problem presented have been retained.

CASE EXAMPLES

Nonattached Attachment

History

Meghan, a 6-year-old girl, is the first-born of two daughters of middle-class parents. Her birth was unremarkable, and her parents assumed she was developing normally until she became a toddler. They noticed a lack of interest in language and had her evaluated when she was 20 months old. She was discovered to have severe bilateral hearing loss. While she could hear loud sounds, she had no ability to hear more moderate levels of sound, including human speech. It took slightly more than a year to fit her with hearing aids. With these aids, her hearing is close to normal, and she is currently attending public school while receiving speech and other resource services for significant language delay.

Symptoms

Meghan is a talkative, friendly little girl whose speech is mostly but not completely understandable. She approaches strangers readily and engages them in interaction. Highly energetic, Meghan tends to move from activity to activity rapidly and has considerable difficulty in school sustaining attention and following classroom rules. While she is eager to play with other children, she is extremely bossy and rarely sought as a playmate. With her parents, she has always been demanding, wanting them to play with her constantly and having tantrums whenever she doesn't get her way. While she can be affectionate, more often she seems detached to the point that her mother wonders if a robot wouldn't be as effective in parenting Meghan as her mother.

Meghan appears to have a nonattached attachment disorder with indiscriminate sociability. She separates easily from her parents with little notice of them on reunion. She shows no apparent desire to please them and, instead, endlessly demands things and playtime from them. Also, she rarely goes to them for comfort. Self-regulation of affect appears impaired as she often presents with rapidly shifting extreme levels of affect, from intense squealing joy to agitated anxiety about dangers and intense angry temper tantrums. Behavioral self-regulation also is impaired, seen in her hyperactive behavior and poor attention span. However, while she appears hyperactive, she doesn't actually meet the criteria for attention-deficit/hyperactive disorder (ADHD) and is better understood as very poorly self-regulated. She frequently shows high levels of anxiety and is particularly upset when startled.

Meghan appears to have experienced relational trauma in her earliest years because of her hearing impairment. It is likely that she was frequently startled by loud noises and by people "suddenly" appearing. Attuned interactions with her parents were rare for several reasons. First, her parents' description of Meghan prior to discovery of the hearing loss was that she was neither demanding nor particularly engaged with them, playing in her crib or room alone. When they did try to engage her, she wasn't consistently responsive. Many of the sounds and words they used to comfort and stimulate her were not perceived. At the same time, she showed pronounced agitated startle responses where she cried vigorously and was difficult to comfort. At age 6, observations of Meghan's interactions with each of her parents, using Marschak Interaction Method (MIM), showed sensitive, nurturing parents who could effectively structure her environment, engage her, and challenge her with playful activities (Lindaman, Booth, & Chambers, 2000). However, in this setting, Meghan was extremely demanding, controlling, and somewhat oppositional. She responded to their attempts at engagement sporadically yet showed no reaction either to separation from or reunion with her parents. Initial play assessment revealed a similar pattern of interaction. While very willing to play with the therapist, she moved rapidly from activity to activity, ordered the therapist to do various things, and, while friendly, remained very superficial in her connection with the therapist.

Dynamic Issues, Treatment Goals, and Play Therapy Techniques

Two aspects of Meghan's behavior presented issues important to treatment. First, Meghan showed a lack of basic trust and a resistance to interpersonal connection. Superficially friendly, she needed to control every aspect of the play setting, including the therapist, yet showed almost no real engagement of the therapist in her play or in a relationship. Second, Meghan showed a pervasive lack of self-regulation. Her affect was extremely labile, marked by extremes of joy, fear, and anxiety. Her behavior was poorly controlled, with minimal ability truly to engage with either the toys or the therapist. Clearly, the initial goal of treatment was to create a relationship between Meghan and the therapist. However, to accomplish this very difficult task, subgoals needed to be articulated that could facilitate her receptiveness to a genuine relationship.

Three relationship goals with related therapeutic interventions were identified to guide the first, rather prolonged phase of treatment. First, the therapist needed to facilitate Meghan's receptivity to interpersonal connection and nurturance. Second, the therapist needed to help Meghan develop self-regulatory skills. Finally, the therapist had to promote Meghan's ability to tolerate, label, and verbalize feelings. Four basic interventions were initiated. First, the therapist focused on being attuned to Meghan. She did this by mirroring and reflecting Meghan's feelings and by inviting bodily expression of feelings. Second, the therapist worked to establish a safe holding environment for Meghan. In Meghan's case, this particularly involved helping her express needs and feelings, especially her fears. Third, the therapist needed to provide safety and to protect Meghan from being startled, clearly an extremely disruptive experience for her. Finally, the therapist also needed to contain Meghan's feelings, especially anxious feelings that she expressed primarily through nervous laughter and rapid shifts in activity. As part of providing safety and facilitating self-regulation, the therapist needed to provide structure and, when Meghan was able to accept it, physical comfort.

The initial phase of treatment was prolonged. It was nearly 4 months before the therapist began to sense she was becoming a genuine person to Meghan. Meghan bumped her ear, hurting herself when the hearing aid was jammed into her ear. For the first time in therapy, she was able to accept comfort from the therapist. The therapist continually reflected Meghan's anxiety, including telling her how the therapist could tell when Meghan was anxious. At first, Meghan showed no reaction to such reflections, but beginning in the 6th month of therapy, she began setting up scary scenes in her play, deliberately scaring the therapist and being scared. She could now talk about scary feelings. Another development at this same point in therapy was a greatly reduced need to control the therapist. She had formed an attachment and secure-base relationship with the therapist. Following this point, therapy focused on challenging her internal working models that others would surprise and hurt her and improving her largely minimal self-understanding or self-regulation. Play focused on safety issues, on saying "boo" and deliberately startling various play figures, and on empowering Meghan to control her emotional reactions and behaviors. It required 7 more months for Meghan to begin to be more controlled, significantly less bossy with other children, and more genuinely attached to the therapist and her parents. Play therapy was augmented with work with the parents primarily focused on controlling Meghan's demandingness and verbally labeling and accepting her feelings, something quite new for her parents.

Secure-Base Distortion with Self-Endangerment

History

Josh, age 3, is the younger of two brothers living with their recently divorced young mother and maternal grandparents. His older brother showed intense sibling rivalry, which included hitting and scratching Josh when he was a baby. At 10 months of age, Josh was briefly (2 weeks) removed from his mother's care by child protective services because she failed to protect him from his brother, who beat him with a toy, requiring his hospitalization. Josh was returned to his mother's care when her parents agreed to provide a home and supervision for her. According to his mother, Josh showed normal development, and she actually came to the clinic to find services for his older brother. Her description of Josh raised sufficient concerns that she was encouraged to bring Josh in for an assessment.

Symptoms

Josh presented as extremely active and indiscriminately friendly, instantly hugging the therapist as she was introduced to him. He seemed attached to some degree to his mother and grandmother and was initially reluctant to leave them, returning to the waiting room several times during the assessment and initial treatment sessions to show them things. The most noticeable feature of Josh's behavior, however, was his self-endangering behavior. He would pick up various objects from the floor or wastebaskets, particularly unfinished food and used gum, and immediately put them in his mouth. He was constantly climbing shelves, cabinets, and any other surface where he could get a foothold. Often, once up on the object, he would simply drop off into the therapist's arms, even though she was frequently unprepared for him to do this. He needed constant monitoring to keep him safe, and often ran away, in the building, in the parking lot, or into the street in front of cars. He was also extremely hyperactive and disorganized, having frequent tantrums when scared by something or when told no. He was impulsive but openly needy of attention and affection at the same time. While he easily met the criteria for ADHD, this diagnosis failed to capture the neediness, fearfulness, and disorganization that characterized this child.

The relational trauma for Josh was twofold. First, he was physically abused in infancy by his older brother and then separated from his primary caregiver, although only briefly. Second, evaluation of the family revealed significant personality problems for this young and overwhelmed mother. She reported significant depression when Josh was a baby and seemed to have little capacity to understand or attune to either of her children. Josh appeared to have developed a disorganized/resistant attachment to her, leaving him extremely needy but unable to trust his mother to meet his emotional and physical needs.

Dynamic Issues, Treatment Goals, and Play Therapy Techniques

While there seemed to be an insecure attachment, with some lack of trust, and poor self-regulation, both issues seen with the nonattached presentation above, there were several other aspects of Josh's dynamics that necessitated quite different therapist behaviors and goals. Foremost among these were his extremely dangerous behavior and his open neediness. Goals for treatment had to begin with increasing his ability to self-regulate and decreasing his recklessness while maintaining his physical safety. Physical contact with the therapist needed to be encouraged to facilitate boundary awareness and enhance his sense of bodily integrity. As in the first case, it was also important to facilitate genuineness in relationships, as his superficial friendliness covered a profound distrust that adults would keep him physically safe.

The primary focus of play therapy initially was keeping Josh safe. He found himself acutely anxious in the playroom, with the result that large portions of the sessions over the first several months were spent outside the playroom exploring the building or its immediate surroundings. While the therapist would have preferred staying in the playroom, it was clear that enormous flexibility on her part would be necessary for Josh to tolerate the relationship building phase of treatment at all. Most of the therapeutic work over these months consisted of Josh trying an unsafe behavior that the therapist would limit while providing both verbal reassurances of her willingness to keep him safe as well as needed physical constraints on his dangerous behavior. At first, he resisted her, saying he was safe. He would also get openly upset if she talked about feelings, especially scared or angry feelings. After several months, Josh began to verbalize that the therapist was keeping him safe and would cue her to hold his hand on the stairs or otherwise invite her help. He became much more tolerant of talk about feelings. At this time, he suffered a minor accident while in therapy, where a large box (fortunately lightweight) unexpectedly fell on him, startling him and making him feel trapped. He became panicked and highly agitated, unable to finish the session. Over the next three sessions, the therapist talked about his being hurt and scared and very angry that she did not protect him. While at first he denied being angry, Josh was then able to talk about not only his anger this time, but his anger at his mother, who still did not fully protect him from his brother.

Therapy continued over the next year, with sustained focus on safety and on the therapist's commitment to keeping Josh safe. He was much more able to accept that help and became more comfortable in the playroom playing themes relating to aggression, danger, safety, and nurturing. Josh continued to have significant problems with his sense of self, almost as if he had not developed a complete sense of himself. Frequently, he would ask to go into the video room and would watch a replay of himself on tape over and over, excitedly identifying himself on the tape. As this work progressed, the dangerous behavior greatly diminished except when he was stressed. For example, when preparing for an extensive summer break in therapy in which he would live with his father, Josh again began running away, climbing dangerously, and needing to watch his video self over and over. When he returned to therapy after the break, he again needed to test the therapist's ability to keep him safe, but it took only a few sessions to reestablish the relationship. Therapy terminated when Josh was able routinely to keep himself safe by controlling his behaviors. He also had a much more positive and organized sense of self and was able to effectively protect himself from his brother.

Disrupted Insecure Attachment with Role Reversal and Hypervigilance

History

There is much missing information in the history of Gavin, almost 5 years old when he entered therapy. He and his older sister were placed in a foster-to-adoption home when Gavin was 2 following their removal from their parents. At that time, the family was living in motels and, finally, a car. The parents were involved in extensive sexual abuse of both children. While it is clear that there was an abrupt disruption in parenting, the nature of the attachment relationship before the removal is unclear. It is highly probable that there was neglect; emotional and physical abuse cannot be ruled out.

Symptoms

Gavin was a superficially friendly child who was fiercely independent and extremely self-contained. He was very controlling with adults and repeatedly stated that he never got mad or scared by anything. He refused help of any kind, whether learning a new skill or dealing with a skinned knee. He was quite obedient when his foster parents were present, although he would hit his sister and break rules when they were not. He was rarely affectionate with his foster parents and often did destructive things around the house. For example, he used scissors he found to cut up his and his sister's clothes. At night, he would get out of his bed and try to hurt his sister, and his foster/adoptive parents had to install a motion detector near his bed for her protection.

While Gavin had been diagnosed with RAD, he did not act like an unattached child. Judging from his behavior, he appeared to be showing a secure-base distortion attachment with significant elements of both the role reversal and hypercompliant/hypervigilant subtypes. Instead of being poorly self-regulated, Gavin was, if anything, overly self-regulated and pseudomature. He showed massive estrangement from his feelings and needs. During the play assessment, Gavin accidentally pinched his fingers in a drawer. He immediately backed up, held his fingers as if they hurt, then quickly reassured the therapist that "it didn't hurt" and returned to his play. According to his foster mother, in the almost 3 years he had been living with her, he had never indicated that he was hurt, despite the usual number of skinned knees and bumps. Also striking was his lack of playfulness and spontaneity. While he seemed to enjoy coming into the playroom, he showed absolutely no thematic play for the first 4 months of treatment, and such play was rare for several more months. He typically engaged in mastery activities, such as building structures, drawing, or making Play-Doh animals using cookie cutters. Finally, whenever he encountered an unfamiliar toy, he would insist on playing with or fixing it, saying "I know" even when there was no way he could have known what to do.

Dynamic Issues, Treatment Goals, and Play Therapy Techniques

Gavin's therapy needed to be quite different from the therapy for Josh and Meghan. His lack of playfulness, extreme defensiveness seen in his denial of any fear or anger, and his intense need to know everything and be able to do everything for himself presented enormous challenges for his play therapist. Superficially friendly, he appeared to distrust all adults, including his foster parents. He showed both the hypervigilance of an abused child and the role-reversal of the parentified child. Not only have children like Gavin developed maladaptive internal working models that say they must take care of themselves as no one can be trusted not to hurt them, but these object relations have become prematurely crystallized and, thus, extremely resistant to change. The primary goal for this child was to develop his ability to connect authentically to others. This would require an increased ability for him to understand the needs and feelings of others, as he lacked the emerging empathy expected at his age. In addition, he would need to become aware of his own feelings and needs and be able to self-soothe when he finally was able to allow himself to be aware of negative feelings. Finally, an additional therapeutic goal was for Gavin to develop the ability to engage in age-appropriate play.

Children like Gavin are very difficult to treat. Play therapy with them needs to be modified considerably in order to get past their defenses and begin to form a genuine relationship with them. Only after this has been accomplished can the working model be challenged effectively. In my experience, it typically takes about a year of quasi-play therapy before the relationship develops sufficiently for therapeutic work to begin. I use the phrase "quasi-play therapy" because, at the beginning, there is very little that is playful about the therapy and usually little or no thematic play.

The primary techniques required during the initial phase of play therapy with role-reversed and hypervigilant children all involve patiently respecting the child's boundaries and supporting his perceived strengths. Basically, instead of challenging the child's ability to be in control and to be able to do everything on his own, the therapist affirms the child's need to decide things and to "do it himself." The therapist also needs to verbalize the hidden and denied feelings, but indirectly and gently, such as, "Most kids would have been hurt if they had fallen like that." Identifying and verbalizing problems and helping the child problem-solve are also important during this part of therapy. The therapist accepts the child's bossy commands unless safety is compromised and allows the child to maintain his claim of invulnerability until he is ready to relinquish it. Gradually, the child will acknowledge troubling feelings and allow the therapist to help do things. In Gavin's case, this gradual change was accompanied by dramatic changes at home. For the first time, Gavin cried when he hurt himself and ran to his foster mother for comfort. He also got up one night and went into his parents' room, saying he was afraid. He also began engaging in thematic play during therapy. He would pretend to be the vet and take care of Teddy, who variously had a sore throat (like Gavin had had recently) or bad feelings that needed to be fixed.

Once this prolonged trust-building phase is completed, play therapy more and more resembles the play of the other children described earlier. The therapist now can be more actively attuned to the child without raising his defenses. He or she can then use child-responsive, invitational techniques to resolve the distorted cognitions, feelings, and traumatic memories and challenge maladaptive internal working models. Gavin responded well to this shift in therapy and gradually worked through the severe abuse of his past.

Disrupted Insecure Attachment with Clinging/Inhibition

History

Karyn, 7 years old at the beginning of treatment, was the oldest of three children born to an intact family. Her parents divorced when she was 4, and she lived with her two siblings and mother, with regular visitation with her father. When Karyn was 6, her mother was killed in a car accident, and Karyn and her younger siblings went to live with their father. Karyn was brought by her father for treatment about 6 months after her mother's death for what initially appeared to be a complicated bereavement.

Symptoms

Karyn was crying frequently in school and often crying herself to sleep at night. She complained of headaches and stomachaches and was clingy with her father. She was also jealous of time her father spent with her younger siblings. When asked about the crying, Karyn would talk about missing her mother and being sad. Karyn's father also reported some symptoms less commonly associated with loss of a parent. Karyn was bossy with other children, had few friends, and was often teased by other children. Also, she talked about her two younger siblings as though she were responsible for taking care of them. She would worry if they were all right when she was separated from them and would often try to direct their activities.

Play assessment was surprising for several reasons. From the beginning, Karyn played family scenes that emphasized an angry, frightening mother and children who were locked in closets for misbehavior. The mother figure in the play would yell at the children or "go into her room." Karyn expressed intense anger at the mother figure. She also would pretend to be the baby, calling the therapist Mommy. At these times, she was very needy, wanting to be held and "fed." This explosion of intense play during assessment quickly shifted to a marked reluctance to enter the playroom coupled with whining, sitting on her father's lap, complaints of not feeling well, and trying to distract both her father and the therapist with various materials in the waiting room.

Karyn appeared to experience two significant relational traumas, the second of which was her mother's sudden death. The first seemed to be an insecure attachment relationship with her mother. Further discussion with her father revealed that her mother had little interest in the activities of parenting and that, before the divorce, the father routinely fed and bathed the children and prepared them for bed. After the divorce, an accurate history was difficult to obtain. However, it is clear that the mother had some problems with both alcohol abuse and interpersonal relationships, with a probable diagnosis of borderline personality disorder. The father, while not aware of any overt abuse, knew that the mother arranged for others to care for the children most of the time. When alone with the children, the mother frequently could not manage their behavior, calling their father to come and take them to his house for the night. He acknowledged that, while they were married, the mother frequently yelled at the children or sequestered herself in her bedroom with "migraines" and showed a high degree of irritability.

It seems probable that the mother's difficulties prevented her establishing a secure attachment relationship with Karyn. The relationship appears to have been one of ambivalence with frequent inappropriate and even frightening behavior on the part of the mother. In this context, bereavement over the mother's death becomes highly complex. In addition to feelings of sadness about her mother's death, Karyn likely experienced considerable anger at her mother even before her death. At age 6, Karyn might have wished her mother to disappear or at least be less frightening and angry. When her mother suddenly died, Karyn, in a way typical of her developmental level, probably felt responsible for her death and guilty for having angry feelings. Her internal working model of her mother seemed characterized by ambivalence and an expectation that her mother would hurt or scare her. Her internal working model of herself, clearly revealed as therapy progressed, was of a bad, unlovable child whom the much needed father would reject if he truly knew how bad she was.

Dynamic Issues, Treatment Goals, and Play Therapy Techniques

The dynamics of Karyn's difficulties went well beyond simple bereavement. She appeared to lack an integrated and positive sense of self. She evidenced limited ability to self-soothe, with a strong tendency to hide her real feelings and needs from others, especially her father. Her coping skills were limited, and she relied on whining or vague physical complaints to get attention. Unfortunately, both behaviors were more likely to irritate her father than gain his positive attention. Her ego development was uneven, with limited stress tolerance and a high level of passivity.

The goals for play therapy with Karyn were colored by the need to resolve her ambivalent attachment relationship with her mother through her remaining parent, her father. She needed help trusting the therapist not to injure her already fragile self-esteem. Therapy had among its goals the need to develop a stronger basis for self-soothing and self-esteem, increasing Karyn's valuing of her own needs and feelings and helping her develop appropriate assertiveness in getting her needs met.

The play therapy techniques in this case were again quite different from those in the previous cases. The basic challenge was for the therapist to remain accepting in the face of strong ambivalence and even rejection by the child. This required providing emotional constancy without either controlling or infantilizing Karyn. It also required containment of Karyn's strong negative affects while modeling both attunement and appropriate boundaries. Therapeutic work with children like Karyn requires a balancing act so that the relationship avoids both the sense of emotional abandonment and engulfment. Providing a constant therapeutic environment was also a central feature of therapy with Karyn. The first play session, Karyn was provided with her own box where she could put toys that were important to her. She latched on to this idea rapidly and took considerable care each week in selecting what she needed kept in her box. Finally, she needed psychological safety, including acceptance of her nearly constant reluctance to enter the playroom. Interestingly enough, once in the playroom, Karyn seemed unable to avoid the intense, emotionally charged play first shown during assessment, and she typically had as much difficulty leaving as entering the playroom.

Play therapy with this type of child does not follow the typical pattern for attachment problems in that building the secure-base relationship occurs slowly alongside thematic play focusing on the distorted emotions and cognitions and traumatic memories. The first two phases are combined so that a secure-base relationship is only fully established near the end of therapy as the relational traumas are resolved and the child is finally able to trust the therapist to be consistently available yet non-threatening. Sessions in the first several months were characterized by Karyn playing the child and the therapist playing the mother role. This play alternated between needy baby play and angry child play, including overt rejection of the "mother," who was forbidden to talk, interact, or even see the child. Gradually, Karyn began to talk more openly about being bad and her dad not loving her. This phase continued to require much patience by the therapist because each such revelation was initially accompanied by intense resistance and rejection of the therapist, whether in the mother role or not. Several sessions, spaced over about 5 months, were intense direct expressions of how frightening the mother character was to the child and how scared and angry Karyn had been at her mother. By the end of therapy, she could begin to see her relationship with her mother in terms of her mother having "grown-up" problems that were not Karyn's fault or because of Karyn's "badness." It was at this point, near termination, that Karyn could experience genuine sadness over her mother's death while retaining a positive sense of self.

CONCLUSIONS

Object relations play therapy, as has been described above, is an approach particularly well suited for treating young children who have experienced relational trauma and/or insecure attachments in the first few years of life. By focusing on the specific modifications of the object relations or internal working models the child has developed in response to the trauma, this approach enables the play therapist to build secure-base relationships with children who, as a group, are slow to trust and impaired in their sense of self and others. Using this secure-base relationship, the therapist can then effectively challenge and, ultimately, modify the maladaptive negative working models of self and others that are the result of the original trauma. The child is thus enabled to return to a healthy developmental pathway.

As has been demonstrated, there are not only many children exposed to relational trauma, but numerous possible relational traumas and several different presentations of attachment problems. Object relations play therapy, relying primarily on child-responsive, invitational, highly attuned therapy techniques, has a variety of specific goals and techniques that can be easily tailored to match each child's specific needs and interpersonal capacities. While therapy with these children is difficult and time-consuming, it is also vitally important if relational traumas are going to be resolved rather than lead to long-term psychopathology. Object relations play therapy has been an effective treatment for many traumatized young children in our clinic. Hopefully, over time, we will be able to gather evidence that it can be an effective treatment for many traumatized children.

REFERENCES

Ainsworth, M. D. S., Blehar, M. C., Waters, E., & Wall, S. (1978). *Patterns of attachment: A psychological study of the strange situation.* Hillsdale, NJ: Erlbaum.

American Psychiatric Association. (1994). *Diagnostic and statistical manual of mental disorders* (4th ed.). Washington, DC: Author.

Benedict, H. E. (1997, September 12). *Thematic play therapy and attachment disorders.* Workshop presented at Southwest Missouri State University, Springfield, MO.

Benedict, H. E. (2003). Object relations/thematic play therapy. In C. E. Schaefer (Ed.), *Foundations of play therapy* (pp. 281–305). New York: Wiley.

Benedict, H. E. (2004a, October 5). *Using play themes in play assessment and for understanding play therapy process.* Pre-conference workshop presented at the 21st Annual Association for Play Therapy International Conference, Denver, CO.

Benedict, H. E. (2004b, October 9). *Play therapy for children experiencing attachment and interpersonal trauma.* Workshop presented at the 21st Annual Association for Play Therapy International Conference, Denver, CO.

Benedict, H. E., Chavez, D., Holmberg, J., McClain, J., McGee, W., Narcavage, D., et al. (1996). *Benedict play therapy theme code.* Unpublished working paper, Baylor University, Waco, TX.

Benedict, H. E., & Hastings, L. (2002). Object relations play therapy. In J. Magnavita (Ed.), *Comprehensive handbook of psychotherapy: Psychodynamic/object relations* (Vol. 1, pp. 47–80). New York: Wiley.

Benedict, H. E., Hastings, L., Ato, G., Carson, M., & Nash, M. (1998). *Revised Benedict play therapy theme code and interpersonal relationship code.* Unpublished working paper, Baylor University, Waco, TX.

Benedict, H. E., & Mongoven, L. B. (1997). Thematic play therapy: An approach to treatment of attachment disorders in young children. In H. Kaduson, D. Cangelosi, & C. E. Schaefer (Eds.), *The playing cure: Individualized play therapy for specific childhood problems* (pp. 277–315). New York: Aronson.

Bowlby, J. (1988). *A secure base: Parent–child attachment and healthy human development.* New York: Basic Books.

Cassidy, J., & Shaver, P. R. (Eds.). (1999). *Handbook of attachment: Theory, research, and clinical applications.* New York: Guilford Press.

Cicchetti, D., Toth, S. L., & Lynch, M. (1995). Bowlby's dream comes full circle:

The application of attachment theory to risk and psychopathology. In T. H. Ollendick & R. J. Prinz (Eds.), *Advances in clinical child psychology* (Vol. 17, pp. 1–75). New York: Plenum Press.

Gil, E. (1991). *The healing power of play.* New York: Guilford Press.

Glickhauf-Hughes, C., & Wells, M. (1997). *Object relations psychotherapy: An individualized and interactive approach to diagnosis and treatment.* New York: Aronson.

Hall, H. (1996). Parental psychiatric disorder and the developing child. In M. Gopfert, J. Webster, & M. V. Seeman (Eds.), *Parental psychiatric disorder: Distressed parents and their families* (pp. 17–41). Cambridge, UK: Cambridge University Press.

Hastings, L. (2001). *Adaptation to relational trauma as reflected in preschoolers' play themes.* Unpublished doctoral dissertation, Baylor University, Waco, TX.

Hinshaw-Fuselier, S., Heller, S. S., Parton, V. T., Robinson, L., & Boris, N. W. (2004). Trauma and attachment: The case for disrupted attachment disorder. In J. D. Osofsky (Ed.), *Young children and trauma: Intervention and treatment* (pp. 47–68). New York: Guilford Press.

Jurkovic, G. J. (1997). *Lost childhoods: The plight of the parentified child.* New York: Brunner/Mazel.

Kaplan, T. (1997). Psychological responses to interpersonal violence: B. Children. In D. Black, J. Harris-Hendriks, & G. Mezey (Eds.), *Psychological trauma: A developmental approach* (pp. 184–198). London: Gaskell.

Kilpatrick, K. L., & Williams, L. M. (1997). Post-traumatic stress disorder in child witnesses to domestic violence. *American Journal of Orthopsychiatry, 67*(4), 639–644.

Kolbo, J. R., Blakely, E. H., & Engleman, D. (1996). Children who witness domestic violence: A review of empirical literature. *Journal of Interpersonal Violence, 11,* 281–293.

Levoy, D., Rivinus, T. M., Matzko, M., & McGuire, J. (1991). Children in search of a diagnosis: Chronic trauma disorder of childhood. In T. M. Rivinus (Ed.), *Children of chemically dependent parents: Multiperspectives from the cutting edge* (pp. 153–170). New York: Brunner/Mazel.

Lieberman, A. F., & Pawl, J. H. (1988). Clinical applications of attachment theory. In J. Belsky & T. Nezworski (Eds.), *Clinical implications of attachment* (pp. 327–351). Hillsdale, NJ: Erlbaum.

Lieberman, A. F., & Van Horn, P. (2004). Assessment and treatment of young children exposed to traumatic events. In J. D. Osofsky (Ed.), *Young children and trauma: Intervention and treatment* (pp. 111–138). New York: Guilford Press.

Lindaman, S. L., Booth, P. B., & Chambers, C. L. (2000). Assessing parent–child interactions with the Marschak Interaction Method (MIM). In K. Gitlin-Weiner, A. Sandgrund, & C. E. Schaefer (Eds.), *Play diagnosis and assessment* (2nd ed., pp. 371–400). New York: Wiley.

Mahler, M. S., & Furer, M. (1968). *On human symbiosis and the vicissitudes of individuation.* New York: International Universities Press.

Mahler, M. S., Pine, F., & Bergman, A. (1975). *The psychological birth of the human infant: Symbiosis and individuation.* New York: Basic Books.

Main, M., & Solomon, J. (1986). Discovery of a new, insecure disorganized/disoriented attachment pattern. In T. B. Brazelton & M. W. Yogman (Eds.), *Affect development in infancy* (pp. 95–124). Norwood, NJ: Ablex.

Prior, S. (1996). *Object relations in severe trauma: Psychotherapy of the sexually abused child.* Northvale, NJ: Aronson.

Schore, A. N. (1994). *Affect regulation and the origin of the self: The neurobiology of emotional development.* Hillsdale, NJ: Erlbaum.

Schore, A. N. (2003). Early relational trauma, disorganized attachment, and the development of a predisposition to violence. In M. F. Solomon & D. J. Siegel (Eds.), *Healing trauma: Attachment, mind, body, and brain* (pp. 107–167). New York: Norton.

Schuder, M. R., & Lyons-Ruth, K. (2004). "Hidden trauma" in infancy: Attachment, fearful arousal, and early dysfunction of the stress response system. In J. D. Osofsky (Ed.), *Young children and trauma: Intervention and treatment* (pp. 69–104). New York: Guilford Press.

Siegel, D. J. (1999). *The developing mind: Toward a neurobiology of interpersonal experience.* New York: Guilford Press.

Sigelman, C. K., & Rider, E. A. (2005). *Life-span human development* (5th ed.). Belmont, CA: Wadsworth.

Solomon, J., George, C., & DeJong, A. (1995). Children classified as controlling at age 6: Evidence for disorganized representational strategies and aggression at home and at school. *Development and Psychopathology, 7,* 447–463.

Stern, D. N. (1985). *The interpersonal world of the infant: A view from psychoanalysis and developmental psychology.* New York: Basic Books.

Winnicott, D. W. (1965). *The maturational processes and the facilitating environment: Studies in the theory of emotional development.* New York: International Universities Press.

Winnicott, D. W. (1971a). *Playing and reality.* London: Tavistock.

Winnicott, D. W. (1971b). *Therapeutic consultations in child psychiatry.* New York: Basic Books.

Wooley, L. M. (1998). *An exploration of the play therapy themes of children who have a parent with a personality disorder.* Unpublished doctoral dissertation, Baylor University, Waco, TX.

Zeanah, C. H., Jr., & Boris, N. W. (2000). Disturbances and disorders of attachment in early childhood. In C. H. Zeanah, Jr. (Ed.), *Handbook of infant mental health* (2nd ed., pp. 353–368). New York: Guilford Press.

Zeanah, C. H., Jr., Mammen, O. K., & Lieberman, A. F. (1993). Disorders of attachment. In C. H. Zeanah, Jr. (Ed.), *Handbook of infant mental health* (pp. 322–349). New York: Guilford Press.

Zero to Three: National Center for Clinical Infant Programs. (1994). *Diagnostic classification 0–3: Diagnostic classification of mental health and developmental disorders of infancy and early childhood.* Washington, DC: Author.

Experiential Play Therapy

CAROL C. NORTON
BYRON E. NORTON

A young child sits in the bathtub, playing with his toys. He hears his mother out in the kitchen cleaning up from the evening meal. The music from the TV show his older brother is watching in the living room reaches his ears, but merely becomes background for his own experience. He does not know where his father is. He pushes a boat around in the tub and makes waves to challenge its stability. Colorful action figures also float along in the waves of bubbles. The bubbles smell too much like flowers to be a part of the action, but he disregards this. He feels the boat bumping into his legs as it moves about wildly in the waves.

From the action of the waves, some bubbles float up from the surface into the air. He notices the rainbow effect on their thin shells. As some of them begin their return to the water, one lands on his nose. He crosses his eyes to look at it more closely. He becomes lost in his fascination of the bubble. Suddenly, he sees himself and his boat inside the bubble. They begin to float over the water, and the seascape slowly changes. The expanse of water is immense. There appears to be no one else around. He feels the breeze blowing on his face. For some reason, he feels no fear at this new adventure. Looking far ahead, he spots a pirate ship on the ocean. It is about to overtake another, smaller ship. The child maneuvers his boat into position to approach the ships. The captain at the helm of the pirate ship looks angry. He presents a large figure and is yelling loudly as he jumps onto the smaller ship and begins to attack the small, fearful, and trembling crew. They cower, feeling their swords are powerless against this giant of a man. The child pulls his boat up next to the two ships. He pulls himself onto the deck of the smaller ship, where he confronts the pirate captain. He knows he is strong and his sword is fast, so he can defeat the hulking menace.

The two fight: this small figure and the powerful giant. The child possesses the power of one who is fighting for good. His sword is true. They battle until the pirate is overcome. Even though he is defeated, he remains loud and threatening. His face is contorted with the shame of his defeat. He loudly protests the crew's treatment of him, continuing his attempts at overpowering them. Having failed at physically conquering them, he now attempts to intimidate them with his verbal strength. The crew of the smaller ship and the child tie his hands tightly with ropes they find on the pirate's ship. They ignore his verbal protests. Together, they force him to walk the plank. The ocean splashes with white plumes as he jumps into the water. The crew celebrates with the child. He is their hero, as he has saved them from sure death.

Abruptly, the fantasy ends as the child hears the front door of his home open. His father roars, "I'm home!" The young boy quickly but quietly climbs out of the bathtub, dries off his small body, puts on his nightclothes, and disappears into his room for the night.

BASIC ASSUMPTIONS
OF EXPERIENTIAL PLAY THERAPY

Fundamental to the developmental of the experiential play therapy model is the belief that children encounter their world in an experiential style as opposed to a cognitive one. That is, children do not think about their encounters; rather, they involve their senses as a means of incorporating information from their environment. This sensory information then elicits an emotional response. For instance, observe the sheer delight of a child upon his first sight of a rainbow or the fear evident in his facial expressions upon his first encounter with a writhing snake. The child does not take time to consider the science behind the formation of a rainbow or the possibility that the snake may be a safe, merely different, form of life. He simply reacts on his initial emotional response.

Exposure to various experiences is believed by developmental experts to be vitally important for children to move from one developmental stage to another (Russ, 2004; Piaget, 1952, 1954, 1962). Through experiences, a cognitive framework is formed with which the child approaches future similar situations. When intense emotional situations arise for the child, he must focus his energy on reaching some level of empowerment over the emotionality associated with the events in order to be able to function in that environment. The child's assimilation and integration of experiences becomes contaminated with intrusive memories of the emotional events, leading to impeded development. He continues reacting to the event while he works on achieving power over his emotionality. He utilizes his play to help him expose himself to the event in a manner in which he has control and does not become overwhelmed. Children cannot become empowered by confronting the reality of the emotional event in its entirety (Perry, 2002). The reality is overwhelming because of the high level of emotionality involved. When they play, they are able to confront the issue in the abstract and therefore on a less invasive level.

Children often will establish certain associations with events, either conscious or unconscious. An example might be a child who hates carousels because his mother took him for a ride on one right after she molested him. During play, children can utilize toys as representations of these associations, distancing their emotionality. As children become more empowered, the toys representing the feared associations will more closely resemble the actual objects or individuals.

Around the age of 2, when a child becomes capable of utilizing a toy to symbolize himself, other individuals, and events or even affect, she is able to communicate her experience of events and the status of her emotional well-being (Seja & Russ, 1999). She will repeat this play until someone understands and responds or until she is able to reach a point where the events no longer overwhelm her. If numerous repetitions are not recognized by significant adults or if these adults merely attempt to control the behaviors, the child accepts an attitude of defeat. The defeat will often manifest itself as withdrawal or more intense acting out.

The relationship between the child and the therapist is the essential dimension in the child's therapeutic process. van der Kolk, Perry, and Herman (1991) found (and summarized in van der Kolk, 1996, p. 198) that "the capacity to derive comfort from the presence of another human being was eventually a more powerful predictor than the trauma history itself of whether patients improved and were able to give up chronically self-destructive activities." When the relationship is nurtured, the child can recapitulate his struggles, test them, watch them crumble, and rebuild them in such a way that he can tolerate, understand, and accept them (Norton & Norton, 2002). The strength of the alliance empowers the child to approach the emotionally laden situation in a more productive fashion. The therapist honors the child in his perception of the event and provides a place of safety and protection where the child may test his own strength in approaching the sensitive issue. Children have a natural propensity to move toward emotional comfort. If facilitated, they will discover a healthy adaptation. If left unattended, they may adopt a style of functioning that creates less tension for them when they are in the situation physically or recreating it psychologically. However, the unattended style of functioning is less adaptive within the broader social milieu. The therapist must allow the child to lead the way and must support the child as, together, they move toward empowerment over the event.

It should be noted here that, if the circumstances that created the distress for the child remain in her environment, the child's therapeutic work will remain focused on emotional and/or physical survival rather than achieving any empowerment over the emotionality surrounding the situation. With the situation in the past and the emotionality in the present, the child may gain empowerment, but when the circumstances are in the present, the child continues to experience a lack of control. In this case, therapeutic work focuses on assisting the child to recognize that circumstances surrounding her do not represent the norm. Through acceptance, modeling, and the power of the therapeutic alliance, the child gains empowerment over her emotional reaction to the circumstances. The child creates an environment in which the therapist feels what it is like to be this child. When the therapist demonstrates, through play, that he or she understands and expresses a similar emotional reaction, the child becomes empowered with the understanding that her perceptions are shared.

Children may incorporate the therapist into their play in several ways. The child will occasionally prefer that the therapist remain an observer. If this is the case, the child will not invite the therapist into the play, but will simply play independently. If the child wishes the therapist to participate in the play but be passive (not even speak), he will find a way to include the therapist in the play but ensure that the therapist remains inactive. For instance, the child will pick up a toy gun, aim it at the therapist, and shoot, saying, "Boom! You're dead!" In this case, the therapist is no longer a clinical observer, but a recipient of the experience. It must be determined from the play whether the experience being communicated is the role of the child, a significant person in the child's life, or the child's envisaged actions toward the perpetrator. On the other hand, the child may wish to have the therapist be an active participant and will indicate this by assigning a role to the therapist. This enables the child to enhance his experience of the event and increases his ability to gain empowerment over the emotionality related to the event. To facilitate empowerment for the child, experiential play therapy encourages active participation by the therapist in the child's play. However, it is important that the therapist not lead the play. He or she may expand the play by active participation in the assigned role but not add another dimension.[1]

The goal of play therapy is for the child to reach a point where she has gained some empowerment over her negative emotionality. Through play therapy, the child slowly reframes the experience, bit by bit, so she can experience the event with a restored sense of empowerment and control (Knell, 1993; Russ, 1995). The sense of being out of control and the feelings of anxiety and fear disappear. Although the child never forgets the event, her reactions to the memories or to the situation are no longer inhibiting her growth. She can proceed with her development.

To accomplish this goal in experiential play therapy, the child proceeds through five basic stages. The stages may vary in intensity and duration, but there is a general pattern children follow in their healing process. Variations may be due to the length of time since the initial traumatic event, the duration of the circumstances, or, of course, the resiliency of the child.

TOYS: THE IMPLEMENTS OF PLAY

To be is to play. Play is the child's introduction to the world, and nothing more expresses his or her being more than play. Toys are the medium for that process, and if children have none, they create some. Since play is the language of children, toys are the words of their expressions. To the developing child, toys are the tools for mastery, interaction, and reciprocation. Toys become representative of the child's identity and provide an avenue toward security to express him- or herself safely. Simply put, toys become extensions of a child's being, projections of the child's thoughts and feelings. To the child, who is less cognitively oriented, toys aid the expression of feelings and experiences. Further, the toys expand to become the symbols that represent his or her existence and meaning in the world (Winnicott, 1999). To the play therapist, toys are the medium by which children express the dilemmas and/or traumas of their experiences. Toys in the hands of a child give him- or her the power to change his or her meaning of life and future view of the world. Through play, children can change their perception of an event, which, in turn, changes their view of their world. Step by step, they feel less emotional about the event. As this occurs, the symbolism of the toys becomes less abstract as they move toward resolutions. Children may play aggressively to portray their struggle in life, but to the play therapist, this struggle or conflict in play is the child's attempt at emotional survival. The child's process of being active in his or her approach to the conflict is referred to as "contact" in Gestalt theory:

> In order to make contact with the environment, in order to get needs met, the child must *aggress* into the environment. To aggress means to

move toward something. This is a healthy and necessary biological and psychological function. Life is not a passive matter. It is aggression that serves the life of the child and which allows distinctions to be made between the child and the environment. From the Gestalt view, it is aggression that enables the self to orient, mobilize, and organize its excitement or energy. Aggression, therefore, is essential for growth and learning. (Carrol & Oaklander, 1997, p. 185)

Without play and toys and the process of play therapy, many of children's meaningful expressions would most likely remain silent. Toys and play become symbolic and metaphorical extensions of the child. Together, the distressed child and the play therapist can enter the child's emotional world and hear his or her pleas for understanding and confirmation.

The play therapist must consider the symbolic meaning of each toy a child selects. A few sessions into the process, play becomes increasingly focused and patterns evolve. At this point, toys are not selected randomly, but to represent various aspects of the child's perception of his or her dilemma. The play therapist must assess the meaning of each toy based on the projective meaning immediately assigned and experienced by the child. In most cases, the meaning will remain constant unless redefined by the child in the context of a new play scenario. For example, the child selects an airplane to fly over a dollhouse. This can have several meanings, which ultimately guide the therapist's responses. An airplane could represent the need to escape the situation because the child needs emotional distance from the intensity experienced at home. It could represent freedom from high expectations or protection from events too powerful to confront directly. To a traumatized child, it may be the flight response to avoid retraumatization. A deeper consideration might be that the child has to dissociate to survive the abusive environment in the home. Other dynamic meanings may be considered, but the therapist should always remember that an airplane is never just an airplane to the child in play therapy.

A few other examples that a play therapist could consider are provided in Norton and Norton (2002):

- Binoculars: perspective, relationship (close/distant), hypervigilance, hunting, stalking, finding, searching, assessing, or surveillance. In trauma, this could represent a flight or an orientation response.
- Costumes: disguise, relationship, power, communication, adult, anonymity, perpetrator, fantasy, or deceit. In trauma, this could

represent a flight response with the ability to fight without being recognized.

- Doctor's kit: healing, injury, repair, respect, power, life/death, pain, body image, crisis, changing, intrusion, internal conflict, or self-confirmation. In trauma, this would most likely represent an immobility or intrusive response.
- Kitchen set: home, nurturing, care, neglect, sibling conflicts, relationships, family, respect, family process, emotional support, or unmet needs. In trauma, this could represent flight (focus on nurturing instead of trauma), fight (anger at disliked food), or immobility (a lack of capacity to confront the trauma), depending on the play context.
- Soldiers: conflict, attack, aggression, protection, force, life/death, struggling, people, survival, grouping, or support. In trauma, this could represent the fight response. (The trauma additions were adapted with consideration from Johnson, 2005.)

The context of the environmental metaphors in which the toy is featured is also highly significant. For example, a family of wolves that lives in the desert connotes a different environment than a family of wolves that live in a jungle. The first may be a neglectful, emotionally impoverished family environment, and the second may represent a chaotic, fearful environment. This is also true for animal representations. Symbolically, living in a dolphin family would be significantly different from living in an alligator family. Again, the first represents a family of support and unity, while the second represents a family of aggression and primitive survival.

A playroom with a broad selection of toys gives the child the ability to speak with directness and without confrontation as his or her story is told. After the failure of repeated attempts to communicate their experiences and perceptions, many children abandon these attempts and begin concealing their inner truths. When they are offered the opportunity to have those truths heard and understood, however, they become readily proficient in revealing their personal narrative.

EXPRESSIVE FANTASY PLAY: WHEN PIGS DO FLY

Most of the literature on fantasy play reviews the role of fantasy play in identification and mastery of the adult world. Axline (1955) recognized fantasy play to be highly significant to the child while viewed as insignificant from the adult perspective. Oaklander (1988) describes fantasy as a central component in therapeutic work with children. She believes that fantasy expression is the reflection of the child's inner world, with perceptions and feelings conveyed through the use of symbolism and metaphor. References to the use of metaphor as the child's style of self-expression in play therapy are limited (Mills & Crowley, 1986). Symbolism has been the cornerstone of the sand tray (Kalff, 1946; Lowenfeld, 1991) and Jungian (Allen, 1991; Jung, 1956, 1964) methods but has been less significantly reviewed in play therapy. The purpose of identifying the symbolism of a child's play is to enhance the meaning of his or her expression. The interactions the child creates among self, toys, and environmental symbols lead to the metaphorical meaning of the child's expressions. This metaphorical communication is motivated and sustained by the energy of the child, and the creation of expression is determined by his or her psychological or emotional press. This concept follows the Gestalt principle of organismic self-regulation identified by Perls, Hefferline, and Goodman (1951). The play therapist must consistently follow the emotional energy of the child. There are times when the play therapist is limited in understanding a child's play, but if the energy of the child is followed, he or she is free to continue the release or movement. The experiential play therapist believes that play is the process *and* the intervention. The child must externalize his or her inner emotionality in metaphorical form to reveal the energy and to release the trauma.

This energy can be expressed in many forms, for example, in drama play (with the child as king and the therapist as servant), in object play (with the lion dominating the jungle), in art play (with the child drawing a monster that frightens the baby rabbit), or in sand play (with a baby whale surrounded by angry sharks). Additionally, this energy may come in the form of dream energy that the child brings to play therapy, for example, a dream about being trapped in the shopping mall and chased by a bear. Children have a variety of creative ways to shift their emotional energy into symbolic and metaphorical representations to convey their inner world and distresses. The medium of play is the preference of the child; understanding the expressive significance is the responsibility of the play therapist. Understanding a child means acceptance of the child's expressions when playing the assigned receptive role in play. This dramatic style of fantasy play creates the experience to be conveyed and the experience the child seeks to change. The child externalizes his or her inner concerns into the fantasy play, wishing to be dominant rather than impotent over emotions related to the trauma situation. During dramatic play, where the child is dominant, gradual shifts in his or her perception occur. Those modifications in the child's perceptual set in turn affect his or her behavior. This relation between the dimensions of fantasy play and emotional understanding was found by Seja and Russ (1999). The form in which the energy is expressed is only the medium; the force or source of the energy remains constant and meaningfully personalized to the child. During the course of therapy, the play context may vary, but the theme(s) expressed in the play will be consistent.

The child's ability to create symbolism and metaphorical expression in play is his or her foremost resource for resiliency. The child who can transform her perceptions of her experiences through the use of symbolism and metaphor can transcend painful experiences when allowed to journey through her pain with a sense of dignity and empowerment provided by the validation of the therapist that the journey is meaningful. To the distressed or traumatized child, fantasy play is a construct of reality, a reality that the child can control and change for her benefit or well-being.

The advantage of the energy of fantasy play is that merely wishing something to be makes it so. Fantasy allows the child a defense against the overwhelming power the world has over him or her. Energy in the use of fantasy play is unlimited (J. L. Moreno, personal communication, 1967). A child can create the energy of any person he or she chooses. To some children, it may be their mother who died during childbirth. To others, it may be the controlling boyfriend who hurt their mother when the child lay in his or her crib. Fantasy energy allows the child to be alive in death and dead in life. Children who are dying often play beyond their death to experiences that are past the realm of ordinary comprehension. This process is extremely meaningful to the disempowered child. Still other children choose to go back 120 million years and play with dinosaurs, identifying with their survival and loss. Others project into the future and protect their great-great-granddaughter from abusive family dynamics. The potential of fantasy energy gives the world of children to a wisdom that few adults enjoy. It is a world that play therapists encounter every day.

The true understanding of fantasy play comes when the play therapist, acting in the nemesis role with the child as director of the play, can face the child in a gun duel, fire a shot at the child in real time, and trust that the child will create the desired results through his empowerment in the play. The therapist/villain fires the shot, and the child slowly pulls out his gun and shoots the bullet in mid-air, showing the villain that his malevolent power is not dominating this experiential moment. Fantasy keeps the child in the power position, allowing an expression of how the perpetrator misused power in the relationship.

The therapist must have an appreciation for the creative fantasy play of the child. The therapist will be required to enter the fantasy play in the capacity that the child ascribes by representing a role necessary for the child to confront some aspect of his or her pain. While most therapists like the role of alter-ego to the child, in experiential play therapy, the therapist is most often the victim/child or the perpetrator/villain. The therapist is the protagonist when representing the child and the antagonist when acting as the perpetrator or some aspect of the traumatic experience. In the child/victim role, the therapist reflects empathy for the pain of the child. In the perpetrator/villain role, the therapist is confronted and disempowered through the play process. The therapist is usually required to play the ineffectual position in the child's play focus. Caution should be given that the therapist only plays these roles in response to the child's expressions and does not lead or initiate dynamics into the play.

METAPHORS OF PLAY: THE CHILD'S LANGUAGE OF EXPRESSION

The literature on metaphors for children has mostly been in the form of stories that attempt to bring about change in the child through introjection. Little has been written on how children express metaphors to adults as a means of communicating experiences that the child has not yet developed the capacity to express through language. The child has the implicit memory or traumatic memory to know what he or she has experienced, but emotional and/or traumatic experiences are not stored in a cognitive framework. Trauma researchers indicate that trauma and emotionality are sensory experiences stored in the body or in somatic experience (Levine, 1997; van der Kolk, 1996). Infants have somatic memory (Paley & Alpert, 2003) and, therefore, store their traumas as implicit memory and bodily experiences. The expression of these events can be conveyed though an experiential play process that articulates the meaning of the experience without the use of words. Children are masters of this process. In play therapy with a traumatized child, the fantasy play is driven by a need to express the internal distress the child is experiencing. Since young children do not have the expressive capacity to articulate complicated feelings, they use play situations to help the recipient of their play experience the feeling associated with the dilemma or distress. The play therapist "re-lives" the child's past traumatic events and, in the therapeutic growth stage, witnesses the change experience.

Every child is in the process of expressing the meaning of his or her life in every moment. This intensifies with distress or with disregard of the child's importance. The behavior of the child will become a metaphor expressing the unacknowledged emotional experience. This can be as obvious as resistance or reluctance or the more forceful expression of a temper tantrum. However, in play therapy, these metaphorical expressions are heard at a much deeper level, and the child is allowed to complete the expression. For example, a 5-year-old boy is playing his conflict with his father who was abusive and has abandoned the family. He expresses the conflict of their relationship by becoming his father and assigns the role of himself to the therapist. The two then swordfight, representing the conflict of their relationship. The boy backs the therapist into the corner of the playroom, where she is trapped and a victim of his power. He then states, "My father stole all my toys." A surface interpretation would be that his father took his toys away from him, but at the deeper metaphorical level, this boy has just stated that his father, in his dominating and intrusive style, stole his childhood from him. The depth and intensity of his communication is far greater than most adults attribute to children's expressions. A verbal example cannot truly convey the experiential metaphor the therapist is feeling when in play with the child. It is the experience or feeling the child recreates through play that is more explicit about the child's emotional status in that moment. Through play, the depth of the child's expression is communicated. The child is no longer viewed as an unknowing or unaware being who does not assimilate the world around him. Almost all children speak at this level of communication once they know their listener is attuned to their expressions. Experiential play therapy is a constant process of metaphorical expression with a therapist who attempts to hear the underlying meaning of the child's play and experiential expressions.

THE STAGES OF PLAY THERAPY

The Exploratory Stage

The exploratory stage occurs in the first session. It is the time when the therapist begins to build a relationship with the child. The child explores the toys and the room to become familiar with and comfortable in the playroom. During this time, the child becomes familiar with the style of the therapist and inserts his or her own personality into the experience. The unstructured format of experiential play therapy allows the child to enter the therapy process in the same manner he or she approaches life.

This immediately gives the therapist information about the child's view of the world and his or her means of coping with these perceptions.

Initially, it is easier for children to examine the toys than to interact with the therapist. Also, they are curious about the room. They will generally spend much of the first session picking up the toys and examining them. It is common for them to ask questions about the toys. Behind each question lies an important disclosure about the child's personality and perception of the world. Common questions might include "Why is this here?" Underlying the question about the toy is a more significant question: "Why am I here?" It is important to answer the underlying question while staying in the metaphor—for example, "That is a very important toy. I'm glad it's here because I love playing with it." Another example might be "How do you play with this toy?" Behind that question lies the child's curiosity about how he or she is expected to act when in the room. One answer might be "There are lots of ways we can play with that toy. In here, toys can be whatever you like." A few broken toys may be found in the playroom as well. If a child questions why a broken toy is kept in the room, the response is, "Yes, that toy is broken, but I love that toy and play with it a lot. It is an important toy."

The therapist honors the child by respecting her pace. The child expresses herself in her own way, dictated by her past experiences and personal style. It is important for the therapist to accept the child's style, whether it is passive, dependent, cooperative, demanding, or aggressive. Acceptance is communicated by verbal responses of an observational and affirming nature. For example, a child moves a shovel through the sand and some sand falls onto the floor. The child glances quickly at the therapist to ascertain his or her reaction. The therapist states, "It's OK if sand gets on the floor in here." At this point in the process, therapist responses are kept at a more superficial level until the child indicates she is ready to enter a relationship with the therapist. How this is indicated will become clear as the stages unfold. Acceptance may also be communicated by mirroring the child's style of play.

By honoring the child's style and respecting the child's pace, the therapist creates an atmosphere where the child comes to understand that he or she is safe in the playroom with this adult. During this time, the therapist observes the child and matches his or her expressions. The therapist does not initiate any direction to the play, as the child will lead the way.

During the child's initial explorations, his comments are an indication of his view of the world. He also discloses, through his comments and approach to the room, his capacity to trust and his need for protection. The child who rushes immediately to the guns and knives, then turns and points one at the therapist, is indicating he does not feel safe in this new environment or in his world in general. The therapist accepts this attitude as reflective of the child's reality and communicates acceptance of these perceptions. A statement like "I'm going to have to be careful to stay at a safe distance from those guns and knives" indicates the therapist's acknowledgment of the child's feeling threatened in his world. (Were this behavior to occur after the child–therapist relationship is established, a different response would be more appropriate.)

Generally the child will move from one toy to another without spending much time on any one. The child will make short, meaningful statements, the meaning of which may not become apparent to the therapist until much later, when the child adds more content to his or her play. Initially, the statement may appear to be merely an innocent comment, but, upon reflection, the significance of a simple statement becomes evident. A child who picks up a telephone, dials it, says, "Hello," then hangs up saying, "No one was there," may later reveal him- of herself to be struggling with abandonment. During this first session, there will be no theme development. However, an overture of themes is presented. As the child becomes more comfortable, he or she will begin spontaneous play, which will begin the theme development.

Upon leaving the room after the first session, the child feels respected and honored. Thus, the primary objective of this stage (i.e., honoring the child's expression of him- or herself) is accomplished. This leads to a spontaneous decrease in symptomatic behavior. It is, however, a temporary improvement based on the therapist's positive reception of the child, an occurrence she may not have experienced in some time. As the acceptance of her perceptions is communicated and understood by the child, trust in the therapist begins to grow. With this foundation, the child will feel secure enough to confront the therapist in order to deepen the relationship. She will push on to determine the therapist's acceptance and understanding of what she perceives to be the less acceptable parts of herself.

Testing for Protection: Building the Relationship of Trust

Critical to the establishment of a therapeutic relationship is the child's trust that the therapist will attend to the child's needs for expression rather than strive for control of the experience. Generally, the play therapist must use the first two sessions to build the relationship. When the child has experienced the play therapist as present and honoring in the initial session, he realizes that this person cares about his activities and expressions. However, the child knows that the experiences stored in his memories are unsettling and disturbing. The child must determine whether this attending and caring person will stay focused on his expressions at all costs, even if he enters the depth of his internal pain. To achieve security in this unique relationship, the child must challenge the therapist. This is not a mere testing of limits as defined by many authors in play therapy (Ginott & Lebo, 1961; Rhoden, Kranz, & Lund, 1981), but an I-and-Thou, here-and-now exchange of trust within the context of the relationship. The basic limits of play therapy are not set in the experiential model of play therapy. Instead, the therapist waits for the child to initiate the development of the relationship by challenging the therapist with a behavior that would usually result in limits being imposed upon the child. The child will confront one of the basic limits addressed by Axline (1947). Whereas Axline would introduce these limits as a form of security for the child entering play therapy, the experiential play therapist allows the child to introduce this dynamic when he or she feels some degree of ownership in the therapeutic relationship. Axline's goal was to provide a sanctuary of security for the child in play therapy by establishing a set of external limits. In the experiential approach, the therapist awaits the child's assessment of the conditions of the relationship. In this way, the security within the therapeutic experience develops from within the context of the relationship and is secondarily associated with the playroom. The relationship between child and therapist becomes the primary sanctuary of security.

The exploratory stage establishes the positive or social boundary of child–therapist interaction. The testing-for-protection stage establishes the depth and security boundary of the therapeutic relationship. The child often introduces this challenge to the relationship near the end of the second session, when the therapist gives the time limit to the child. At this point, the child will frequently challenge the therapist by selecting an oppositional challenge in response to having to leave the security of the therapeutic relationship in the playroom. The therapist must not frame this challenge as a power struggle but as an opportunity to provide understanding, meaning, and assurance to the child that she can be any way she wants to in the playroom. (Note: The clinical limits that no one gets hurt or violated remain constant at all times.)

The most common limit contested by children in experiential play therapy is leaving the playroom. This validates that the security and trust are being assimilated by the child and it is now the play therapist's responsibility to prove understanding, meaning, and respect for the child by honoring his or her assertion of defiance. The therapist does not over-power the child but fosters the child's expression of empowerment. This expression of power will be crucial to the child's ability to confront and challenge violations and injustices that the child has had to endure as part of his or her life. The therapist must assume a nonpower position and reflect the meaning of the child's stance. This may be accomplished by stating one or more of the following: "The playroom has become an important place for you"; "You like the way you can play here and know you are safe"; "It's so hard to think of leaving the playroom because your play here is so important"; "I really enjoy our time together, and I know how hard it is to end our time together"; "You like the way you play in the playroom and want to stay and play more." The purpose is not to make the child leave the playroom but to express the meaning of what is currently being experienced. After the child realizes that the therapist will stay with him even when he is oppositional to the request, and the thera-pist focuses on responding to his needs, the child will be ready to sepa-rate. Notice that the expressions are focused on the immediacy of the rela-tionship rather than the oppositional stance. After the child capitulates, the therapist can say, "We can play again next week at our special time." Trust in the relationship with the therapist is established.

Critical to this stage of therapy is that power was not used to control the child; instead, respect was the essential dynamic. The child can now enter the depths of the dependency stage of therapy, dependent on the therapist for emotional protection and security as he or she confronts the situations and behavioral expressions that brought him or her to therapy.

The Dependency Stage

The most critical stage after the relationship is established is the depen-dency stage. The child is now free to express the emotional pressure that results from the trauma or situation that disturbs his sense of well-being. This stage is the beginning of the healing journey. In this stage, the child's play has distinct characteristics that enable him or her to confront the emotional constrictions that have contained expressions of the trauma or area of concern. The first change is that the child enters into fantasy play focused on personally poignant content. The purpose of fantasy play is to serve as the child's disguise or defense against the world that is over-whelming. In fantasy play, the child determines the content and pacing of her personal confrontation with her world. At this point, the child can engage the process of change with assured security and control over pre-vious experiences. The child is now the director of her play, which allows her emotional energy to move toward conquering the injustices that consume her experiences.

The second element significant to the dependency stage is the development of theme play by the child. The child has expressed behaviors and attitudes that have brought him to play therapy. However, these manifestations of his internal conflict have been random and unproductive in relieving the pain he experiences. In the play process, the child can express this internal conflict by moving his pressured emotional energy toward symbols that represent his struggle or anguish. The child plays in a manner that confronts the persons or unresolved situations that have contributed to his conflict. The theme and style of the play is the child's externalization of the inner pain he carries (Clegg, 1984).

The next critical aspect of the dependency stage is the regression of the child to the point where the onset of the issue or trauma occurred. When asked at intake to describe their child's behavior when she is expressing her struggle, most parents will know exactly the developmental age that this behavior represents. When parents confirm this repeated behavior, it conveys that this is the developmental age when the child's emotional security was disrupted. In the playroom, the child will also indicate a developmental age that the distress or enactment play is occurring in. A child may express the regressive level in several ways. Verbally, a child may blurt out an infantile expression such as "goo-goo," without any awareness of the expression, or the child may begin speaking in an immature or baby voice. These meta-expressions tell the therapist the developmental age the following play will represent. Other examples are the child who rolls on the floor like an infant in a crib and the child who crawls into the playroom rather than walking. Many children will walk by the baby bottle and reach out and suck it for a few seconds while they are selecting toys for the session. These are very important messages to the therapist as to how the fantasy play that follows will progress.

When the therapist is asked to express emotionality for the child, the expression must represent the developmental age the child indicated. If the child indicates an event that the therapist must play, the expressive style must be from the identified developmental age. For example, if the child puts the therapist to bed and then indicates that something scary is happening, the therapist must respond within the indicated developmental stage. This may be expressed through crying, whimpering or sucking the thumb, and shaking the body as the child approaches the therapist representing a monster or scary person. This reenactment of his experience validates for the child that his experience is being understood. When play is used to acknowledge the child's expressions, it is not uncommon for the child to stop for a moment, watch the expressions portrayed by the therapist, and then give a recognition response in the form of a smile. This smile shows appreciation that his or her expressions are understood and have meaning. Accurate empathy is communicated through the play experience rather than language expression. Therefore, children can express events that remain in their implicit memory even if they have no associated language to express these events.

The next significant element of the dependency stage is the child's invitation of the therapist to join the fantasy play. With trust in the therapist, the child can now include the therapist in his or her journey. This is highly significant because the child needs this relationship to provide security and protection as he or she confronts aspects of his or her dilemma that are overwhelming. The therapist cannot assist the child in healing without the content of the play, and the child cannot confront the content without the security and validation of the therapist. The journey toward healing requires a mutual relationship of trust and play. The child is the director of the play and paces it according to his capacity to integrate elements within it. If the therapist were to direct the play, it would only reaffirm the child's lost belief in himself. Instead, the acknowledgment and acceptance of the child's expressions by the therapist confirm the meaning of these expressions. The child now knows that he is not alienated by his expression but that his expressions are confirmed by a significant other whom he trusts. Fantasy play becomes the process of expression and discharge of the emotional energy.

The dependency stage comes together as the child, most commonly, has the therapist play the victim's or child's role in an intrusive or traumatic event, while the child metaphorically enacts the event or perpetration from his or her memory. This process may also be expressed from one toy to another, with the therapist expressing the anguish or cries of the victim toy. The first purpose is to demonstrate the event, with pain and fear being identified. The second is for the child to be validated. The third is for the child to gain power over the person or event. The final process in the dependency stage is to control and conquer the situation or the fear of the perpetrator's power. This is usually completed by metaphorically annihilating the perpetrator in play. To the child, this is a spiritual victory that ends the self-alienation he or she has been experiencing since the onset of the trauma.

Completion of this dynamic process dissipates the internal emotional pressure experienced by the child. Therefore, the intensity of the child's play returns to a more normalized level. Once the pain has significantly dissolved, the child recognizes she has alienated a part of herself. She then experiences grief and loss of her alienated self. The emotional energy of the child shifts to reclaiming the fragmented self that was abandoned in the trauma.[2]

Therapeutic Growth Stage: The Integration of Self

When the child expends an enormous amount of energy surviving a dysfunctional or traumatic environment, he loses the time and energy he normally would have spent on developmental tasks. Once he has confronted and resolved those issues, he notices a void in his life. He no longer has to think about protecting himself or consciously organizing his world so that he can function. During this time, the therapist will notice a lull in the child's play. He will no longer confront the perpetrator or struggle with the chaos surrounding him. His play seems uninvolved, with little emotionality and no intensity.

With the pressure of the trauma removed the child begins to re-experience her identity, which had become lost. She discovers a renewed capacity to experience and integrate her surroundings. The lost identity is that which was developing when the trauma caused the abandonment and disruption of the integrated self. The abandonment occurred in the last developmental stage where growth was secure. The child revisits this last developmental period to reclaim her development and the self-growth experiences that were interrupted.

During this time in the play process, the child enters the playroom in a manner similar to his or her first session (exploratory) but explores developmentally oriented toys rather than intensely dramatic activities. This process usually occurs in a somewhat detached style and with flat affect. The play is basically unfocused and lacks a meaningful theme. Time in the playroom seems meaningless and unproductive. Outside the playroom, the child will have episodes of intense rage, usually focused on the nonoffending parent, or on both parents if the violation was external to the family. This anger is the child's way of confronting the caregiver who did not protect him or her from the perpetrator or traumatic event. At this time, it is important for the parent(s) to apologize to the child for not protecting him from the frightening and painful events he endured. For best results, the apology should be generic and not recapture specific details of the event(s). Typically, a parent might say, "Mommy (Daddy) should have protected you from the scary things that happened to you. It's Mommy's job to keep you safe, and I didn't keep you as safe as I should have. I love you so much and you are so valuable to me that I never want anything to hurt you. I will work hard to keep you safe from now on because you are so precious to me." (Caution: Do not say, "You should have told me." All children who were sexually abused told an adult, especially the caregiver. The problem is, they communicated the message in metaphors or play, and the adult did not understand the meaning of the message.) When children are violated outside the family of origin, each parent must give an individual apology. The expression of rage at this juncture of the therapy is the parent's cue to apologize. Children usually only ask for one or two apologies, and then the rage episodes disappear. Failure to respond and complete this process will elicit strong anger responses and delay the positive growth that is about to emerge.

Following this period of calm, apparent indifference, the child comes to realizes she is free to pursue her own interests. She becomes aware of enjoyable pursuits, ones she was unable to engage in previously because she was always in a state of upheaval. With her newfound sense of well-being, she can now approach the developmental tasks she either missed or only accomplished superficially. In addition, she has gained a sense of empowerment she never experienced before. With those tools in hand, she can return to the time when she last felt safe and proceed from there. During this time, it is not unusual for a child to talk baby talk and want to suck a baby bottle. She may ask to be cuddled and rocked. From there, she will progress to exploring the world with a restored sense of wonderment. She notices more of the toys in the room and is able to use them to expand her play and her world. She becomes creative with the toys, using previously utilized toys in new ways. Her speech will progress from baby talk to easier articulation of her thoughts. She will become interested in various types of relationships and how they work. Also, at this time, her dependence on the therapist decreases. Her focus slowly moves toward appropriate dependence on her caretaker. The therapist's role during this time is to remain involved in the play as he or she is assigned. Responses to the child's work will be within the context of the play with emphasis on how good it feels now to be capable of doing things she could not do before, for example, while building with blocks, a simple statement of "I never knew before that this could be done with blocks."

The Termination Stage

In a dramatic shift from play that had been driven with intense emotional energy fueled by fear and helplessness, the child's play becomes more interactive and cooperative. Time in the playroom is enjoyable, with creativity, silliness, goofiness, and laughter. These are the characteristics of a child using his or her play to move through normal development with the confidence that comes only from a child who feels valued and protected. Usually simultaneously with this change comes a time when the child no longer eagerly anticipates his time in the playroom. Instead, he may ask if he "has" to go. He expresses a desire to remain engaged with his friends in their activities. Even if this does not occur, reports from home and school are such that it is obvious that the child is functioning well in both arenas. He is no longer disruptive or withdrawn. He now has friends with whom he enjoys time both in academic pursuits and in social activities. Life in the family has become smoother because the child is no longer creating the tension he had been. These changes become apparent in the playroom with the much more relaxed atmosphere and casual camaraderie.

As this occurs, these changes should be discussed during consultation with the child's parents. A parent or the therapist may introduce the question of termination. It is important that both parties agree that termination is appropriate.[3] When they are in agreement, the therapist is the one to introduce termination to the child. Actually, the therapist recognizes the approaching time while the child is in the latter part of the therapeutic growth stage and may mention a general idea of a time when the two will no longer be playing together. When the therapist and parent have agreed that termination is appropriate, a plan can be set into place and introduced to the child. Termination is, in itself, a process, just like the progression through the stages. Therefore, a minimum of two sessions is recommended for termination. The length of termination depends on the length of the therapeutic process. If a child has been seen for 2 years, termination may appropriately take four sessions. Therapeutic responses to the child at this stage will emphasize the capability of the child to perform on his or her own. For example, while the therapist and child are painting together, the therapist may point out how the child is able to use so many colors or individual items and pull them together into a new creation. If playing with the dolls, the child will now be the caretaker, and the therapist can remark on how important the baby is and that the child is working hard to take very good care of him or her.

The child may choose to use the termination time to revisit her past. She may return to toys and styles of play she has not utilized since beginning therapy. It is not unusual for a child to do a chronological review of her progress through toys and play she made use of along the way.

The end of the therapeutic alliance signals the end of a highly significant relationship. Even though termination may be appropriate, the loss of this relationship is still experienced and must be mourned; thus, the child and therapist working together toward closure is essential. Trust in the therapist may, once again, become an issue for the child and must be addressed. Introduction of termination should occur in the first 10–15 minutes of the session so that any issues that arise out of this loss may be immediately addressed. While self-disclosure on the part of the therapist is unusual in play therapy, this is a time when it is appropriate. The child will be encouraged to know how important this relationship has been to the therapist as well as to him or her. The feeling of mutual appreciation and respect builds self-esteem for the child. It is important to follow up this disclosure with reassurance for the child through the therapist's confidence in the child's ability to survive and thrive without this relationship. The end of the relationship should be complete, with no promises made for the future. It is difficult for the busy therapist to remember to send birthday cards or make calls to past clients, and it is not therapeutic to do so. The child must be allowed to move forward with his or her life. If, by chance, there is future contact with the therapist, both therapist and child can be delighted in the occurrence, exchange their continued appreciations for each other, and move on. If, at termination, the child is fearful of encountering future difficulties without the therapist, he or she can be reassured that the therapist will remain available if it becomes necessary.

Unfortunately, circumstances may necessitate premature termination. If this is the case, it is still recommended to have as much time as possible for closure to the therapy and to the relationship. The parents must be informed of the ramifications of the disruption, as trust issues will reawaken. The child will be angry about the sudden loss of someone upon whom she was so dependent. She will feel betrayed. If abandonment was an issue for her, this incident will certainly renew that struggle. If it is not possible to have a terminating session, request alternative means. A phone call where the two may discuss this loss is better than nothing. It is important to emphasize to the child that this situation is not due to anything he or she has done or said. This is not something that either therapist or child (and often the parents) would have chosen. If the child is expected to resume with another therapist, good wishes and encouragement can be forthcoming from the therapist so that the child understands there is no resentment on the part of this therapist toward the future therapist.

While termination can be a happy time, with a tinge of sadness, it may also be an unfortunate time. Nonetheless, it must be handled with respect for the child and his or her future. How well termination occurs determines how well the experience of therapy is integrated.

THE IMPORTANCE OF PLAY IN TRAUMA RESOLUTION

When children play, their action has two characteristics, activity (movement) and purpose. To many adults, play is viewed as more activity than meaning. In trauma play, the child is very focused and deliberate in conveying the trauma experience (Terr, 1981). The play therapist must remember that trauma is a somatic experience and, therefore, the traumatized child will be either extremely active or extremely constricted in play. Most children will be focused in their intent, but some will be chaotic and disorganized to convey their loss of control in relation to the event. One consistency is that the child will most likely be active and highly anxious when expressing and confronting the trauma experience (Pynoos, Nader, & March, 1991). The child must be given control of the pacing and expression of the content of his or her experience. Since trauma memory is a somatic experience, the use of body and movement is crucial in playing out the event. According to van der Kolk, McFarlane, and Weisaeth (1996) "The first task of treatment is for patients to regain a sense of safety in their bodies" (p. 18). Children cannot resolve trauma by sitting still nor by listening to an authority figure tell them what to do. Since trauma is a fight, flight, or freeze response, the child must confront his modality of response in order to regain his sense of dignity, empowerment, and control. Most likely, the maladapted style of functioning has consumed him to this point. By playing and applying the lost attributes (dignity, empowerment, and control) to the play process, they become assimilated into the child's identity. Experiential play therapy focuses on the four S's in trauma resolution. The S's represent the focus on *sensory* responses as the child creates the experience. As the child integrates and focuses on the trauma experience, energy builds in his or her body. This activates the *somatic* experience associated with the trauma. This buildup of emotional or trauma energy leads to an emotional *surge* or discharge in the child's play. This expression can become very focused and intense. Most often, these expressions occur over several episodes in the process of play therapy. The final step is *soothing* of the emotionally discharged energy so the child can play a corrective or more empowered play style.

This process of resolving trauma may be completed in several small steps during the course of play. In the dependency stage of therapy, each scenario of the play the child creates is an important component of the larger view of the trauma. All play in a session of play therapy is an interwoven part of a larger picture. What may seem disconnected in the play process to the therapist is integrated for the child.

The play therapist working with trauma must perceive the play process from a sensory level. Since trauma is somatic, responses to the child must be focused on sensory reflections. A statement like "That just exploded" should be replaced with an intense explosion sound with the child and therapist falling backwards from the impact. Now the sensory experience has been activated for the child. Once this level is active, the experience moves into the body or somatic level. At this level, the child's body becomes active in the play. Common movements include sword-fighting, crawling and ducking, throwing balls or bombs, or running to escape. Movements usually consist of increased activity in legs and arms to protect the body or self. This process is supported with auditory sensory input of sounds and guttural expressions by the child and validated by the therapist when appropriate or required. Visual input is usually provided by the child in describing the setting (e.g., a swamp of alligators or walking a tightrope over an erupting volcano). Children do not usually give a direct visceral response since their purpose is to power the situation and overwhelming emotional experience. Consideration must also be given to olfactory or gustatory responses. In play therapy, the child regains the empowerment that was lost in the traumatic event. Dignity is restored, and the need for control becomes developmental in nature. Developmentally empowered children are able to listen and integrate. Disempowered children must resist and rebel to discount the devaluating system and experiences.

CASE EXAMPLE

One September morning, Kevin, a 5-year-old boy, was visiting relatives with his parents in New York City. On that day, the relatives were gathered on the high-rise balcony overlooking the water and the Manhattan skyline. As they admired the panoramic view, they noticed the low-flying commercial airplane approaching the city. In horror, they watched the tragedy. Overcome with awe and curiosity, the family watched the day unfold with the second airplane and the fires and sounds of rescue and panic. With disbelief, the group watched the collapse of each tower and the plume of ashes that covered the skyline. The television blared with news alerts and coverage.

Family members talked of the horrific events they were witnessing. Kevin observed and experienced the intense dismay that prevailed with his parents and relatives. Little focus was directed toward Kevin's reaction to the events that were transpiring. For the next few days, the apartment was filled with anguish and concern for the rescue and survival of the victims of the catastrophic event. Kevin continued to observe and become consumed with the concerns of those he loved and relied on for security. Kevin left New York City in the midst of the chaos to return to his life in his hometown, many states away from New York.

Kevin resumed his regular activities, playing with his friends at school and being the active boy that he customarily was. However, playing wasn't as enjoyable as it once was. Thoughts of fear and possible death began occupying his mind. In the middle of his favorite play activities, he would stop as if frozen, thinking of that day in September. Several of Kevin's normal patterns became irregular. Sleep was restless and interrupted, food didn't seem important, and happiness seemed distant and foreign.

Kevin's parents noticed his shifts in emotional style and performance. Concerned about such a distinct change in his attitude and behavior, they took Kevin to a play therapist. After examining her playroom and building a trusting relationship, Kevin entered the dependency stage of play therapy. Kevin built a Lego tower and then started flying a toy airplane around the playroom. The plane then made a course toward the tower, crashing into it. The therapist, by identifying with what Kevin would have experienced, made a loud explosive sound. Kevin's body shivered in a startle response. He continued his play with another airplane crashing into the tower. Again the therapist expressed the loud explosion. Kevin, now kneeling in front of the tower, stared motionless at the site. After a few moments, Kevin rose up on his knees and flung his body over the tower, causing it to crash into a pile on the floor. Kevin lay over the debris and began to cry intensely, identifying with the anguish and pain of the event. The therapist held Kevin as he wailed for some time. As the intensity of his crying began to wane, the therapist began to soothe Kevin by slowly rocking him and stroking his arms and head. As Kevin became more conscious of himself, he acknowledged the soothing he had received. Once soothed to the point he needed, Kevin moved into action and stated that they needed to get all the fire trucks, ambulances, and police cars to the scene to help the people and save their lives. With the trauma expression and energy discharged, Kevin was now able to be proactive and was no longer helpless in the fearful experience that had immobilized him emotionally. As he played his rescuing play, his fears of threatened survival diminished and his emotional focus could move toward the developmental experience of being 5 years old.

SUMMARY

Experiential play therapy focuses on the experience of the child as communicated by the child. The expressions of the child are viewed as valid and representative of his or her emotional state. Children have a natural wisdom about themselves, and when life does not provide a sense of security and a respectful self-identity, there is a need to express their distress. The tools to communicate experience are toys or symbolism used within the toys. The language of expression is through the use of play and metaphor, the natural modality for children. When children are heard, the purpose of their play is to heal themselves from their unsettling experiences. The play therapist becomes a personal expansion in the healing journey. Without knowing the content of the journey, the play therapist listens and experiences with the child. Children have a keen sense of finding their well-being. This is integrated and assimilated into their functioning, and life begins anew. With this satisfaction and the joy of life's experiences, the purpose of life becomes theirs to share with the world. And with these new skills and the ability to use them, children will not inflict the trauma onto the next generation.

NOTES

1. Active participation is the major departure point between experiential play therapy and child-centered play therapy. When the therapist plays with the child, under the child's direction, it allows the child to keep the overwhelming material on an experiential level and allows him or her to maintain control over how it is presented. A verbal response directly to the child, even though it is responding to affect, does so in such a manner as to bring the disguised content into consciousness and pushes the child to acknowledge the event in a conscious, cognitive manner. In this way, the child loses control over presentation of the affect. While the verbal response may be completely accurate, the child must struggle to accept or reject its impact. When the child controls the experience, he or she gains mastery over the emotionality at his or her own pace.
2. The next stage in the progress is the therapeutic growth stage. For the purpose of distinction in describing these two stages, they have been characterized as distinct and linear. However, it is not uncommon for some children to interweave these two stages, with focus on the dependency stage initially predominating. As therapy progresses, the growth stage becomes predominant.
3. When children have experienced severe trauma, it is possible for them to reach a point of resolution for themselves that is appropriate for their age and stage of development. However, it is important to point out to the parents that

as the child progresses through her development, it may be necessary for her to return to therapy briefly to work on issues related to the original trauma that are specific to this age. For example, the child who is sexually assaulted at the age of 3 may find himself, at 4, no longer overwhelmed by fears of being overpowered again. But he may also find it necessary to readdress the issue of sexual relationships as he approaches puberty and his budding interest in sexual relationships leads him to question how they can occur in a positive manner.

REFERENCES

Allen, J. (1991). *Inscapes of the child's world.* Dallas: Spring.

Axline, V. (1947). *Play therapy: The inner dynamics of childhood.* Boston: Houghton Mifflin.

Axline, V. (1955). Play therapy procedures and results. *American Journal of Orthopsychiatry, 25,* 618–626.

Carrol, F., & Oaklander, V. (1997). Gestalt play therapy. In K. O'Connor & L. Beaverman (Eds.), *Play therapy theory and practice: A comparative presentation* (p. 185). New York: Wiley.

Clegg, H. (1984). *The reparative motif in child and adult therapy.* New York: Aronson.

Ginott, H., & Lebo, D. (1961). Play therapy limits and theoretical orientations. *Journal of Consulting Psychology, 25*(4), 337-340.

Johnson, J. (2005). *Fight, flee, or freeze: Identifying and responding to the stress response during play therapy.* Paper presented at the Colorado Association for Play Therapy Conference, Denver, CO.

Jung, C. (1956). *The collected works: Vol. 5. Symbols of transformation.* Princeton, NJ: Princeton University Press.

Jung, C. (1964). *Man and his symbols.* Garden City, NY: Doubleday.

Kalff, D. (1946). *Sand play.* Glencoe, IL: Free Press.

Knell, S. M. (1993). *Cognitive-behavioral play therapy.* Northvale, NJ: Aronson.

Levine, P. (1997). *Waking the tiger: Healing trauma.* Berkeley, CA: North Atlantic Books.

Lowenfeld, M. (1991). *Play in childhood* (2nd ed.). New York: Cambridge University Press. (Original work published 1935)

Mills, J., & Crowley, R. (1986). *Therapeutic metaphors for children and the child within.* New York: Brunner/Mazel.

Norton, C., & Norton, B. (2002). *Reaching children through play therapy.* Denver, CO: White Apple Press.

Oaklander, V. (1988). *Windows to our children: A Gestalt therapy approach to our children and adolescents.* Highland, NY: Center for Gestalt Development.

Paley, J., & Alpert, J. (2003). Memory of infant trauma. *Psychoanalytic Psychology, 20*(2), 329–347.

Perls, F., Hefferline, R., & Goodman, P. (1951). *Gestalt therapy.* New York: Gestalt Journal Press.

Perry, B. (2002). *Identifying and responding to trauma in children up to 5 years of age.* A video series: Understanding Childhood Trauma. Barrington, IL: Magna Systems.

Piaget, J. (1952). *The origin of intelligence in children.* New York: International Universities Press. (Original work published 1936)

Piaget, J. (1954). *The construction of reality in the child.* New York: Basic Books. (Original work published 1937)

Piaget, J. (1962). *Play, dreams, and imitation in childhood.* New York: Norton.

Pynoos, R., Nader, K., & March, J. (1991). Post-traumatic stress. In J. Weiner (Ed.), *Textbook in child and adolescent psychiatry* (pp. 339–348). Washington, DC: American Psychiatric Press.

Rhoden, B., Kranz, P., & Lund, N. (1981). Current trends in the use of limits in play therapy. *Journal of Psychology, 107*(2), 191–198.

Russ, S. (1995). Play psychotherapy research: State of the science. In T. H. Ollendick & R. J. Prinz (Eds.), *Advances in clinical child psychology* (Vol. 17, pp. 365–391). New York: Plenum Press.

Russ, S. (2004). *Play in child development and psychotherapy: Toward empirically supported practice.* Mahwah, NJ: Erlbaum.

Seja, A., & Russ, S. (1999). Children's fantasy play and emotional understanding. *Journal of Clinical Child Psychology, 28,* 269–278.

Terr, L. (1981). Forbidden games: Posttraumatic child's play. *Journal of the American Academy of Child Psychiatry, 20,* 741–760.

Terr, L. (1988). What happens to early memories of trauma?: A study of 20 children under age 5 at the time of documented traumatic events. *Journal of the American Academy of Child and Adolescent Psychiatry, 27,* 96–104.

van der Kolk, B. (1996). The body keeps the score: Approaches to the psychobiology of posttraumatic stress disorder. In B. van der Kolk, A. McFarlane, & L. Weisaeth (Eds.), *Traumatic stress.* New York: Guilford Press.

van der Kolk, B., McFarlane, A., & Weisaeth, L. (Eds.). (1996). *Traumatic stress.* New York: Guilford Press.

van der Kolk, B., Perry, J., & Herman, J. (1991). Childhood origins of self-destructive behavior. *American Journal of Psychiatry, 148,* 1665–1671.

Winnicott, D. (1999). *Play and reality.* London: Tavistock. (Original work published 1971)

CHAPTER 3

Dynamic Play Therapy

STEVE HARVEY

A 5-year-old boy, Michael, enters the playroom with his father, John. They have the intention of playing together. The boy and father have been told that they will play as part of a mental health intervention. Michael's parents asked for assistance because he has had constant trouble attending his first year of school due to his difficulties separating from them. At school, Michael takes a long time to become involved in his classroom activities or with his friends. At home, he often sleeps with his parents and has nightmares when he is alone. He has been aggressive toward his younger brother. Both parents report that no discipline plan seems to help change their son's behavior.

Once in the playroom, Michael refuses to draw with his father when asked to by the therapist. While he sits in his father's lap, he grabs hold of John's neck tightly, preventing further activity. The therapist encourages John to be patient and carry Michael over to some large pillows and stuffed animals in another part of the room. Michael leaves his father, runs to the pillow pile, and begins to wiggle into the pillows to hide from the watching adults. The therapist suggests to John that he begin a game of trying to find his son. John tries initially to reach Michael by grabbing him while Michael crawls farther into the pillows. Michael claims he is making a house; John then knocks on a pillow as if it were a door. When Michael invites him in, John crawls toward his son. At this point, Michael bounds out of the pile and begins jumping from pillow to pillow. The therapist hands John an elastic rope and they both try to "catch" Michael by throwing the rope around him. After some chase, the rope lands around Michael's waist. John and Michael then begin a tug-of-war until they both fall into the pillows laughing.

Michael leaves his father, crawls under the pillows again, and asks to be buried with all the large soft props, looking as if he wants to repeat the interaction. The therapist labels this activity as a game of "getting Michael to school" with the object of trying to get Michael out of his home (the pillows) and to school (another pillow across the room) using the catching rope. John continues trying to catch his son as Michael crawls farther under the pillows, which he calls his "cave." The therapist suggests that Michael may find some animals or other friends in the cave, referring to several of the stuffed animals and puppets mixed among the pillows.

Michael finds a tiger and he pretends to roar loudly. The therapist then helps John set up a series of other animals along a "road" leading to the school. The tiger looks out from his cave and roars, and the father begins to use a large dog to bark back. John, as the dog, invites his son to come along the road with him. Both father and son, as the tiger and dog, move along the road chasing the other animals away from them by using loud animal sounds as they find their way to the school pillow. John and Michael complete the session by drawing a map of the journey to the school and using small clay figures they have just made to move along the path showing the various encounters with other animals. The therapist suggests that John and Michael take their drawing and continue their storytelling before bedtime following the session.

Over the next 2 months, Michael has play sessions with his mother, younger brother, and entire family. During these playtimes, he and his play partners continued to play hide and chase using the pillows and ropes. As these games became more elaborate, Michael's pillow houses and the resulting stories of the tiger's journey to school became more complex during play improvisations. Such enactments were videotaped and viewed at home. Michael and his parents use these times at home to come up with new ideas to bring into the sessions. Additional characters and plot turns are drawn and included during these later sessions.

The parents and therapist find a new stuffed tiger that Michael can use in his stories and take home with him after the last session. A ritual conversation and play episode between the tiger from the playroom and the new tiger occur in a final farewell. These conversations include the subject of Michael's becoming older and more able to do things for himself, such as go to school. The tigers agree on this development as Michael smiles at his parents. Concurrently, Michael becomes more able to separate from his parents to attend school and sleep by himself with his new tiger, and his aggression decreases. Family-oriented play therapy is successfully completed after 6 sessions with a final viewing of a tape of the sessions, which includes the talking tigers.

These sessions highlight the resources children of any age and their families have to interact creatively with each other to address the emotional difficulties they encounter. Clearly, in this example, Michael is having a problem becoming 5 and being an older brother. Such conflicts are influencing his ability to attend school independently. When looked at in another way, Michael's problems with separation can be seen as a metaphor for leaving the felt sense of security he had established with his parents before the inclusion of his younger brother and his new task of spending time at school. Likewise, his parents were unable to find a way to support this change with empathic understanding or flexibility toward their son's new situation. They had resorted to discipline practices, which were not effective, and their communications with Michael had become one-sided, excluding more attunement to his emotional conflict despite their verbal statements about their intention of helping him become an older brother.

In their play, however, Michael and his father were able to use their interactions to create a different emotional state or playspace with each other. Once in this imaginative give and take, John and Michael could generate an active imagination, initially in movement, then using more physical dramatic storymaking to create a metaphor about this family shift. Emotional sharing was achieved by active mutual participation in the play metaphors.

The activities of chase, house making, mapping the journey, video making, and the dramatic action of father and son using the tiger to fend off more dangerous animals became a way for this family actively to engage the important event of their oldest child's going to school. The play facilitated episodes of emotional mutuality in which the father helped his son defeat (or master) his fears related to growing up. The playstate also helped Michael and his father concretely experience fun together after weeks of feeling only anger and frustration. Such shared moments led to father and son becoming more hopeful that they could again become intimate even during this difficult time, and their play developed a restorative quality. Michael could become a student with more ease and trust in his situation.

DYNAMIC FAMILY PLAY

Dynamic family play (Harvey, 1990, 1993, 1994a, 1994b, 1994c, 1997a, 2000a, 2003a, 2003b, 2005; Harvey & Kelly, 1993) is an intervention style in which family members are helped to engage in mutually developing play episodes using movement, dramatic, storytelling, and artistic expressions together to address child- and family-related concerns. These episodes can be videotaped and important scenes can be elaborated into a ritual enactment for more symbolic meaning. All family members become included at some time during the intervention, while various parent–child groupings are seen together to develop more specific scenes. Children are often seen for individual play-related sessions as well.

The main goal of this intervention is to help the family members to develop and use the creativity they share to be better able to adapt to their current conflicts with more flexibility and emotional responsiveness. The central premise is that this creativity is naturally generated within the context of important basic emotional family relationships to some degree and that such creativity is activated in play. This natural creativity contains problem solving and facilitates emotional closeness as family members enter into and more fully experience a state of play with each other.

ATTACHMENT, ATTUNEMENT, AND NATURAL PLAY

Michael and John easily used the creativity they experienced in their shared play to generate metaphorical experiences. They also were able to share positive emotional states that emerged in their mutual play. Because of Michael's previous positive experiences with his parents, he had developed a secure attachment with them, and their experiences with play developed relatively soon in this intervention. Play in this instance helped to restart their naturally occurring flexible adaptation to a temporary conflict related to the adjustment of the family's development.

Other families have a great deal more difficulty recognizing and generating creative play with the concurrent restorative emotional effects, and their expressive episodes break down quickly. In these situations, simple play activity can generate ongoing emotional isolation and conflict.

Such difficulty with play expression occurs frequently in families that have experienced more intense emotional conflicts such as those associated with psychological trauma, significant loss, abuse or violence, and family transitions. The task of the family play therapist in intervention is to support families in beginning to play together and guide such play to become mutual, intrinsically motivated, and effective in addressing a family's central concerns. Most often, this will include developing play in which a family's basic emotional issues of attachment, loss, separation, and transition are addressed in some metaphorical manner.

Two of the underlying assumptions of this intervention style are that playful interactions are pleasurable and intimate and that family members generate this mutual play in an intrinsic manner. Family play is closely related to the development of basic family attachment (Bowlby,

1972, 1973, 1980) as well as affective attunement (Stern, 1985, 1990). "Attachment" refers to the close, lasting, and specific emotional relationships that develop among family members. "Attunement" refers to a style of specific and ongoing nonverbal emotional communications.

Attachments initially develop between an infant and primary caregiver, usually the mother, and become generalized to the larger family system (Byng-Hall, 1991) of other adults and siblings as children enter the preschool and early primary school years. Attachments emerge as the main caregiver responds to an infant's distressed states using interactions that help the infant return to a physically felt sense of security by using nonverbal communications responsive to the infant's expressions of distress. These interactions are primarily nonverbal and develop patterns that are immediately recognized by both caregiver and infant during the course of their daily time together. Such communication patterns produce varying qualities of physical/emotional experiences, with many parent and child dyads feeling secure and others experiencing greater insecurity and disorganization following their attempts to change the initial distressing state. As children enter primary school, their emotional experiences of basic security/distress are closely reflected by and generated in the ongoing interactions among their important family members.

Affect attunement (Stern,1985, 1990) is a concept closely related to family attachment. While attachment interactions involve those patterns in which high levels of distress are addressed by a caregiver (or family at older ages) and a child, attunement refers to the nonverbal patterns of interaction that become generalized around specific high-intensity emotional states, including joy or positive feelings. As attunements become more generalized, these "dances" or mutual expressive episodes allow these feelings to become shared events. Attunement between a young child and parent can become especially observable during the toddler years and occurs across expressive modalities. For example, when a young 2-year-old child starts to show happiness in his bodily movement and his mother responds verbally, matching her vocal rhythm to the toddler's smiling and other physical expressiveness, attunement is occurring. As similar events occur on several occasions, this vocal/physical attunement develops a mutuality that can generalize in ongoing daily interaction, and parent and child begin to have shared emotional experiences.

The ongoing nonverbal interactions involving attachment and more specific attuned emotional events influence the shared emotional environment of a family. The qualities of different nonverbal interactive patterns give evidence of how it feels to live in a particular family on a moment-to-moment basis and such nonverbal exchanges can be observed. Major events, such as the experience of developmental shifts within a family (e.g., Michael and John) or events involving strong emotional reactions, such as psychological trauma, loss, and separation, contribute to a family's inner emotional experience and are reflected in its attachment-related and attuned interactions. If there is a death of child or a parent experiences a traumatic event, for example, the attachment and attuned interactions reflect and influence levels of distress and the quality of shared emotional experience. The resulting emotional atmosphere of the family can be observed in repeated nonverbal communication episodes. Importantly, such episodes also continue to create the emotional atmosphere in the pattern of the moment-to-moment communications. Unfortunately, when a family experiences conflict and the atmosphere becomes negative, such emotional exchanges can become static and lose spontaneity. A negative emotional atmosphere can be carried on for years after a traumatic event.

Episodes of shared family play are also highly related and contribute to attachment and attuned communication. While not exactly the same thing as attachment, family play certainly contributes to and reflects the basic communication patterns discussed above. From infancy onward, children and parents (and siblings) generate play interactions spontaneously. Such play develops greater complexity as children grow older and their parents change in their responsiveness. For example, an infant will seek out her mother's smile to play a game of laughing with her while face to face, a toddler will engage his father in a game of run and chase upon his father's return from work, a 5-year-old will tell and show dramatic stories using stuffed animals with his mother and older sibling, a 10-year-old might produce Lego creations with his family members, and even teenagers and parents can use humor. All such events can be considered shared play and contribute to a shared emotional atmosphere.

These play episodes offer a way to see attachment and attunement in a very clear and understandable way. The play of families with problems lacks the same quality of spontaneous flow as that generated by those families who have been more successful in developing family security and clear attunement with each other. The play themes also differ in that play episodes with problematic families contain images of stress and the play expression becomes disorganized easily. Whereas the flow of interactive play of more secure families generally leads to successful resolutions, the play scenes of problematic families lead to greater conflict and lead the players to the experience of conflict with and alienation from each other. The play within families experiencing problems feels different and lacks the interest, fun, and intrinsic flow of positive exchanges and activity that helps restore family members after a hard day with each other.

Play episodes reflect the emotional atmosphere generated by the attachment and attunement. Expressive interactions contribute to change in very natural ways. The spontaneous experience of playing together can generate shared pleasure and hopefulness even after very conflictual events in a family. In this way, episodes of play can serve as healing events that restart attuned communication and reintroduce flexibility and creative problem solving in a spontaneous manner. Such events can be simple, such as an 8-year-old playing and winning a card game with his parent after a tantrum, or more complex, such as two brothers making a movie together about an imagined space attack after an intense conflict about their mismatched needs.

In the example of John and Michael, the interaction of Michael holding his father's neck was anything but fun for them and quickly created the feel of the emotional conflicts that led them to therapy. As this father and son began to develop an attuned playstate with each other that was enjoyable, solutions to the family problems with Michael's separation emerged with only a small amount of coaching from the therapist. As the play episode developed a life of its own, John and Michael generated activities in which they could share pleasure and positive emotion and creatively developed images and story meaning. Their play became about the main emotional conflict as Michael went on a journey of becoming more independent. The therapist was able to help craft this play experience to better define the experience and meaning for the family. The final play episodes contained solutions that the family generalized. In addition, the family members were able to share positive emotions with each other again.

Put simply, in this style of intervention, the goal is to help families develop or restart play that has broken down within them. Such play is thought to be a natural antidote to emotional difficulty. Dynamic play is a form of intervention in which strong emotional events in families can be developed in play episodes that contain an experience of shared mostly pleasurable experience and make images and story themes that can develop meaning. The therapist initially facilitates or coaches family members to develop play that is attuned and organized and has elements of shared positive emotion. As this play becomes ongoing and self-generating, family members are helped to elaborate it to become meaningful for them. In this way, difficult emotional themes are made more manageable in play behaviors.

BACKGROUND

Dynamic play developed from the creative art therapies including the dance, drama, and art modalities. Though much about these practices has been written, this material is unfortunately not often mentioned in the literature surrounding play therapy. This is particularly true for the contributions from dance and drama therapy. A brief review of some of the main practices from these areas is presented to illustrate how interactive movement, dramatic improvisations, and ritual making can be integrated into interventions that draw on a family's natural play resources to develop creative responses to conflict.

Dance therapy emerged in the 1940s and 1950s as pioneers from creative dance began to apply improvisational movement to groups of people with identifiable psychiatric difficulties. One of the most important of these early innovators was Marian Chace (Chaiklin, 1975). Ms. Chace began using movement with psychiatric inpatients at St. Elizabeths Hospital in Washington, DC. Her basic assumption was that every person had a desire to communicate and that dance could fulfill this need. Basic components of her work included body action, symbolism, therapeutic movement relationship, and rhythmic activity.

In this work, the dance therapist begins by following the movement patterns in a group setting, using the natural gestures and postural changes of each individual as he or she responds to others. Interactions involve the therapist in movement relationships with patients as a way of deep emotional acceptance and communication. Such movements are then guided into more organized dances in which the whole group participates, especially through the use of rhythmic movement. Verbal imagery provided by group members helps define emotional themes relevant to the participants as they arise on a moment-to-moment basis. In this approach, the therapist maintains a role of observer/participant by carefully watching and attuning to the movement of the patients, then joining these movements so that relationships can be established on a movement level. The therapist uses the movement deviations and variations produced as cues to transform and change the activity into an emergent flow connecting the movement of one person to another from one gesture to the next. As the group proceeds, the therapist identifies and verbalizes basic themes that have emotional relevance, particularly through the use of verbal imagery.

Mary Whitehouse (1979) developed another way of using spontaneous movement as a vehicle to explore an individual's less conscious emotional states. In this form, both spontaneous and simple movement structures are a way for individuals to use their movement as a form of active imagination to explore archetypal images that emerge. The movements generated in therapy are deeply personal. One such style that evolved is called authentic movement. During authentic movement, participants' expressions are thought to reflect deeply physically felt emotional experience. The therapist more often is in the role of a witness who observes and attunes to emotional experiences of the movers. One goal of this practice is for the client to have an experience of being seen or understood on a basic physical and less defended level.

Movement has also been applied to therapeutic work with children and families. Adler (1968) and Kalish-Weiss (1974) describe using their own movement to establish a relationship with autistic children. Leventhal (1974) reports using more structured movement to help children with hyperactivity and learning disabilities begin to organize their movement and apply thinking to control their bodies and their behavior in general.

Dulicai (1976) and Bell (1984) began to apply movement observations to work with families both in evaluations and in helping to make interventions to change basic communication patterns. Such techniques involved using various structures to observe a family's nonverbal communication to identify underlying emotional themes. Bell reports using simple movement structures, such as having one family member show his or her understanding of interactions using physical placement of other family members and then change such placements to how he or she would like them to be.

Johnson (2000) extended the concept of Chacian dance therapy to include the use of dramatic play through improvised character, story, and enactments of conflict in the drama therapy method of developmental transformations. In this style, expressive action is organized around a developmental continuum from more purely physical action to sounds, imagery, personified roles, and then enactment of scenes and more verbalization. Expressions early in the sessions demand less complexity in task, interpersonal relatedness, and emotional expressiveness and increase in emotional, personal, and expressive demands as sessions progress. In developmental transformations, therapeutic activity begins with body action and moves ahead through the use of a flow of movement and imagery in interactions with others.

In this activity, the therapist is a participant and maintains an empathic mirroring of the participant's movement, mood, and affective tone. Developmental transformations achieve more dramatic enactment than does the dance therapist through the active use of the playspace in which both therapist and participant become aware and agree that the interaction, imagery, and role enactment are indeed play. Symbolism becomes emphasized in the playspace to differentiate roles, plot, a story-line, and enactments of conflict. Dramatic enactments are improvised freely by the therapist and participant as the therapist follows the client's lead.

James, Forrester, and Kim (2005) describe a drama therapy case study in which an 8-year-old boy with a history of abuse and family separation begins to engage with a drama therapist in the playspace by initially introducing dramatic role playing in which he is in total control of the therapist. The case proceeded with the boy introducing more stereotypical roles from TV shows for both him and the therapist to play, then more fantasy characters of monsters, and eventually roles in which the boy finally confronts his abuser in direct dramatic action. Throughout this evolution, the drama therapist takes on the roles assigned him by the boy and clearly defines entering into a "placespace" to use the various roles and improvised scenes as symbolic communication about the inner experiences related to the boy's past. The therapist's role is one of full participation in the dramas in an attuned manner to the expressive flow of the boy.

Hoye (1997) describes using a psychodramatic approach of entering into the metaphors of children's dramatic play in an experiential manner. After children are encouraged to develop dramatic play in an engaged and intrinsic manner, they enter into what is described as "surplus reality," where the experiential world emerging in the play has more emotional expressiveness than is present in normal daily interaction. The therapist then can begin communication and understanding of the emotional world by becoming actively involved in the roles and this drama. As the drama is expanded and elaborated though techniques such as doubling, mirroring, and maximizing, surprises and spontaneity emerge, and the therapist helps the child use the resulting metaphors as reciprocal communication.

Kindler (2005) also reports the advantages of emotional meeting and understanding that occur during moments of mutual co-created dramatic role playing. Dramatic interaction between therapist and child proceeds as the therapist attunes to the dramatic role-playing offers by the child. During such play episodes, and often at surprising moments, the playing pair experiences new emotion. These moments are particularly relevant, as they occur within metaphors related to the child's strong emotional life. It is during these experienced moments of meeting and emotional understanding within the shared metaphor that change occurs. Old expectations around past events such as loss or trauma can be dropped, and more positive experiences of intimacy, empathy, and a felt understanding can be experientially added. Such moments are beyond mere verbalization and require the shared experience of a "now moment" in which old expectations are changed in the co-created spontaneity required by both the dramatic improvisation and the shared emotional meeting (Process of Change Study Group, 1998).

Riley and Malchiodi (1994) describe using conjoint art making in families as helping to encourage sharing of meaning and metaphor making. In ways similar to drama and dance modalities, art is useful in helping family members express inner states that are too difficult or inaccessible to express verbally. However because art making requires less physical involvement than either dance or drama, families can develop symbolic representations that have more psychological distance. In this way, the active imagination can be less threatening and can help with more insightful and/or cognitive planning of the expressive experience.

Levy (1988) describes how art, movement, and dramatic activities can be integrated to elaborate the metaphor development of expression, with each modality contributing to different aspects. While symbolic communication occurs in all these activities, movement in general contributes to relationship development and basic empathy, drama facilitates basic emotional expression, and art can help with more cognitive reflection when metaphors are being developed. The use of video and story making in dynamic play contributes to further elaborate the mutual creativity. Not only do these media provide more psychological distance from the more physically felt sense of movement and drama, the making of movies and stories can be used to help families begin to plan and organize their joint expression.

A final background source for dynamic play has to do with ritual. Imber-Black (Imber-Black, Roberts, & Whiting, 1988) described how rituals contribute to the enrichment of family life and how they can be used therapeutically to address significant conflict. As with other expressive techniques, metaphor is central to ritual. Metaphor can be used to address conflicting and complex feelings within a single image or action in a ritual. Rituals are constructed so that parts of a family's life are imbued with particular significance. In therapy, ritual actions are used to symbolically unite aspects of a family's life together in a way to help develop resolution and a shared meaning to situations that were more isolating. Rituals are particularly useful when addressing death and loss, trauma, transition periods, and acceptance of new relationships while simultaneously accepting the loss of older attachments.

APPLICATIONS TO FAMILY PLAY

Several central ideas that concern how change can be achieved when expressive modalities are used emerge from this material. These ideas can help explain how the mutual play experience between family members can be crafted into interventions and include:

Metaphors for Emotional Experience

Expressions of movement, drama, art, video, and storytelling can develop into special experiences that reflect inner emotional states of both individuals and families in a metaphorical manner. In dynamic family play, the therapist identifies and uses the dramatic themes that emerge in mutual play. Themes and images related to strong emotions such as anger, loss, death, grief, fear, protection, and hope, as well as events involving change, leaving, and transition are particularly relevant, especially when they emerge in a child's play in direct relationship to and in the presence of an emotionally significant parent.

Such images are considered "hot spots" in dynamic play. Special attention is paid to them, and they are often creatively elaborated within interventions. A hot spot developed in the play episode described at the beginning of this chapter when Michael first started to move away from his father. Even though Michael's action was on a movement level, this behavior clearly suggested leaving or separation as it was enacted in his father's presence. By further developing the activity using movement games, dramatic play, art representation, and movie making, this image could be used to better direct natural play to address this important family emotional event.

Attunement

Attuned communication that has an element of empathy for the physical felt sense between therapist and client is essential. While this physical sense forms the basic element in dance therapy interventions, improvised drama, story, and art making stress attunement as well. This element is called "attuned play" in dynamic family play. Unlike the more individual interventions described above, in dynamic family play, the development of attuned play among family members is an essential goal. Though the therapist must be able to attune with individual family members, interventions are primarily directed to help the parent follow the child's play, particularly in its physical aspects. The therapist's action when Michael continued to run from his father was to help John join the play physically by using the elastic rope and turn the action into a game of chase to achieve play that could develop attunement.

Play Flow

Play flow is created when a parent has an awareness of the child's play initiatives and responds in a moment-to-moment fashion. The therapies described above stress the goal of developing expression that has a flow (in both movement and dramatic role playing). This principle is applied to dynamic family play as "flow/break." As mentioned previously, as families begin to play together, their play flow stops when they begin to experience the interactive aspects of their emotional conflicts. "Break" in this context refers to any behavior that functions to stop the easy flow or play action.

Examples of play breaks include breaking the preestablished play rules (implicit as well as explicit), small injuries or aggression (verbal or physical) toward play partners when in the playspace, stopping and refusing to continue play action when clear expressive development is available, and/or strong emotional state changes that are out of context with the play action. In addition to helping establish attuned play, therapeutic action to redirect breaks into another style of play flow is an essential intervention. Redirecting John and Michael to more physical play after Michael refused to draw with his father is an example of using the break as a cue to move the expressive activity toward flow.

Use of Structure, Organized Activity, and Spontaneity

A closely related concept to the use of moment-to-moment play flow and play break is the use of structures in combination with spontaneous expression to organize expression better. In dynamic family play, this is called "form/energy balance." In any improvisational expression, a balance needs to occur in which the general organization and point of the expressions need to be balanced with the energy of spontaneity. When too much form is present, the expressions are meaningless and soon stop, but when too much energy is present, activities can go off in so many directions that they lose communicative value. Balance of form and energy is achieved by adding rules, game structures, more defined roles, preplanning expressive activity, or switching expressive mediums (particularly to art or video) when more form is needed. The use of free movement, nondirective play, or encouraging what is already occurring to be maximized and extended are ways to help achieve more energy in a play episode.

John was encouraged to play games with rules such as chase and, later, tug-of-war with Michael to add more form to Michael's highly energetic movement. The use and encouragement of loud animal noises between John's dog and Michael's tiger added energy and interest to the interaction when the boy could have stayed in the pillows, away from his father.

Meeting within the Metaphor

Important change occurs when therapist and child interact fully and empathically within the experience of the metaphor. This meeting occurs on several levels (in the play action and within emotional communication) once the child is fully engaged in play and the images are symbolically directly related to important emotional states. These moments are called surplus reality in psychodrama and "now moments" in psychoanalytical play and occur when spontaneity increases within the playspace of transformations.

This level of engaged play occurs in dynamic family play when "expressive momentum" develops within attuned family episodes. Expressive momentum emerges when the players become intrinsically engaged, curious, and committed to the experience of the play moment. Often this is recognized as the fun of the play. It is during these times that the players can develop joint creative leaps and find pleasure in each others' initiates. John and Michael's play developed expressive momentum as these players spontaneously began to enact the journey from the pillow house to the school, chasing away the fearful animals along the road by making loud animal noises, in order to arrive at school. In the moment of joint pleasure, the father and son were totally involved in the play and allowed new expressions to emerge naturally. This was particularly relevant as the play was symbolically related to Michael mastering his fears of going to school. The father and son met in these moments of surprise, and their experience of each other was distinctly different and more positive.

Ritual

Certain metaphors address several emotional experiences simultaneously in a single conjoint event of a ritual. Such rituals develop after conflicts have been identified. Michael and his family developed a ritual when

Michael had a conversation with the two stuffed tigers at the end of the intervention about saying goodbye as well as discussing becoming an older brother and leaving his younger self behind.

ADAPTATIONS FOR FAMILY PLAY

Two other components of dynamic family play have been developed that are unique to this style and seen as necessary in work with family groups: (1) the use of a playroom, which facilitates moving from one expressive modality to another and (2) the use of play home activity.

Playroom

One advantage of using several of the expressive modalities is that interactions between parents and child can be used to help the development of symbolic and dramatic play from all the action that occurs between them. By having both parent(s) and children in the playroom together, virtually everything that occurs in interaction is emotionally meaningful and has the potential to be shaped into symbolic play. The selection of play material is designed to make use of this assumption. This is particularly true for props that children can use easily to shape their movement.

For example, when Michael ran from John, he was guided toward the pile of large pillows. As he crawled into them to get away, his more oppositional actions were used as an entrance into the playspace when the pillows were labeled as his house. In this way, such props produce a "nonfailure" environment, where almost all nonverbal action moves into metaphor effortlessly. As Michael initially tried to leave his father's presence, his actions could be seen as an emerging dramatic event of him entering his home with his father outside needing to knock on the door to visit him. By having art and video material readily available, these actions could be creatively extended and elaborated into drawing and movies. Use of these basic props can be very useful in addressing breaks in play action.

Another principle addressed in the design of the playroom is that props are selected to be relatively neutral so that play partners are encouraged to use imaginative leaps to project their play ideas. These ideas can change in a moment-to-moment, flexible fashion to keep up with interactive behavior. One moment, the pillows can be a house, the next a mountain to climb, and the next a shore next to a lake designated by a large parachute. Different characters can be added to the dramas quickly with drawings and other art productions. More set toys used in other play therapy forms prove to be too limiting to allow this more fanciful approach in the moment-to-moment projection that arises when movement and dramatic role taking are central to the play action.

The most advantageous playroom for dynamic play to accomplish this free flow of movement to drama, art, and storytelling is one in which a variety of expressive and imaginative activities are encouraged. It is best if such play is conducted in a relatively large open space where family members can use whole body movements in an open way. There should be potential for activity such as chase games, tug-of-wars, and hide and seek. Stuffed animals of varying sizes help suggest imagined dramatic play scenarios. Large, soft pillows can be used to make physical play safe as well as incorporated in making houses or walls. Colorful scarves and elastic ropes are easily employed in simple physical play and as props for dramatic activity. Large newsprint paper and varying types of markers, crayons, pencils, and clay should also be available.

In general, the play materials are relatively nonspecific and designed to help family members use their physical, dramatic, and artistic imagination to turn these materials into what their play demands in the moment, then easily transform it a few minutes later. A large pillow might be used by a mother and preschooler as a safe place to fall into together at the end of a chase game only to be used as a wall for an imaginary house filled with stuffed animals signifying both parents and children a few minutes later. It is very helpful to have a video camera and monitor in the room so that action episodes can be videotaped and reviewed shortly after the performance.

Play Homework

Families are often asked to continue to complete play-related activities at home between in-office sessions. The main goal of these exercises is to help families begin to accommodate in-office "natural play" into their home environment. One expectation of interventions is that families will introduce episodes of playful interactions spontaneously into their everyday life and that such play will have the beneficial effects of being restorative and producing mutual pleasure. Additional goals of using home play are that play episodes can be more directly linked to real home events and that the symbolic nature of these expressions can be made more overt. Often, home activities are used during the initial phase around real scenes from the family's daily events as a directed step in applying metaphor making to give play expression real-life meaning. Once this step has been accomplished, more spontaneous unique play usually develops or is restarted and does not require as much therapist direction.

For example, after a session early in the intervention, a mother and her 9-year-old daughter were asked to draw a picture of their family together as a therapeutic task. They jointly agreed to produce a positive scene involving a family holiday. As parent–child conflict was part of the original referring problem, they were asked to draw a positive and a more conflictual scene from the next week at home. After a few days, the girl had a heated conflict with her mother about schoolwork. This interaction was so negative that it left them unable to communicate with each other. They did not even attempt to finish their art assignment. In the next session, the therapist set up a story in which the mother and daughter enacted surviving an anger dragon by working together to find their way around it to get to a safe home, fighting the dragon only when they needed to. They were then assisted in completing a drawing about chasing away the dragon together. The therapist added statements to the drawing from the home argument as well as verbalizations concerning underlying feelings of helplessness and rejection that may have been related to their original home confrontation. This new picture was then given to the mother and girl, and they were asked to add details to their drawing from their next week. As the week went well, they were able to add several new positive images and statements to their drawing. This use of homework was helpful for this family to begin to see their play expression as related to their family experience. They were also able to actively experience metaphor making as helpful in changing the emotional feelings they shared.

Other homework activities often involve the viewing of video material of play scenes generated in session with the task of mutually creating a name for the movie, developing a more positive ending or next scene, or adding lines for their play characters that relate to emotional content their character might have in the drama. These ideas are then brought to the next session to be incorporated into a new video. In a similar way, children who are experiencing problems with separation have been asked to create a positive artistic image with their parent to take with them when they are required to be separated. They can also be asked to complete a small part of a positive drawing only to complete the whole thing when their parents return. Often, when a family develops a play scene that successfully addresses significant fears, they are helped to create and illustrate a book for their play story and then use this book to tell stories before going to bed. When preparing for in-session rituals, families are also often asked to use art to make props for the enactment.

STRATEGY AND METHODS

The general strategy for maximizing the beneficial effects of family play is to have the family first develop mutual play, then use this play to communicate and resolve important emotional issues while experiencing the pleasure and restorative nature intrinsic to play. In order to accomplish this, the therapist needs to help the family appreciate the metaphorical qualities of play, develop attuned play with each other, be able to generate expressive flow with each other by incorporating their play breaks, have parents be responsive to their children's emotional experiences while in the surplus reality of their play, and use metaphor within rituals to find family meaning for difficult life events. Each of these stages requires different strategies and use of play interventions. These phases are (1) evaluation and introduction to play, (2) use of initial games to address specific problems, (3) addressing the "core" scene, and (4) use of ritual and termination.

Initial Evaluation and Introduction to Family Play

During the initial evaluation, the therapist observes a family's expressive style in several different play situations using preset evaluation activities. A verbal interview is conducted to review presenting emotional and behavioral concerns and obtain a clinical history of attachment, loss, separation, and emotional trauma. Evaluation activities might include asking the family to play a game of follow the leader with everyone being leader, having them complete a drawing together, or having them use large stuffed animals to improvise a story about a family. Another valuable task is for a family to play freely with each other for a brief time (10 minutes) and then for the adults to leave the children to play freely for another 10 minutes. A final play episode then occurs in which the parents return to complete another 10 minutes together with the children. A comparison of play style and themes between episodes is then done. A family's performance of such activities can be observed by the therapist or videotaped to be viewed by the therapist and family together at a later time.

The main task during these initial sessions is to help family members make connections between the content and style of their play and the emotional–behavioral themes they verbally report. Therapy goals are then defined in play as well as verbal terms. The therapist is primarily an observer in such sessions. Verbalizations are more reflective, summarizing information and asking questions to better define problems and relevant history. The therapist assists the family in seeing how their play expression can be seen as metaphorical communication. A more complete listing of evaluation activities and more thorough presentation of how such play material is integrated into verbal clinical material is presented elsewhere (Harvey, 1991, 1993a, 1994a, 1995, 1997a, 2000a, 2003a, 2003b, 2005).

Initial Games: Developing Attuned Play

Following the evaluation and introduction period, the therapist introduces organized initial games to help families begin to improvise their play together around specific themes that seem problematic for them. The aim of this stage is to help develop attuned play. These games have simple rules initially set by the therapist that help families focus on developing successful play. It is expected that such play will break down and that such breaks will be reflective of basic emotional conflicts. For example, families who have difficulties with the insecurity arising from a child's overwhelming fear (such as could occur when a child has experienced psychological trauma) could be asked to chase away a monster together (Harvey, 2000a). Typical traumatized children and their parents are unable to accomplish this play actively together, and the therapist can help coach them to solve this problem first with their spontaneous play and later with in-home activities. The play performances can then be used to help the parent(s) and children begin to talk about their fears and need for safety.

Other examples of initial games include: "volcano" (Harvey, 2000b), in which large pillows are placed on a child or child and parent, and they "erupt" by kicking the pillows off. This physical activity is followed by having the participants draw a volcano and develop a label for what kind of feeling might be inside it during the explosion. Related homework activities include having the family find "volcanic" moment in the family life during the next week to be further elaborated on during in-office sessions. Another series of activities includes dividing the room into "lands" and having family members move from one land to another. The lands are defined with labels relevant to the family's life, such as "good land" and "bad land" (for behavioral problems), "angry land" and "calm land" (for problems related to emotional control), and "mom's house" and "dad's house" (for children whose emotional difficulties follow parental divorce). (This list is very partial list and is used for illustration only.) While parents and their children are moving between these areas in the room, it is expected that interactive patterns will emerge and affect the process of the game in unexpected ways or breaks. Such breaks are then incorporated into the new scene.

A main aim of coaching in this phase of treatment is to help parents and children begin to enjoy more organized improvisation in short scenes together and begin to generate expressive momentum in small ways. Also, the metaphor-making possibilities of the various play modalities are explored. The goal of such coaching is to facilitate family members in their natural play in relatively short play scenes by finding a play form for the more difficult feelings the family is having. The main goal of this phase of intervention is to help families become more proficient in play improvisation.

Such coaching is often quite directive, as family members in conflict often do not know how to play together. Play props such as elastic ropes or scarves are often introduced to help extend play breaks into more expressive activity (e.g., tug-of-wars). The therapist becomes a participant and observer of the play, sometimes modeling or leading positive play expression, sometimes suggesting variations, and always observing mutual expression and the emotional states generated. Verbal strategies here consist of labeling emotional states and connecting such states to expressive activities. Connections between play and home behavior also occur during this time. Play homework activities are often used to emphasize the connections between play expression and real family events. Specific lists of initial games related to specific issues are presented in Harvey (1991, 1993, 2000b), and several case studies describing how the therapist coaches the play breaks into more meaningful metaphors are presented in Harvey (1993, 1997a, 1997b, 1997c, 2000b, 2003a, 2003b, 2005).

Meeting in the Metaphor: "The Core Scene"

In the next phase of treatment, the therapist helps the family identify its core scene or central emotional issues as they are generated in free play. In this stage, families are able to appreciate the metaphorical quality of their play, and homework is not used as often. It is during this stage of treatment that surplus reality, "now moments," and/or spontaneity in communication between parents and children within the metaphor occur more readily. This is accomplished as the therapist helps identify repetitive themes in a family's more freely generated play improvisation in combination with the family's verbal presentation of the emotional experiences within the play. Often, during this stage of treatment, children are seen individually or in interactions with one or the other parent. Play is more often spontaneously generated by the family members themselves rather than being therapist directed. The therapist becomes more of an observer, and therapeutic verbalizations are more reflective of emotional content emerging from the play.

During these play episodes, the therapist also uses verbalizations to encourage and coach more play theme development and the elaboration of images that emerge. It is also during this phase of treatment that play images and themes often reflect highly stressful emotional themes associated with loss and trauma with more clarity. The therapist attempts to discuss such themes with families to help clarify their meaning.

Use of Rituals

Finally, families are helped to devise their own ritual play to develop some correction of their core issues. Various ritual activities are presented in Harvey (1993, 2000b, 2003a, and 2003b). Termination is dealt with during this phase. The therapist helps families reflect on their metaphors with insight at this point in verbal discussion, and the final session of treatment usually becomes a goodbye ritual.

In the making of a ritual, the therapist helps families connect images generated in the play experience to the complexities of their family life. Importantly, the action of a ritual is completed by parents and children in a mutual manner so that no matter how difficult the experience the families are confronting, they are confronting it in a shared way.

A core issue for one family involved the impending death of a parent due to a serious illness. After a series of several play sessions in which the family expressed significant grief, the family members decided to make a book together that contained pictures of important family events: letters, poems, and drawings from the children to the parent and a final collage of family events. During the ritual, the family reviewed this book together and decided to make a copy and place it in the parent's coffin during the funeral. All family members were fully involved in the design of this event.

CASE EXAMPLES

Examples of a family with a young toddler and a family with a 10-year-old boy follow. These cases were chosen to highlight the similarities in use of attachment/attunement to guide play activity and the clear differences of complexity of metaphor due to the age and developmental level of the children involved.

Toddler and Family

Melinda, a girl of 20 months; her mother, Keri; and father, Randy, were referred due to Melinda's inability to gain weight, eating concerns, and developmental delays. Melinda had shown signs of failure to thrive at 6 months. She was very small for her age and had not begun to crawl. Her language development was also delayed. Keri had developed a depressive disorder following her daughter's birth, and Randy was now very involved in his daughter's care, having taken time off work recently.

During the first session, Keri was asked to engage Melinda in face-to-face play. Melinda was very reluctant and would not look at her mother's face even when Keri was clearly inviting. Melinda was more interested when Randy attempted to play with her, though she would look at her father's eyes only briefly. Melinda produced very few noises when in close physical contact with her parents but was more vocal when on her own. After these observations, Keri and Randy noted that the lack of interaction while in close contact could well be part of Melinda's problem. Keri was able to see that if she could develop a more animated approach to Melinda, it might help her daughter engage with her more easily and that such engagement was important to Melinda's interest in eating. Keri and Randy were quite agreeable in trying to develop more face-to-face play as part of the plan to address their daughter's overall delay.

As Melinda was becoming mobile with her crawling and physical movement on the floor, Randy, Keri, and the therapist spent several sessions on the floor with her, rolling when she did, crawling next to her, and vocalizing and singing along with all the mutual movement. Melinda enjoyed these episodes and soon began to start such movement as soon as she came into the playroom. Keri began to use the scarves in front of both her and Melinda's face while singing with her during the floor play. Soon, Melinda began to look for Keri, and face-to-face time increased along with the accompanying vocalizations. Keri reported that she was able to enjoy this time with her daughter.

During the last series of sessions, the therapist used the pillows to build small tunnels through which Melinda would crawl. Initially, Randy helped his daughter begin her journey through the pillows, and Keri would look through openings and use her voice to encourage Melinda all the way through. After a few times, Melinda eagerly moved through the pillows looking for Keri, expressing her enjoyment physically and vocally. Throughout this session, Melinda would take small breaks to have a bottle offered by her parents. Over the sessions, her length of feeding increased along with her participation in the movement games.

Ten-Year-Old and His Mother

Jamie, a 10-year-old boy, participated in family-oriented play therapy with his single adoptive mother, Sandy, for more than a year. Jamie had been removed from his parents' care when one of his younger brothers died due to probable family violence. Jamie's other two brothers were sent to different long-term care arrangements. There were reports that Jamie and his siblings had been exposed to long-term physical and sexual abuse as well. Sandy reported that she genuinely liked Jamie, but he was very moody and uncommunicative. He could also be quite aggressive toward property and threatening to her, though he had never actually harmed her.

During initial play interactions, Jamie participated very little with Sandy. When Sandy and Jamie were asked to draw themselves doing something together, Sandy produced a lively, colorful picture of herself attempting to play catch with Jamie, while he added a small stick figure of himself and little else. During a game of follow the leader, Sandy tried to engage Jamie with several props and then picked up a large stuffed bear and tried to wrestle with him. Jamie participated only briefly. When it was his turn to lead, Jamie became animated, moving quickly with little regard to Sandy's efforts at following him and then performed several physical flips on the pillows and aggressive actions that Sandy could not even attempt to follow. Jamie's play was clearly meant for him. Jamie and Sandy agreed that they participated very little together in their play and that this was much like home when Sandy would try to have Jamie talk with her about his feelings and he would withdraw. Often, he would go into his room and throw things at the walls during these times. Sandy stated that she wished that there could be more interaction in play as well as at home. Jamie wasn't so sure, but he did say he would come if he could continue play fighting.

After a few sessions of conjoint play in which the episodes were very much like the initial play action, Jamie was seen individually in order to help him develop a play game that he could teach to Sandy. Jamie then began a long series of sessions in which he would play the initial game of volcano (see above). The therapist helped Jamie extend this game in many different ways, by adding the concept of eruptions lasting for certain time periods and eruptions in which he would try to kick a specific number of pillows across the room or to the roof. After a few months, Jamie was ready to ask Sandy to come back to play volcano with him. During these versions of the game, at times Sandy was asked to join Jamie and erupt while the therapist attempted to throw the pillows back on the two of them, while at other times Sandy stayed on the therapist's side and tried to win by throwing more pillows onto Jamie than he could kick off. Jamie began to complete a series of volcano drawings, and Sandy and Jamie kept track of their volcanic moments (episodes of conflict) at home.

Finally, after a particularly energetic game of volcano, Jamie said that he wanted to be buried. Sandy and the therapist buried Jamie several times in various ways until he asked to be buried with all the scarves so that he could see. At this point, Jamie crawled out and spent a very long time preparing a way to create a cage with a single large scarf connected to the wall and the floor in such a way that he could move behind it. He began to enact being a lion prowling in his cage. As he had used a light scarf, Sandy was able to watch and witness Jamie as the lion for the rest of the session.

In a session following this, Sandy told Jamie that she finally understood his feeling to be that of a wild animal being watched in a cage. They agreed that this was how it was when Sandy had kept asking him to tell her about how he felt and especially about how he felt about the death of his brother. Jamie's angry outbursts decreased, and he and Sandy said they became closer.

They were able to develop a ritual of gift giving in one of the last sessions, in which Sandy prepared a collage of pictures of lions both in the wild and in cages while Jamie wrote Sandy a letter about what he remembered about his experience of living with his birth family and some of the things that had happened to him. They both reported that the image of Jamie moving like a lion in a cage was the most significant of the intervention.

In both these cases, these families created new episodes or patterns of interactions once they developed attuned play. Melinda began to look for her mother, while Keri could begin to have more positive experiences with her. Jamie finally slowed down enough to create a way he could be seen so that his adoptive mother would stop asking him to express painful feelings from his past verbally. Both children became caught up in their expressions in ways their parents could join them in important metaphorical experiences. These new experiences (the "now moment") became pivotal in establishing a new meaning around family intimacy. Clearly the symbolism involved with Jamie's expression had more complexity and the ritual communication between him and Sandy had an emotional balance and maturity to it. Both interventions were very important in facilitating behavioral change as well as creating a more positive feeling in the family situation.

REFERENCES

Adler, J. (1968). The study of an autistic child. In *Proceedings of the American Dance Therapy Association third annual conference* (pp. 43–48). Columbia, MD: American Dance Therapy Association

Bowlby, J. (1972). *Attachment and loss: Vol. I. Attachment.* London: Hogarth Press.

Bowlby, J. (1973). *Attachment and loss: Vol. II. Separation.* New York: Basic Books.

Bowlby, J. (1980). *Attachment and loss: Vol. III. Loss.* New York: Basic Books.

Bell, J. (1984). Family therapy in motion: Observing, assessing, and changing the family dance. In P. Bernstein (Ed.), *Theoretical approaches in dance-movement therapy* (Vol. II, pp. 177–256). Dubuque, IA: Kendall/Hunt.

Byng-Hall, J. (1991). The use of attachment in understanding and treatment in family therapy. In C. M. Parks, J. Stevenson-Hynde, & P. Marks (Eds.), *Attachment across the life cycle* (pp. 199–216). London: Tavistock-Rutledge.

Chaiklin, H. (1975). *Marian Chace: Her papers.* Columbia MD: American Dance Therapy Association.

Dulicai, D. (1976). Movement therapy with families. *APA Monograph, Special Education,* 1104.

Harvey, S. A. (1990). Dynamic play therapy: An integrated expressive arts approach to the family therapy of young children. *The Arts in Psychotherapy,* 17(3), 239–246.

Harvey, S. A. (1991). Creating a family: An integrated expressive arts approach to adoption. *The Arts in Psychotherapy,* 18(3), 213–222.

Harvey, S. A. (1993). Ann: Dynamic play therapy with ritual abuse. In T. Kottman & C. Schaefer (Eds.), *Play therapy in action: A case book for practitioners* (pp. 341–415). Northvale, NJ: Aronson.

Harvey, S. A. (1994a). Dynamic play therapy: Expressive play intervention with families. In K. O'Connor & C. Schaefer (Eds.), *Handbook of play therapy, Vol. 2: Advances and innovations* (pp. 85–110). New York: Wiley.

Harvey, S. A. (1994b). Dynamic play therapy: Creating attachments. In B. James (Ed.), *Handbook for treatment of attachment-trauma problems in children* (pp. 222–233). New York: Lexington Books.

Harvey, S. A. (1994c). Dynamic play therapy: An integrated expressive arts approach to family treatment of infants and toddlers. *Zero to Three, 15,* 11–17.

Harvey, S. A. (1995). Sandra: The case of an adopted sexually abused child. In F. Levy (Ed.), *Dance and other expressive arts therapies: When words are not enough* (pp. 167–180). New York: Routledge.

Harvey, S. A. (1997a). A dynamic play therapy: A creative arts approach. In K.

O'Connor & L. Braverman (Eds.), *Play therapy theory and practice: A comparative presentation* (pp. 341–368). New York: Wiley.

Harvey, S. A. (1997b). The scarf story. In H. Kaduson & C. Schaefer (Eds.), *101 favourite play therapy techniques* (pp. 45–50). New York: Wiley.

Harvey, S. A. (1997c). The stealing game. In H. Kaduson & C. Schaefer (Eds.), *101 favourite play therapy techniques* (pp. 150–155). New York: Wiley.

Harvey, S. A. (2000a). Dynamic play approaches in the observation of family relationships. In K. Gitlin-Weiner, A. Sandgrund, & C. Schaefer (Eds.), *Play diagnosis and assessment* (pp. 457–473). New York: Wiley.

Harvey, S. A. (2000b). Family dynamic play. In P. Lewis & D. Johnson (Eds.), *Current approaches in drama therapy* (pp. 379–409). Springfield, IL: Charles C Thomas.

Harvey, S. A. (2001a). Monster. In H. Kaduson & C. Schaefer (Eds.), *101 more favourite play therapy techniques* (pp. 183–187). Northvale, NJ: Aronson.

Harvey, S. A. (2001b). Volcano. In H. Kaduson & C. Schaefer (Eds.), *101 more favorite play therapy techniques* (pp. 188–192). Northvale, NJ: Aronson.

Harvey, S. A. (2003a). Dynamic play therapy with adoptive families. In D. Betts (Ed.), *Creative art therapies approaches in adoption and foster care* (pp. 77–96). Springfield, IL: Charles C Thomas.

Harvey, S. A. (2003b). Dynamic play therapy with an adoptive family struggling with issues of grief, loss, and adjustment. In D. Wiener & L. Oxford (Eds.), *Action therapy with families and groups* (pp. 19–44). Washington, DC: American Psychological Association.

Harvey, S. A. (2005). Stories from the islands: Drama therapy with bullies and their victims. In A. Weber & G. Haen (Eds.), *Clinical applications of drama therapy in child and adolescent treatment* (pp. 245–260). New York: Brunner/Routledge.

Harvey, S. A., & Kelly, E. C. (1993b). Evaluation of the quality of parent–child relationships: A longitudinal case study. *The Arts in Psychotherapy. 20*, 387–395.

Hoye, B. (1997). *Who calls the tune?: A psychodramatic approach to child therapy.* London: Routledge.

Imber-Black, E., Roberts, J., & Whiting, R. (Eds.). (1988). *Rituals in families and family therapy.* New York: Norton.

James, B. (1994). *Handbook for treatment of attachment-trauma problems in children.* New York: Lexington.

James, M., Forrester, A., & Kim, K. (2005). Developmental transformations in the treatment of sexually abused children. In A. Weber & G. Haen (Eds.), *Clinical applications of drama therapy in child and adolescent treatment* (pp. 67–86). New York: Brunner/Routledge.

Johnson, D. (2000). Developmental transformations: Toward the body as presence. In P. Lewis & D. Johnson (Eds.), *Current approaches in drama therapy* (pp. 87–110). Springfield, IL: Charles C Thomas.

Kalish-Weiss, B. (1974). Working with an autistic child. In K. Mason (Ed.), *Focus on dance VII: Dance therapy* (pp. 38–40). Reston, VA: AAHPERD.

Kindler, R. (2005). Creative co-constructions. In A. Weber & G. Haen (Eds.), *Clini-*

cal application of drama therapy in child and adolescent treatment (pp. 87–106). New York: Brunner/Routledge.

Leventhal, M. B. (1974). Movement therapy with minimal brain dysfunction children. In K. Mason (Ed.), *Focus on dance VII: Dance therapy* (pp. 42–48). Reston, VA: AAHPERD.

Levy, F. (1988). *Dance movement therapy.* Reston, VA: AAHPERD.

Process of Change Study Group. (1998). Non-interpretive mechanisms in psychoanalytic therapy. *International Journal of Psycho-Analysis, 79*(5), 903–921.

Riley, S., & Malchiodi, C. (1994). *Integrative approaches to family art therapy.* Chicago: Magnolia Street.

Stern, D. (1985). *The interpersonal world of the infant: A view from psychoanalyses and developmental psychology.* New York: Basic Books.

Stern, D. (1990). *The diary of a baby.* New York: Basic Books.

Tortera, S. (1994). Join my dance: The unique movement style of each infant and toddler can invite communication, expression, and intervention. *Zero to Three, 15,* 1–10.

Whitehouse, M. (1979). Jung and dance therapy: Two major principals. In P. Bernstein (Ed.), *Eight theoretical approaches in dance movement therapy.* Dubuque, IA: Kendall/Hunt.

Narrative Play Therapy

ANN CATTANACH

Knowledge proceeds from:
"What am I?"
To: "I do not know what I am."
To between "Perhaps I am not" and "I will find myself";
To between "I will find myself" and "I am"
To "I am what I know myself to be,"
To "I am."

—ABU-HASAN AL-SHADHILI, "I" (1968)

When children come to play therapy, they usually have a story to tell about themselves and what has happened to them. "What am I?," "Perhaps I am not," and "It's my fault" are constant themes. The stories are often overwhelmingly negative, with children taking the blame for their life circumstances. Alan was 7, trying to adjust to living with his adoptive parents. It was a struggle to adapt, and he found school difficult. When I asked him to tell me about himself he said that he was a naughty boy and had naughty behavior. He said he was talking all the time, wriggling, shouting, not doing his work at school, fighting the children, and not listening to the teacher. His story was negative, and he couldn't think of anything to say about himself that was positive. He thought he was "naughty," and sometimes in the dark at night he felt especially vulnerable as he tried not to wet the bed; "Perhaps I am not" was his overriding fear. He thought he disappeared in the dark. Jake, another 7-year-old, found it hard to make friends at school. He always introduced himself by saying, "Don't play with me. I'm bad. My mommy killed my sister." This history defined his identity. It was so overwhelming that he was unable to discover any other aspect of himself and felt obliged to tell everyone he met that he came from a terrible family.

The dominant stories these children presented were not helping them at school or at home as they continually sought through their behavior and talk to have their opinions of themselves reinforced by those around them. They constantly set up situations to prove the dominant story that they were "naughty" or "bad." In play therapy, the themes the children presented in their social world also appeared in the imaginative stories they expressed. In therapy, we played together with these stories, expanding themes, changing and shifting meanings, exploring alternative plots and solutions until the stories developed and new ways of being emerged. Alan's stories moved from themes of the child abandoned to the child adventuring and eventually going home to waiting parents. There were many twists and turns, but the theme of the child coping alone shifted, and, as his stories developed, some of the responsibilities of caring for the child were managed by adults taking on parenting roles. He explored what it meant to be a child in his new family and what he could expect from his new parents. His dominant story changed and he no longer presented himself as just a "naughty boy."

Jake also told stories of abandoned children, lost in the world, lacking love and care, and taking responsibility for the actions of adults. As his play developed, he learned to tolerate his feelings of grief. After one session, he asked me if I could find out what had happened to his sister because he wasn't really sure of the details of her death. We were then able to investigate the life and death of his sister and understand the circumstances of his early life so that the burden of responsibility for his sister's death was lifted from him. He could then begin to explore his present situation and describe himself as part of a loving family. He shifted the dominant story, which had limited his sense of self-worth and given him a narrow focus in which to explore his social world.

NARRATIVE THERAPY IN PLAY THERAPY

Narrative therapy can be used in play therapy as a way of helping children express and explore their experiences of life. Engel (1995) states that every story a child tells contributes to a self-portrait he or she can look at, refer to, think about, and change; this portrait can also be used by others to develop an understanding of the storyteller. The stories we tell, whether they are about real or imagined events, convey our experience, our ideas, and a dimension of who we are.

The therapist and child construct a space and a relationship together where the child can develop a personal and social identity by finding stories to tell about the self and the lived world of that self. The partnership agreement between child and therapist gives meaning to the play as it happens. The stories created in this playing space may not be "true" but often will be genuine and powerfully felt and expressed.

THE SOCIAL CONSTRUCTIONIST STANCE

This way of working uses themes developed in social construction theory. Burr and Butt (2000) state that postmodern thought proposes that we will never be able to penetrate the real with our imperfect perceptions and constructions, but we are naturally sense-making beings who interpret events and confer meanings upon things. They posit an objective world that is revealed to us through our senses. There is a split between the objective world and our subjective reality; the world we experience is between subject and object. What we experience is both made and found. So we are limited both by events in the world and by our constructions of those events. We might describe this as the "lived" world. The perceived world is not a more or less perfect replica of objective reality. We produce constructions that serve our purposes and help us in our projects.

THE HERMENEUTIC APPROACH

The social constructionist view of the world is a hermeneutic approach. Hermeneutics is the activity of interpreting and explores how meaning is constructed through language discourse, story, and narrative. In this form of analysis, the world appears as we interpret it, and the search for meaning is ongoing. Knowledge is a socially interpreted event constructed through relationships and conversation with others. Anderson and Goolishian (1992) state that a therapist working in a hermeneutic way lets the client's story unfold until a coherent theme or new meaning emerges from the dialogue. It is the therapist's curiosity to know more about what is being said—that is, how a client makes meaning—that engages the future or not-yet-said narrative. Therapeutic conversation involves a mutual search for understanding in which the therapist and client talk *with* not *to* each other. This not-knowing hermeneutic stance is the therapist's expertise to support the client in finding his or her own meaning in understanding his or her own problem.

The basis of narrative therapy when used in play therapy is to explore the stories children present in play and facilitate an exchange of ideas and thoughts about the stories. This approach means that the relationship between child and therapist is one of co-construction, sharing ideas and listening to each other to find the story that best supports the child in what he or she wants to say. This is a hermeneutic stance because the therapist's listening response is a continuous inquiry toward the material presented in a play session. This developing narrative always presents the therapist with the next question. This is a not-knowing position; the therapist's understanding is always developing.

THE NARRATIVE FOCUS

White (2005) lists a series of concepts that describe his key ideas of narrative therapy. He states that the primary focus of a narrative approach is the expression of the client's experiences of life. The narrative expressions of both adults and children act as interpretations through which people give meaning that seems sensible to themselves and to others to their experiences of life. He states that meaning does not exist before the interpretation of experience.

He considers that expressions are constitutive of life, the world that is lived through; they structure experience and inform future understanding. Expressions have a cultural context and are informed by the knowledge and practices of life that are culturally determined. The structure of narrative provides the principal frame of intelligibility for people in their day-to-day lives. It is through this frame that people link together the events of life in sequences that unfold through time according to specific themes.

Narrative therapy is about options for the telling and retelling of the preferred stories of people's lives, rendering the unique, the contradictory, the contingent, and (at times) the aberrant events of people's lives significant as alternative presents. White and Epston (1990) make the assumption that individuals experience problems when the narratives in which they are storying their experience and/or in which they are having their experience storied by others do not sufficiently represent their lived experience and that in these circumstances there will be significant aspects of individuals' lived experience that contradict these dominant narratives.

NARRATIVE THERAPY
AND TRADITIONAL PSYCHOLOGY

Dunne (1992) compares narrative therapy and traditional psychology in three areas: theory of self, client problem, and therapist stance.

- *Theory of self in narrative therapy.* The self is relationally defined, and persons continuously construct their lives and identities.
- *Theory of self in traditional psychology.* The self is enduring, objectively discovered through assessment measures.
- *Client problem in narrative therapy.* The client presents a problem-saturated story. This old story blinds him or her to other stories and resources.

The problem concerns the client's beliefs about who he or she is and associated interpersonal patterns.

- *Client problem in traditional psychology.* The problem is inside the person. The person, their dysfunctional personality profile or "disease," is the problem.
- *Therapist stance in narrative therapy.* The therapist is nonexpert and should orient to the effects of the problem in the life and relationship of the client. The therapist invites the client to compare the old story with the new to see which direction suits him or her better. The therapist invites the client to reflect and build on exceptions to problem behavior in constructing a new story.
- *Therapist stance in traditional psychology.* The therapist is the expert. The therapist discovers historical facts that cause or determine the current personality profile and diagnosis. The therapist prescribes a treatment plan based on the similarity of behavior to other clients, reinforces positive behaviors and confronts dysfunctional behavior or denial, and interprets the meaning of the client's behavior and teaches the client more effective life skills.

THE PLAY THERAPY CONTEXT FOR NARRATIVES

The play therapist can offer a context for many forms of telling and retelling children's narratives of their lives. Humans story experience through the creative process of co-construction. An individual or group identity is fluid, not solid, because it is continually reconstituted through social interaction. The therapeutic space and the relationship between child and therapist is an interaction in which the child can explore and experiment with aspects of his or her identity and the roles played by other dominant people in his or her life.

In narrative therapy, it is thought that the stories told by influential people are likely to dominate and subjugate the stories of less influential people; these dominant stories can become cultural themes for all of us. Less influential people may be portrayed negatively, often internalizing the dominant view of themselves as inferior. This is often true for a child's stories when adults assume they know what the child is thinking and feeling. The child then feels inferior because he does not experience what the adult assumes he should. It is often difficult for a child to tell how he feels about an adult who has harmed him because those influential people—the social worker, the teacher, the parent—express a view of the perpetrator that is not experienced by the child. If the child's story is heard and acknowledged, then he can become empowered. If the therapist and child co-construct the narrative together through their therapeutic relationship, the child can use the therapist to be heard and is free to explore alternative stories in the safety of the therapeutic space.

CASE EXAMPLE OF A NARRATIVE IN PLAY THERAPY

James was obsessed with Elvis Presley and at 10 years of age described himself in this way:

My Life in Elvis Presley Songs

Age 4 years, 5 months	"Girls, Girls, Girls"
	"GI Blues"
	"Crying in the Chapel"
	"Flaming Star"
Age 6 years, 4 months	"All Shook Up"
	"My Baby Left Me"
	"Wooden Heart"
	"It's Now or Never"
	"Heartbreak Hotel"
Now	"Don't Be Cruel"
	"Pot Luck"
	"Such a Night"
	"Teddy Bear"
	"Loving You"
	"Treat Me Nice"
	"King Creole"
	"Don't Cry Daddy"

James was adopted but still longed for his birth mother. Elvis was her favorite singer. We used a hermeneutic approach to tease out meaning as he told me about the structure of his lists. We were able to explore his understanding of life through Elvis and his songs. It was a powerful auto-biography, spanning past and present to make a kind of integration at that moment in his life, with Elvis connecting him to his birth mother and his adoptive family. He liked the coded nature of his presentation, yet each song also held layers of meaning he could express. He was singing his life story, transforming his love of Elvis to give meaning to his own life.

James could explain how each song held specific meanings for a particular time in his life; it took many sessions for him to establish the order of the songs. He wove his life around incidents mirrored in the songs so that his life story became coherent. He liked to perform the songs in Elvis's style. There was also a fluidity in his list, with songs moving from section to section and his interpretation of the meanings in the songs changing. He could connect the songs to people in his life and how he viewed them now and in the past.

EXTERNALIZATION

One interesting concept of narrative therapy is the way the therapist can use the linguistic practice of externalization. This separates the person from the problem. The problem is seen as the problem; the person is not seen as the problem. This shifts the child from the role of client to the role of consultant, with the capacity to find a solution. This is helpful to the child's formation of identity, for example, Alan and Jake were able to shift the stories they had been told about themselves and find new ways to think about who they were. This exploration of identity is what children do as they play. They can explore roles and behavior as they make up stories with toys, paint pictures, dress up and act, play games, or listen to the therapist read or tell a story. James as Elvis was the story of James and his life but also the story of Elvis Presley and his songs.

USING NARRATIVE IN PLAY THERAPY

In my play therapy with children, I use the concept of co-construction as the basis of the relationship. As therapist, I have the task of keeping the child and the space safe for the relationship to develop. I take a stance of not-knowing knowing and follow the narratives the child presents.

I encourage imaginative stories as a form of externalization and what the arts therapist calls "distancing" through arts/play processes. I offer the child sensory materials like sand, water, slime, Play-Doh, and clay. I have small figures and other objects for projective play and story making and toys and objects for role playing. I use sensory materials for embodied play that many children use to get themselves into the frame to tell a story with the toys or to role-play. We might begin by making a pile of slime and putting creatures in it, which could lead to a story.

> There was once a monster who was greedy.
> His name was Justin.
> He ate slime, and his friend ate a ball.
> Then he spitted it out.
> Then he was sick.
> He ate purple slime.
> This was naughty because it tasted disgusting.

This is a typical early story and helps the child create a narrative form with a beginning, middle, and end.

It is often very hard for children to explore painful events, especially at the beginning of a relationship with the therapist. The following story told to me by Peter describes the anxiety:

> There was once a whole crowd of goofy people, and there was a bossy woman who tried to get them to be sensible, but they wouldn't.
> They just stayed goofy because it saved them having to play football or talk because. . . .

There the story ended, and I was challenged to respond. I asked about the strategy of staying "goofy" and whether it worked and what was the price the goofy people had to pay to avoid doing the things they found difficult. Did being goofy stop bossy people, or did it make them bossier? There was a silence, and then we made a slime river together. We returned to the theme of goofy people versus bossy people many times in later sessions.

Peter is 12 and still shocked by the life he led when he was a baby. His mother lived chaotically, experiencing the world through a haze of drugs. When he was born, Peter was left with his aunt, but then his mother took him away to live with her and he experienced the chaos of her life dominated by her need for drugs. Peter's relatives tried to help him, and eventually he left his birth mother to live permanently with his aunt, who has cared for him since he was 4. But his insecurity remains, and he struggles to attach himself to anyone who shows he or she cares about him. He doesn't trust adults and blames them for his troubles.

Peter finds school too difficult and has special help to cope. He is impulsive and lives for the moment with an intensity that uses all his energy. He sees the world and people as good or bad, bossy or goofy, with nothing in between. Play has a calming effect on him, and his aunt says it has helped him cope better in the family. Peter is attracted to danger and is unable to think about consequences, so I tell him stories he enjoys. We use stories as a way of externalizing his problems so he can tolerate a few moments of reflection. The co-constructed relationship means that I can bring my narratives to share and we can deconstruct my stories as well as Peter's stories. All can be accepted, rejected, turned on their heads, or shaped to our satisfaction. He especially likes Mr. Miacca because of the gruesome nature of the story, and we use it to think about dangerous behavior.

Mr. Miacca

Tommy Grimes was sometimes a good boy and sometimes a bad boy, and when he was a bad boy, he was a very bad boy.

Now his mother used to say to him, "Tommy, Tommy, be a good boy and don't go out on the street or else Mr. Miacca will take you."

But still, when he was a bad boy, he would go out on the street, and one day sure enough he had scarcely got round the corner when Mr. Miacca did catch him and popped him into a bag upside-down and took him off to his house.

When Mr. Miacca got Tommy inside he pulled him out of the bag and set him down and felt his arms and legs. "You're rather tough," said he, "but you're all I've got for supper and you'll not taste bad boiled. But, body of me, I've forgotten the herbs and it's bitter you'll taste without herbs. Sally, here I say, Sally," and he called Mrs. Miacca.

So Mrs. Miacca came into the room and said, "What do you want, my dear?"

"Here's a little boy for supper and I've forgotten the herbs. Mind him while I go for them."

"All right, my love," says Mrs. Miacca and off he goes.

Then Tommy Grimes said to Mrs. Miacca, "Does Mr. Miacca always have little boys for supper?"

"Mostly, my dear," says Mrs. Miacca, "if little boys are bad enough to get in his way."

"And don't you have anything else but boy meat? No pudding?"

"Ah, I love pudding," says Mrs. Miacca. "But it's not often the likes of me gets pudding."

"Why, my mother is making a pudding this very day," says Tommy, "and I'm sure she'll give you some if I ask her. Shall I run and get some?"

"Now that's a very thoughtful boy," says Mrs. Miacca. "Only don't be long and be sure to be back for supper."

So off Tommy peltered and right glad he was to get off so cheap and for many a long day he was as good as good could be and he never went round the corner of the street.

But he couldn't always be good, and one day he went round the corner and as luck would have it he hadn't scarcely gone round it when Mr. Miacca grabbed him up, popped him in his bag, and took him home.

When he got there Mr. Miacca dropped him out and when he saw him he said, "Ah, you're the youngster who tricked me and my missus leaving us without any supper. Well you shan't do it again. I'll watch over you myself. Here, get under the sofa and I'll sit on it and watch the pot boil for you."

So poor Tommy Grimes had to creep under the sofa and Mr. Miacca sat on it and waited for the pot to boil.

And they waited and waited and waited and still the pot didn't boil until at last Mr. Miacca got tired of waiting and he said, "Here, you under there, I'm not going to wait any longer; put out your leg and I'll stop you giving us the slip."

So Tommy put out a leg, and Mr. Miacca got a chopper and chopped it off and put it in the pot.

Suddenly he calls out, "Sally my dear, Sally," and nobody answered.

So he went into the next room to look out for Mrs. Miacca and while he was there Tommy Grimes crept from under the sofa and ran out of the door. For it was the leg of the sofa that he had put out.

So Tommy Grimes ran home, and he never went round the corner again until he was old enough to go alone.

Peter recognizes that there are dangers "round the corner," and although he still impulsively follows his nose into danger, he has learned the value of the cell phone to keep in contact with his family. We decide Tommy Grimes should get a phone.

THE CO-CONSTRUCTED RELATIONSHIP: NOT-KNOWING KNOWING

There is a very special quality to a relationship based on storytelling. There is a storyteller, a listener, and the story in the middle as a way to negotiate a shared meaning between the two.

I have stated elsewhere (Cattanach, 1997) that in play therapy children tell stories as containers for their experiences, which are constructed into the fictional narrative of a story. There is a playfulness in the communication, whatever the horror of the story, and the roles of storyteller and listener have an equal function as the story emerges in the space between the two. There has to be a spark of recognition between storyteller and listener as the story unfolds. The equality in the relationship facilitates the unfolding of the story. Together, therapist and child share the drama of the story as the meaning emerges. The not-knowing–knowing therapist does not displace this process with a hierarchy of professional knowledge but learns to listen in a way that supports the unfolding of the tale. The story can be acknowledged by the therapist, who as listener values what is presented, or the child and therapist can deconstruct and reconstruct the story to the satisfaction of the child if new options seem desirable. This is defined as a polyvocal collaboration. The aim is not to locate a solution or a new story but to generate a range of new options. Mary, age 4, liked to play with a witch doll, the bad witch. At the end of the story, Mary thought of many endings: the bad witch can be dead never to come to life again, be dead but come to life, go to prison, or change into a good witch. She didn't have to make a choice just to tell me what might happen; there were options.

Goolishian (1990) states that maintaining a position of openness and uncertainty in a therapeutic conversation requires the skill and patience of an experienced therapist. The therapist's not knowing does not mean the dissolutionment or abandonment of prior knowledge, but rather its questioning. Not knowing refers to what I do with what I know.

A therapist's knowing comes from a variety of sources: theory, training, clinical and life experiences, empirical research, intuition, empathy, and colleagues. This knowledge base has to be used hermeneutically so that it enriches the client's understanding rather than closing it off by imposing an expert opinion. So, knowledge is brought to the therapeutic conversation as part of the desire to understand more.

FACILITATING STORY MAKING IN PLAY THERAPY

Before beginning work with a child, the child's caregivers, the child, and the referrer have a meeting. In the United Kingdom, much of play therapy's work is done through child and family psychiatry, social services, or in schools. These services are free.

At the first meeting, we discuss the reasons for the referral and work out a program, which might include support for the caregivers with other professionals as well as play therapy for the child. Some of the children I see for therapy are being looked after in foster care while decisions are made about their future (whether a return to the family, long-term foster care, or adoption). Other children have had their future determined and are living in a permanent placement with long-term caregivers, are waiting, or have been adopted. I often see children through the process of leaving their birth family to finding a new family. If children are in foster care or adopted, I often see them at their home, which can be a safer place to meet with them. When children are locked into the care system, they see so many professional people in clinics, medical centers, and social service offices that playing at home feels safer to the child.

I negotiate a safe place in the house where we won't be disturbed and set out my blue mat, where the child and I sit to play. This mat is delineated as the playing space where we can play what we like and say what we like but without hitting or hurting each other. I have bags of toys that offer a variety of playing experiences: slime, Play-Doh, clay, and sand for sensory play and a box of small figures, including family figures, magical figures like dragons and witches, and animals for stories. I have dolls and puppets for drama and materials for drawing and painting. The materials change as we get to know each other, and I am often asked to find a particular small figure or something special like pink Play-Doh, which I try to do. I write the children's stories in a book if they want me to, which they mostly do.

Mary is 4 and is in foster care. She has lived a chaotic life so far; her mother is an alcoholic, and Mary and her brother and sisters were severely neglected. Mary's mother will not cooperate with social services. Mary sadly told me that she thinks her mother won't be able to stop drinking. She loves playing and remembers every small figure and every object I bring for her. She was pleased when I found pink Play-Doh. She loves to make stories with the small figures. This is one of the first stories she made up.

> Once upon a time there was a wicked witch and a wicked dragon.
> They lived together.
> They put the birdie in the cage.
> They hurt the birdie and hit it.
> They drank a lot.
> They hurt the dog and the baby.
> The wicked witch is dead.
> Mary killed her.
> She put the animals in the cage and shot the animals.
> They are all dead.

This story expresses the pain and confusion Mary feels about her family and the responsibility she feels for leaving them. I ask if they are dead forever or if they will come to life again. Mary is not sure. We talk about what it means to be dead. It was at this point that Mary offered the variety of options for the ending I previously described. The witch could be dead forever, dead and come to life, go to prison, or change into a good witch. The introduction of the good witch was developed in the next story. Mary placed a set of figures in a lake of slime.

> This is a nasty place it is hot.
> The wicked witch is boss of the place and the dragon.
> There is a pig there who was caught by the wicked witch.
> The babies are there without their moms.
> The wicked witch touched the pig and the babies.
> The babies have nice moms but the wicked witch has taken the babies away but there is one mommy still there.
> She can't look after the babies.
> The witch has put the little girl in the bin.
> "Stay with me," said the witch and she put the little girl in the sand and carried her.
> The little girl was very very scared and she began to cry.
> The wicked witch buried her in the sand and the good witch put her back with her mom.
> "I'm sorry," she said and gave her a cuddle.
> There are two good witches and they fly everywhere in the whole world.
> They do nice things for people.

We think about witches, both good and bad. We also think about the powerlessness of the babies snatched from one place to another because their mothers aren't strong enough to challenge the wicked witch. We do not explore the pain of the little girl being dragged along the sand. Mary holds that sadness in this imaginary story, and I have listened and acknowledged the fear.

It is difficult for the therapist to hold the pain of a small child caught up in circumstances over which she has no control. We cannot make it better, but we can really hear what the child is saying and acknowledge how it might feel. There are no easy answers. Mary is resilient. She makes up another story, then asks for the pink Play-Doh. She squeezes it and smells it, and we scrunch it up together. The session ends. We put the toys away. Mary puts on her shoes and runs to join her friends playing outside. As I leave she waves goodbye. The sun shines; Mary is swinging on the rope swing. She had told me that she had learned to use the swing that week. She swings and sings and laughs and shouts, "See you," and I wave agreement.

THE THERAPIST AS STORYTELLER

When I listen to the stories children make up in play, I am often reminded of folk tales or stories that are congruent with what the child has invented. I might then tell the story to the child because to know that other people have told stories with similar themes can help the child feel like everyone else rather than the only person in the world who has particular life experiences or who can tell such stories.

I see two boys who are 9 years old. They are at the stage of telling gruesome stories and trying out shock tactics. They have been in trouble for swearing at the wrong people in the wrong places. We explore these issues as they play, and they make up gruesome stories to shock themselves and me. I told them the story of the boy on the ice. They were impressed and asked if the story was true. "Who knows?" I said. "It's a story." We all laughed. There were others out there who had our sense of the gruesome.

Keep a Cool Head

He was a great lad for telling stories. He had a great lot of stories, and there was a New Year's Day. Ice came on the loch, and all the young boys came down there skating.

They were all out there, ice on the loch, and they were skating and then one of the boys got a bit too far out, and in the middle of the loch the ice was soft, and it broke with him and he went down, down in a hole, and the other edge of the ice just catched him under the chin.

He slid away under the ice 'til he came to another hole, and his head did the same on top of the ice, and when they came together there his head just stuck on again . . . the frost was that strong it just froze his head on again.

In the evening then they were sitting around the hearth telling stories, and the boy was there too, and he was getting rid of some of the cold with his dip in the cold water, you know, and he starts to sneeze.

As he was going to blow his nose (they just blew their nose with their fingers then you know), as he was going to blow his nose and with the heat, it kind of thawed the ice about his neck, you know, and he aimed his head and it shot right into the fire.

I enjoy the story of "A Pottle o' Brains," which I often tell to children who are impulsive or confused about their world for whatever reason. I think we all need somebody who likes us for who we are, and this story shows that there are ways of managing after many struggles if you can find someone to help.

A Pottle o' Brains

Once in these parts, and not so long ago, there was a boy who wanted to buy a pottle o' brains, for he was always getting into scrapes because of his foolishness and being laughed at by everyone.

Folk told him he could get everything he liked from the wise woman that lived on the top of the hill and dealt in potions and herbs and spells and things. She could even tell the future.

So the boy asked his mother if he could seek the old woman and buy a pottle o' brains.

"Yes, you can," said his mother. You are in great need of them and if I die who would take care such a fool as you who has no more idea of looking after yourself than a newborn baby. But mind your manners when you speak to her because such wise folk are quickly displeased."

So off he went, after his tea, and there she was, sitting by the fire, stirring a big pot.

"Good evening, missus," he says. "It's a fine night."

"Aye," says she, and went on stirring.

"It'll maybe rain," says he and fidgets from one foot to the other.

"Maybe," says she.

"And happen it won't," says he and looks out of the window.

"Happen," says she.

And he scratched his head and twisted his cap.

"Well," says he, "I can't mind nothing else about the weather, but let me see, the crops are getting on fine."

"Fine," says she.

"And the beasts is fattening," says he.

"They are," says she.

"And, and, and," then he comes to a stop.

"I reckon we'll tackle business now having done the polite like. Have you any brains to sell?"

"That depends," says she, "if you want a king's brains or a soldier's brains or a schoolmaster's brains, I dinna keep them."

"Oh no," says he. "Just ordinary brains, same as everyone has around here, something clean, common like."

"Aye so," says the old woman, "I might manage that if you'll help yourself."

"How do I do that, missus?" says he.

"Bring me the heart of the thing you like best of all, and I'll tell you where to get your pottle o' brains, but you'll have to read me a riddle, so as I can see you've brought the right thing, and if your brain is about you."

"But," says he, scratching his head, "How can I do that?"

"That's not for me to say. Find out for yourself, my lad."

So the boy went back home and told his mother what had happened.

"I reckon I'll have to kill the pig," says he, "for I like fat bacon better than anything."

So he killed the pig and next day set off for the old woman's cottage.

"Good-day," he said. "I've brought you the heart of the thing I love best."

"Aye so," said she and looked at him through her spectacles. "Tell me this then: what runs without feet?"

He scratched his head and thought and thought but couldn't tell.

"Go thy ways," said the old woman. "You haven't fetched me the right thing yet."

So off the boy went to tell his mother, but as he got to his house, out came folk running to tell him his mother was dying.

When he got in, his mother smiled because she thought he had his brains and then she died.

The boy was very sad because he remembered how kind his mother had been to him and how she had looked after him so well and put up with his foolishness.

Then he realized that his mother was the one he loved the best but he couldn't cut out her heart to bring to the old woman.

So he put his mother into a sack and carried her body to the old woman's cottage.

"Good-day, missus," says he. "I think I've fetched the right thing this time."

"Maybe," said the old woman, "but read me this: now what's yellow and shining but isn't gold?"

He scratched his head and thought but couldn't tell.

"Thou hast not hit the right thing yet," said the old woman. "You are more foolish than I thought."

The boy left and sat down by the roadside.

"I've lost the only two things I care for. What else can I find to buy a pottle o' brains?" And he began to cry.

And up came a girl who lived nearly and asked him what had happened and he told her about the old woman and the pottle o' brains and that he was now alone in the world.

"Well, I wouldn't mind looking after you," said the girl. "People like you make good husbands."

They got married and decided to wait a bit before going to see the old woman again.

The boy and girl were very happy together and after a while, the boy told the girl that she was now the person he liked best of everything

"But I'm not going to cut out your heart for a pottle o' brains."

"I'm glad to hear it," said the girl. "You take me to see the old woman and I'll help you read the riddles."

"I reckon they are too hard for womenfolk," said he.

"Well, let's see now. Tell me the first."

"What runs without feet?"

"Why, water," says she.

"And what is yellow and shining and not gold?"

"Why, the sun," says she.

"That's right," says he. "Come, we'll go to the old woman."

So off they went.

The old woman was sitting outside twining straws.

"Good-day missus," says he. "I reckon I've fetched the right thing at last."

The wise woman looked at them both.

"Canst tell me what that is as has first no legs and then two legs and ends with four legs?"

And the boy scratched his head but couldn't tell. And the girl whispered in his ear,

"It's a tadpole."

The boy told the old woman, who nodded her head.

"That's right, and you have your pottle o' brains already."

"Where be they?" he asked, searching in his pockets.

"In your wife's head," says she.

So they went home together, and he never wanted to buy a pottle o' brains again, for his wife had enough for both.

At the end of a hard day, I console myself with *Meditations* by Marcus Aurelius (2003). I especially like at such a time Book 9, Meditation 32:

You can discard most of the junk that clutters your mind—things that exist only there—and clear out a space for yourself:

> by comprehending the scale of the world
> by contemplating infinite time
> by thinking of the speed with which things change—each part of
>   everything;
> the narrow space between our birth and death; the infinite time
>   before; the equally unbounded time that follows. (p. 125)

REFERENCES

Abu-Hasan al-Shadhili. (1968). I. In *I. Shah, The way of the Sufi* (p. 248). New York: Penguin Books.

Anderson, H., & Goolishian, H. (1992). The client is the expert: A not knowing approach to therapy. In S. McNamee & K. J. Gergen (Eds.), *Therapy as social construction* (pp. 25–39). London: Sage.

Aurelius, M. (2003). *Meditations* (G. Hays, Trans.). London: Weidenfeld & Nicolson.

Burr, V., & Butt, T. (2000). Psychological distress and postmodern thought. In D. Fee (Ed.), *Pathology and the postmodern* (pp. 186–206). London: Sage.

Cattanach, A. (1997). *Children's stories in play therapy*. London: Jessica Kingsley.

Dunne, P. B. (1992). *Narrative approaches to drama therapy*. Los Angeles: Possibilities Press.

Engel, S. (1995). *The stories children tell*. New York: Freeman.

Goolishian, H. (1990). Family therapy: An evolving story. *Contemporary Family Therapy, 12*(3), 173–180.

White, M. (2005). *An outline of narrative therapy*. Available online at: www.massey.ac.nz

White, M., & Epston, D. (1990). *Narrative means to therapeutic ends*. New York: Norton.

PART II

RESEARCH

Evaluating the Effectiveness of Theraplay

HERBERT H. G. WETTIG
ULRIKE FRANKE
BESS SIRMON FJORDBAK

Theraplay[®1] is a directive, interactive short-term play therapy, the aim of which is to help behavior disordered, attachment disordered, developmentally disabled, resistant, or traumatized children on their relevant level of development to change the symptoms of their interactive behavior. Theraplay can help children raise their self-esteem, gain trust in themselves and others, regulate their affect, and adapt themselves to their caregivers and others.

THERAPLAY

Directive Play Therapy

When hearing the term "play therapy," many therapists first think of nondirective play therapy as described by Axline (1947) or Moustakas (1953, 1973); role playing with puppets or drawings (Oaklander, 1978); the sand tray as play medium (Lowenfeld, 1969); or client-centered play therapy (Landreth, 2002; Goetze, 2002). Therapists may imagine puppets, sand trays, or toys with which children can express themselves and their problems. This kind of play has the aim of substituting for therapeutic talking, as young children cannot express their problems or traumatic events by verbalizing them or may refuse to talk. The therapist participates in the child's play and interprets his or her feelings or thoughts. Theraplay is different from this kind of play therapy.

Theraplay is *directive*, led by the therapist who is responsible for the course of the therapeutic play. Theraplay is *interactive*, so no sand tray or toys are used. The therapist interacts playfully with the child, offers rituals and surprising elements, seeks eye contact, and communicates both verbally and nonverbally, using gesture and pantomime to engage emotionally the right hemisphere of the child's brain. The therapist uses play to initiate and maintain a relationship with the child, reacting with warmth and empathy based on the needs of the child. The therapist shares positive affect, improves attachment behavior, is vivid and nurturing, and touches the child while playing like parents do (Jernberg & Booth, 1999). The activities are introduced at the child's developmental level and fit his or her affect. The therapist regulates the arousal of the child by quieting, soothing, comforting, and structuring or through exciting or challenging games. Counting the number of sessions, Theraplay is a *short-term play therapy*.

Model

Ann M. Jernberg, PhD, a Heidelberg-born clinical psychologist, developed Theraplay in the 1960s, having in mind the model of a "healthy mother–child relationship" (Jernberg, 1979) and what Winnicott (1958) called "a good enough mother." After observing more than 400 mother–child dyads as reported by Munns (2003), Jernberg found five essential dimensions of interactive behavior in the natural mother–child dyads: structuring, challenging, engagement (stimulation), nurturing, and play. Theraplay is based on these dimensions. As a therapeutic treatment, Theraplay fosters an active, empathic, and playful relationship between child and therapist. The child changes perspective, learning to see him- or herself as being worthy and lovable and to see the world as a positive and interesting place. Parents have an active role in Theraplay and are encouraged to continue at home the interactive games they have seen and experienced.

History of Theraplay

Theraplay and The Theraplay Institute in Chicago were developed by Jernberg. Since 1967, Theraplay has been used extensively within the framework of the American Head Start Program, in early intervention, in day care, in special education, in parenting skill programs, with hospital-ized patients and in outpatient clinics, and especially in family therapy, not only in the United States but also in Australia, Canada, Finland, Germany, Great Britain, Hong Kong, Israel, Japan, South Korea, and South Africa.

Indications for Theraplay

Theraplay has been shown to be particularly effective with children suffering from adjustment disorders, attachment disorders (e.g., adoptive or foster children), attention-deficit disorder and attention-deficit/hyperactivity disorder, social behavior disorders, autistic-like lack of social mutuality, mutism, shyness, and social anxiety. Theraplay has also been shown to be effective as an initial treatment to help developmentally disabled or difficult to treat children—for example, with diagnoses such as oppositional-defiant or those who are noncooperative, aggressive, reticent, or socially withdrawn—become more open to functional therapies designed to meet their specific problems.

THEORETICAL BACKGROUND

On the one hand, a meaningful explanation as to why Theraplay works comes from the ethological research of Harlow and Harlow (1966), who described the important role of the mother, her way of emotional interaction, and their consequences on the development of young rhesus monkeys (even though the results cannot be directly applied to humans). On the other hand, there have been many scientific findings in neurobiology in the last decade, broadening what is known about the influence of positive emotional interaction during early childhood, about the close attachment and bonding between child and caregiver, and about the importance of positive emotion, play, and touch on the healthy development of the child. Research-based evidence allows formulation of hypotheses to explain why Theraplay is effective.

Neurobiology

Currently, imaging methods such as positron emission tomography (PET) or functional magnetic resonance imaging (fMRI) offer evidence to suggest where information is encoded in the brain of a child as positive or negative events are experienced, as new knowledge is developed, and as the child learns to regulate his or her affect (Schore, 1994, 2003). It is hypothesized that Theraplay changes the neural networks of a child. The plasticity of the child's brain and the related socioemotional functions play an important role in early childhood. Schore describes the ability of a child to regulate affect as originating in interaction with a responsive, regulating caregiver. In the absence of such attuned caregiving, the child is unable to achieve self-regulation; and disorders of the self occur that result in social interaction disorders. In *The Developing Mind* (1999), Siegel explains the importance of interpersonal relationships in the development of the growing infant's ways of thinking, experiencing, and behaving. As Schore (2003) also explains in his theory about the hierarchical change of the neural network, early childhood experiences that create negative interactive behavior may be turned around by later therapeutic intervention. Siegel and Hartzell (2003) offer a useful and easily understood description for parents: positive emotional interactions between caregiver and child may allow for development of new neurons in the hippocampus and more synapses in the prefrontal and orbitofrontal cortex of the right (emotional) hemisphere of the brain. New positive experiences lead to new positive behavior patterns. Learning in the context of positive emotional support, for instance by fun and play, is more effective than learning and exercising without emotional support. This fact gives further credence to the idea that Theraplay may effect positive and lasting change to the interactive behavior of children.

Attachment and Bonding

Attachment theory (Bowlby, 1988, 1995; Brisch, 2003; Stern, 1974, 1986, 1995) explains how a child develops attachment to his or her caregiver who offers bonding, allowing an interpersonal relationship to develop between caregiver and child. Extensive research describes the positive influence of early attachment on later development (Goldberg, 2000; Hughes, 1998; Rutter, 1994; Waters, Weinfield, & Hamilton, 2000; Ziegenhain & Jacobsen, 1999). Reports of secure and insecure attachment of children are found in all cultures (van IJzendoorn & Sagi, 1999).

Play

Early childhood play between a child and his or her caregiver is seen as an important element of healthy development and influences the pattern of later interactive behavior and relationships. Theraplay offers play, language, and interaction to the child at his or her respective levels of social and emotional development, a mental starting place by which the child can become healthier (Munns, 2003). Theraplay replicates the typical interactive behavior of a mother during the early development of her child so that the emotional feelings and experiences of bonding between mother and child will be reactivated and positively changed in a nurturing atmosphere. The games offered will change with the growth and development of the child to more age-appropriate activities.

Touch

This is another characteristic feature of Theraplay. Based on Jernberg's observations (Munns, 2003), touch has a fundamental importance in normal, healthy interactions between parents and their child. Brody (1978) practiced touch in her relationship-focused program of Developmental Play. The positive effect of loving, nurturing, and soothing touch has been confirmed by researchers (e.g., Montagu, 1986), especially by Field's extensive studies about the effect of touch (2001).

METHODS TO EVALUATE THE EFFECTIVENESS OF THERAPLAY

Two research projects were carried out to evaluate the effectiveness of Theraplay in the German-speaking part of Europe. Both are field studies, and diagnoses, observations, and interviews were carried out in the usual therapeutic situation, rather than in a laboratory experiment.

Methodologies

Two different studies were undertaken after conducting pilot studies in 1997. The first was a controlled longitudinal study (CLS) started in 1998 in Germany. A randomized sample of $N = 60$ clinically symptomatic children with dual diagnoses was investigated and compared with a matched control of nonsymptomatic children of the same age and sex (CGN). Initially, the clinically symptomatic children were referred to the Phoniatric Paed-Audiologic Center in Heidelberg due to language or speech problems. In addition to communication disorders, the children were diagnosed with severe behavior disorders, which could have seriously hindered treatment of the speech–language disorders. Therefore, the children involved in this study were treated first with Theraplay to reduce the symptoms of behavior disorders and to prepare them for the subsequent functional treatment of their language problems. The aim of treatment with Theraplay was to increase their attention, cooperation, and approachability.

The CLS children were evaluated repeatedly, and their parents were interviewed at different points of administration during the research period. A randomized half of the sample was diagnosed and their parents interviewed at the beginning of a 16-week waiting period. The other half of the sample was diagnosed and their parents interviewed, and treatment began immediately. Data for all subjects were gathered before, during, and after treatment with Theraplay and in a follow-up 2 years after discharge from treatment. The parent–child interaction was repeatedly observed using the Heidelberg Marschak Interaction Method (Ritterfeld & Franke, 1994) via videotape for systematic analysis by clinicians. All therapy sessions treating the children with Theraplay were videotaped in their entirety and were analyzed scaling each sequence by 42 operationalized criteria of interaction behavior. Each analysis was done by two trained clinicians, scaling independently to ensure inter-rater reliability. The parents were interviewed repeatedly and extensively at the same intervals of time as their children were tested.

The CLS was completed in January 2005, and the results were clinically and statistically highly significant. Due to the homogeneity of the speech–language-disordered population and the consistent therapy setting with the same therapist, the results show a very high internal, but also a low external validity. The high internal validity of the results indicates how effective Theraplay has been in these cases. Due to the low external validity, however, the results may not be generalized to other populations of patients.

Therefore, in 2000, a second project was undertaken, a multi-center study (MCS) in Germany and Austria. The research targeted replication of the CLS to evaluate the effectiveness of Theraplay on a wider scale of populations of patients. The patients of nine quite different therapeutic facilities were investigated for the MCS, including a center for handicapped children, a center for early intervention, an outpatient facility for ear, nose, and throat medicine, a special education facility for early intervention for language-delayed children, a kindergarten in a socially impoverished area, a family therapy psychological practice, and several practices of speech–language pathologists. By the end of 2004, 14 Theraplay therapists completed the treatment of $N = 319$ children. The net sample of the MCS resulted in $N = 291$ toddler and preschool children, ages 2 years, 6 months to 6 years, 11 months, with dual diagnoses of behavior disorders and speech–language deficits or delay. The attrition of $N = 28$ is explained in the section below about sample size.

Informed Consent

All parents and caregivers received detailed information about Theraplay and the research project before giving informed written consent for their children to take part in the research project.

Research Questions

The results of both studies, the CLS and MCS, answer a number of scientific questions. Out of these, only the results about the symptom-reducing effect of Theraplay and the duration of the therapy will be reported here. The following questions were addressed in evaluating the effectiveness of Theraplay:

- What kinds of symptoms were the children experiencing before treatment with Theraplay?
- How severe were the symptoms of these children before treatment using Theraplay in comparison with clinically nonsymptomatic children of the same age and sex?
- Are the disordered behavioral symptoms reduced by treatment with Theraplay? How much reduction was observed?
- Is the reduction of the symptoms clinically and statistically significant?
- Is the effect of the treatment with Theraplay maintained for at least 2 years after the end of the therapy?
- How many Theraplay sessions are needed to reach the therapeutic aim?

Sample Size

The initially accumulated sample of the MCS contained $N = 319$ clinically symptomatic children with dual diagnoses of behavior and speech–language disorders. The data were collected from nine different therapeutic facilities. Of these 319 children, 22 were eliminated from the sample because they were younger or older than the target group age of 2 years, 6 months to 6 years, 11 months at the start of treatment. In another six cases, the data about the psychopathological symptoms were not completely recorded. Therefore, the number of cases was reduced by $N = 28$

from $N = 319$ to a net sample of $N = 291$ children. Most of the diagnoses were given by physicians, not by the Theraplay therapists. However, in some of the private practices, where no diagnosis was given by a physician, therapists who had been trained in assessing symptoms diagnosed the type and severity of the disorders.

The initial sample of the CLS included $N = 68$ clinically symptomatic children with dual diagnoses of both developmental language or speech and severe behavior disorders. In eight cases, parents in the waiting-time control group (CGW) canceled the arranged therapy before it started. The remaining net sample contained $N = 60$ toddler and preschool children up to 6 years, 11 months of age diagnosed with multiple disorders.

Sample Structure

Participants in the CLS were randomly assigned to one of two sub-samples, between which there was no significant difference. The variance of the investigated characteristics guaranteed the homogeneity of the two groups. Children in one of these two subsamples were assigned to a waiting-time control group (CGW). Children in this group waited 16 weeks after initial identification before beginning Theraplay treatment. In this way, the researchers could control for symptom change during the process of normal aging and development of disordered children. Participants in the other subsample began Theraplay treatment immediately. The accumulated sample of the MCS was also randomly divided into two subsamples to assess the homogeneity of the relevant characteristics. There was no significant difference found in relevant criteria of both samples, CLS and MCS.

Table 5.1 shows the size and the structure in sex and age of both samples: the MCS containing $N = 291$ and the CLS containing $N = 60$ clinically symptomatic children out of which $N = 30$ were randomly selected for the waiting-time control group (CGW). There was also a control group of $N = 30$ clinically nonsymptomatic normal children (CGN) matched in sex and age. The sex distribution was proportionately the same in all samples, about 70% boys, 30% girls. However, in closer analysis of certain symptoms, the proportions changed (e.g., in cases of oppositional defiance or aggressiveness, more boys were represented, compared with an increased portion of girls experiencing anxiety). The mean age of the children in all three samples (CLS, MCS, CGN) was around 4 years, 5 months at the beginning of the treatment.

Table 5.2 describes some social demographic characteristics of the mothers and their children in the samples of MCS, CLS, and CGN. The

TABLE 5.1. Sample Size, Sex, and Age of the Toddler and Preschool Children Treated with Theraplay

Sex	MCS (clinically disordered children)		CLS (clinically disordered children)		CGN (nonsymptomatic children)	
	N	%	N	%	N	%
Total sample	291	100.0	60	100.0	30	100.0
Boys	199	68.4	43	71.7	21	70.0
Girls	92	31.6	17	28.3	9	30.0
Age (in months)	N	M_{month} SD	N	M_{month} SD	N	M_{month} SD
Age of all	291	53.6 14.5	60	51.8 15.2	30	53.6 15.4
Age of boys	199	53.3 14.6	43	52.5 14.4	21	54.5 15.9
Age of girls	92	54.1 14.4	17	50.2 17.4	9	51.6 14.8

Note. MCS, multicenter study; CLS, controlled longitudinal study; CGN, control group of nonsymptomatic children; N, number of children/sample size; M, mean; SD, standard deviation.

TABLE 5.2. Sociodemographic Sample Structure of Toddler and Preschool Children Treated with Theraplay

Criteria	MCS (clinically disordered children)		CLS (clinically disordered children)		CGN (nonsymptomatic children)	
	N	%	N	%	N	%
Mother's marital status	291	100.0	60	100.0	30	100.0
Married	202	69.4	54	91.5	29	96.7
Unmarried, living with partner	28	9.6	—	—	—	—
Single parent	61	21.0	5	8.5	1	3.3
Birth status	291	100.0	60	100.0	30	100.0
Children living at least with one biological parent	268	94.4	57	95.0	30	100.0
Adopted and foster children	16	6.6	3	5.0	—	—
Upbringing of the child	291	100.0	60	100.0	30	100.0
Both parents	225	79.8	49	87.5	28	96.6
Single parent	57	20.2	7	12.5	1	3.4
Attendance at kindergarten	291	100.0	60	100.0	30	100.0
Yes, in kindergarten	231	80.5	40	69.0	27	93.1

Note. Single parent, divorced, separated, widowed, and unmarried mothers; children living at least with one biological parent, legitimate and illegitimate natural children. Other abbreviations as in Table 5.1.

marital status of the mothers in the studies differs, as a higher percentage of mothers in the CLS sample were married than in the MCS, and the difference may be reflected by the patient population in these two studies. Many of the participants in the CLS cohort were identified with developmental language and speech disorders, having been presented to the ear, nose, and throat (ENT) phoniatric specialist by parents who were worried about the language problems of their children. Some of the children in the MCS cohort were living under difficult social situations, such as neglect and poverty.

Points of Administration

The results of the psychopathological findings of the clinically symptomatic children in the CLS cohort are reported here for only three of the possible eight data collection points $(t_0–t_7)$ investigated in the study:

- t_1 = at the beginning of the Theraplay treatment
- t_6 = at the end of the Theraplay treatment
- t_7 = 2 years after the end of the Theraplay treatment

The data gathered at the beginning of the waiting time (t_0) and during the therapeutic process $(t_2– t_5)$ will not be reported here. The MCS was designed as a pre–post-intervention study, and the data reported here include only:

- t_1 = before Theraplay treatment
- t_6 = after the period of Theraplay treatment

For purposes of comparison, the data of the control group (CGN) of clinically nonsymptomatic children were collected:

- t_1 = at the beginning of a 16-week period
- t_6 = at the end of a 16-week period

This model allows for analysis of comparable data from all three samples to evaluate the effectiveness of Theraplay on the severity of the symptoms and the change from the beginning (t_1) to the end of the therapy (t_6) and also for the CLS 2 years after the discharge from the treatment with Theraplay (t_7).

Data Sampling Instruments Used

The CLS was designed to address a wide spectrum of research questions; correspondingly, varied instruments and data collection methods were necessary:

- To observe repeatedly the parent–child interactive behavior
- To assess repeatedly the type and severity of the child's symptoms
- To quantify the change of symptoms across the course of the therapeutic process
- To interview repeatedly the child's parent or caregiver

Many of these data sampling instruments were designed as practice-based observational tools because, at the time of the pilot study, there were either no relevant standardized and valid instruments in the German language or the tools available were not practically useful because of a time-intensive administration. Some of the instruments used in the CLS were also used in the CGN to compare the data collected from clinically symptomatic and nonsymptomatic children matched in age and sex and from their parents.

The goal of the MCS was to replicate the data of the CLS in different populations for the purpose of generalizing the results evaluating the effectiveness of Theraplay. Therefore, the only data collected in the MCS included medical history, sociodemographic structure, psychopathologic assessment at the beginning and end of the treatment, and data about the number of sessions needed to achieve the therapeutic aim.

Table 5.3 shows which research instruments were used for sampling the data of the MCS, CLS, and CGN and at which points of administration each instrument was used. The research instruments included for this report are printed *italicized and bold*.

Q12 is a questionnaire to gather sociodemographic data of the child, the mother and father, and, in the case of adopted or foster children, the primary caregiver. The parents were also asked for the country of birth and mother tongue of the child, his or her bi- or multilingual use of language, and if he or she attends a kindergarten. Other data gathered by questionnaire Q12 are not reported here, for example, about the course of pregnancy, problems of the child's birth, congenital defects, early development of the child, number and sex of siblings, sequence of siblings, upbringing of the child, educational style and method, education and professional training, occupation or profession, and religious denomina-

TABLE 5.3. Research Instruments Used and Points of Administration

		Points of administration							
		MCS		CLS				CGN	
Research instruments		t_1	t_6	t_0	t_1	t_6	t_7	t_1	t_6
Basic interviews with parents/caregiver									
Q11	History of disorder	×		×				×	
Q12	*Sociodemographic data*	×		×				×	
Q13	Out-of-the-ordinary events			×					
Observation, assessment, and tests to diagnose the child's disorder									
O14-1	Diagnosis: Communication ability				×				
Q14-2	Parent's report: Communication				×				
T18	*CASCAP-D Psychopathology*	×	×	×	×	×	×	×	
T21-1	Diagnosis: Language ability			×	×	×		×	
Q21-2	Parent's report: Language usage			×	×	×			
T23	Receptive language ability test			×	×	×	×		
T24	Development test (WET)			×	×	×	×	×	×
S31-1	Diagnosis: Child's home behavior			×	×	×			
S35-1	Diagnosis: Effect of the therapy					×			
Observation and evaluation of the parent–child interactive behavior									
O16	Parent–child separation and reunion			×					
O/S251	Diagnosis: Mother–child interaction			×	×	×	×	×	×
O/S252	Diagnosis: Father–child interaction			×	×	×	×	×	×
Repeated interviews with each parent									
S31-2	Parent's report: Child's criteria			×	×	×		×	×
S32	Parent's report: Child's behavior			×	×	×		×	×
S33	Parent–child relationship inventory			×	×	×	×	×	×
S34	Parent's report: Child's change					×	×		
Q35-0	*Number of therapeutic sessions*					×			
S35-1	Diagnosis: Effect of the therapy					×	×		
S35-2	Parent's report: Effect of the therapy					×	×		
Q36	Parent's report 2 years after concluding therapy						×		

Note. Instruments in **bold and italics** are those whose results are reported in this chapter. O, observation; O/S, observation and later analysis with scale; Q, questionnaire; S, scale; T, diagnostic test; ×, point of usage. Points of administration: t_0, beginning of the waiting time; t_1, beginning of the therapy; t_6, end of the therapy; t_7, 2 years after the end of the therapy; t_2–t_5 during therapy are not included. Other abbreviations as in Table 5.1.

tion of the parents, illnesses and out-of-the-ordinary events in the family, and the medical history of the child's disorder.

T18 is a tool used repeatedly to assess and scale the psychopathological symptoms of the child and to scale symptoms reported by the caregiver. The instrument is based on the German version of the Clinical Assessment Scale for Child and Adolescent Psychopathology (CASCAP-D; Doepfner, Berner, Flechtner, Lehmkuhl, & Steinhausen, 1999). In 1997, when the CLS was planned, the CASCAP-D was preferred instead of the Child Behavior Checklist (CBCL; Achenbach, 1991) or other similar scales because of its simple assessment and dimensional scaling of the type and severity of the child's symptoms and because it was well known and used daily as part of the basic diagnostic documentation in outpatient clinics for child and adolescent psychiatry and children's hospitals. Like the CBCL, the CASCAP-D assesses symptoms rather than disorders as classified in DSM-IV or ICD-10. The clinically marked symptom is scaled as 1, nonsymptomatic; 2, mild; 3, moderate; or 4, severe.

CASCAP-D was empirically validated in Germany by Doepfner et al. using the Cologne studies 1 and 2 (Doepfner, Berner, Schwitzgebel, & Lehmkuhl, 1994; Doepfner et al., 1999, pp. 89–107). The assessed symptoms can be aggregated to solid symptom scales. The intercorrelation among corresponding symptom scales was $r = .54$ through $r = .96$, and the empirically defined symptom scales were sufficiently independent from each other. The intercorrelation was statistically significant with $p < .05$, $N = 597$. The original set of 96 diagnostic symptoms was reduced on practice-based evidence to 53 relevant symptoms indicated to treat interactive behavior with Theraplay.

Q35-0 is a questionnaire in which the number of therapeutic sessions was indicated by the therapist, as well as the number of sessions during which the mother, father, or relevant caregiver took part.

Therapy Setting

All reported therapies of the CLS were carried out in the Phoniatric Paed-Audiologic Center in Heidelberg in a therapeutic playroom, with an adjacent observation room. The simply furnished playroom was well lit and there was a large, soft mat on the floor. A few things necessary for the session were placed near the therapist and hidden by a cloth; all other materials were hidden in closets. Parents could observe the reactions of their child through a built-in one-way mirror from the adjoining room. Two built-in video cameras and a microphone were used to tape the whole therapeutic process for later clinical analysis. In the MCS, the different playrooms for Theraplay sessions in the different therapeutic facilities were similarly furnished to meet the same criteria. Parents or caregivers could observe entire therapy sessions by video. In most cases, the therapeutic setting of the MCS was similar to the CLS.

Therapy Procedure

Theraplay was carried out by certified Theraplay therapists with various professional backgrounds: psychiatrists, psychologists, speech–language pathologists, voice teachers, occupational therapists, and special education teachers. The structure and course of the therapeutic session was very similar in all settings. Often, the children, especially aggressive ones, were treated by both a therapist and a co-therapist. The latter kept the child in her lap, giving him or her warm support and the feeling of being secure, while at the same time protecting the therapist from spitting, scratching, biting, kicking, and other painful injuries that may be inflicted by an aggressive child. The therapist sat or knelt in front of the child to guide him or her through the course of the therapy, and the parent either observed the course of the therapy from the adjoining room or directly participated in place of the co-therapist.

RESULTS OF THE EVALUATION OF THE EFFECTIVENESS OF THERAPLAY

The results are based on repeated assessment of the psychopathological symptoms of toddler and preschool children between the ages of 2 years, 6 months and 6 years, 11 months. Although all the children had received medical diagnoses that warranted treatment, it is important to emphasize that the intervention focused on symptoms, not clinical diagnoses. The effectiveness of Theraplay was demonstrated by a reduction in symptoms or symptom level rather than changes in diagnosis as classified in DSM-IV or ICD-10.

Type and Frequency of Symptoms

The set of 53 symptoms to be treated with Theraplay (instrument T18) was selected out of a total of 96 symptoms of the German-validated CASCAP-D based on clinical experience of their relevance to Theraplay treatment. At the beginning (point t_1 of administration), all of the children had dual or multiple diagnoses of the relevant symptoms to be treated with Theraplay. The frequency of some of the symptoms differed in the two studies, which may be explained by the different structure of the samples. The sample of the CLS was exclusively gathered from children treated in the Phoniatric Paed-Audiologic Center in Heidelberg who were referred due to speech–language disorders. That may explain why the percentage of children diagnosed with receptive language disorder is high (86.7%) and why children experiencing affective disorders or anxiety are seldom diagnosed (5%). On the other hand, the sample of the MCS is populated with patients from very different therapeutic facilities. The spectrum of diagnoses from these facilities is much wider than that of the CLS, and even though nine facilities were included, this by no mean covers the whole spectrum of symptoms that could be successfully treated with Theraplay; hence, the type and frequency of the symptoms found in these two studies may not be seen as an epidemiological distribution of those symptoms in the investigated age spectrum in the German-speaking population.

Table 5.4 shows a high percentage of children diagnosed with attention deficit (MCS: 74.9%; CLS: 83.3%) and being noncooperative (MCS: 68.4%; CLS: 75.0%) at the beginning of the treatment with Theraplay. Inattentive, noncooperative, and hyperactive behavior was found in the sample of the CLS more often than in the MCS, which may be explained by the relatively high percentage of receptive language–disordered children in the CLS sample (86.7%), as noted above. Oppositional defiant, aggressive, and play-disordered behavior was found more frequently in the sample of the MCS, as this more clinically diverse population included children from socially impoverished living areas, children with behavior disorders, and children diagnosed with other handicaps. Conversely, the percentage of shy, withdrawn, and selectively mute children was higher in the speech- and language-disordered sample of the CLS than in the MCS. The different frequencies of certain pathological symptoms to be found in the different samples is understandably influenced by the sample structure. That may also explain why the percentage of affective-disordered, anxious children is quite small in the sample of the CLS. Typically, a lack of language comprehension doesn't cause anxiety in children of this age, and the referral for intervention was more likely due to their parents' worry that their children might not be mature enough to start school. The percentage of children diagnosed with autism, an autistic-like lack of social mutuality, and selective mutism was relatively small in both studies. The following sections discuss the effectiveness of the treatment with Theraplay in reducing the symptoms listed in Table

TABLE 5.4. Type and Frequency of Symptoms Treated with Theraplay

Symptoms	MCS		CLS		CGN	
	N	%	N	%	N	%
Net sample size	291	100.0	60	100.0	30	100
Symptoms of attention, activity, and social behavior disorders						
Attention deficit	218	74.9	50	83.3	3	—
Attention deficit hyperactivity	105	36.1	25	41.7	2	—
Noncooperativeness	199	68.4	45	75.0	1	—
Oppositional defiance	161	55.3	23	38.3	1	—
Aggressiveness	69	23.7	7	11.7	—	—
Playing disorder	118	40.7	21	35.0	—	—
Symptoms of affective and anxiety disorders						
Shyness, bashfulness	149	51.2	21	35.0	3	—
Lack of self-confidence	111	38.1	3	5.0	—	—
Social anxiety	59	20.3	3	5.0	1	—
Performance anxiety	51	17.5	2	3.3	1	—
Selective mutism	38	13.1	9	15.0	—	—
Symptoms of language and pervasive developmental disorders						
Receptive language disorder	193	66.3	52	86.7	—	—
Lack of social mutuality	56	19.2	14	23.3	—	—

Note. N, number of cases of the net sample; %, percentage of the net sample.

5.4, or, in other words, how effective Theraplay is in positively changing the interactive behavior of these children.

Symptom Severity before Treatment Using Theraplay

Again it is noted that the severity of the symptoms before treating the children with Theraplay is scaled either as mild (2), moderate (3), or severe (4). The data given in Table 5.5 are mean values of those differentiated assessments. Each mean value (M_{t_1}; SD_{t_1}) is also dependent on the percentage of children in a sample demonstrating severe, moderate, or mild degree of a symptom.

The highest possible value on the scale to assess the severity of a symptom using CASCAP-D is $M = 4.0$. A large proportion of the clinically disordered children in the MCS (and CLS) scored a mean of $M_{t_1} > 3.0$, very near the highest possible scaling, which may be seen as an indication of the severity of the social behavior of many of these children (see Table

5.5). In the following data, M_{t_1} scores without parentheses refer to the MCS, and those within the parentheses refer to the CLS:

- $N = 218$ ($N = 50$) Attention-deficit $M_{t_1} = 3.20$ ($M_{t_1} = 3.04$)
  disorder
- $N = 105$ ($N \doteq 25$) Attention-deficit/ $M_{t_1} = 3.17$ ($M_{t_1} = 2.96$)
  hyperactivity disorder
- $N = 199$ ($N = 45$) Noncooperativeness $M_{t_1} = 3.13$ ($M_{t_1} = 3.00$)
- $N = 161$ ($N = 23$) Oppositional $M_{t_1} = 3.15$ ($M_{t_1} = 3.09$)
  defiant disorder
- $N = 118$ ($N = 20$) Play disorders $M_{t_1} = 3.02$ ($M_{t_1} = 3.05$)

The explosive nature of the unrestrained, externalizing behaviors is particularly clear if the severity of the clinically symptomatic children is compared with the low scores ($M_{t_1} = 1.00$–1.30) of the same symptom in clinically nonsymptomatic children in the CGN (see Table 5.5).

The children experiencing internalizing behavior disorders are contrasted to the ones demonstrating externalizing behavior disorders. Shyness and social anxiety are examples of internalizing symptoms. Generally, internalizing symptoms of children were scored on a lower level of severity than externalizing symptoms. This difference in scoring, even by trained clinicians, may be because shy, withdrawn children are less disturbing to the caregiver and don't attract the attention of the clinician as much as aggressive children.

- $N = 149$ ($N = 21$) Shyness, bashfulness $M_{t_1} = 3.04$ ($M_{t_1} = 2.52$)
- $N = 111$ ($N = 3$) Lack of self-confidence $M_{t_1} = 3.11$ ($M_{t_1} = 2.33$)
- $N = 38$ ($N = 9$) Selective mutism $M_{t_1} = 3.11$ ($M_{t_1} = 2.56$)
- $N = 51$ ($N = 3$) Performance anxiety $M_{t_1} = 3.02$ ($M_{t_1} = 2.00$)
- $N = 59$ ($N = 3$) Social anxiety $M_{t_1} = 2.83$ ($M_{t_1} = 3.00$)

In Table 5.5, the data of the CLS are notable for the fact that only a few children were diagnosed with a lack of self-confidence, social anxiety, performance anxiety, or selective mutism. This may be explained by the fact that the children of the CLS were presented to the speech–language pathologist with suspected diagnoses of developmental language delay or other language or speech disorder, as compared to the children of the MCS, many of whom were indicated for treatment with Theraplay because of behavior or interactive disorder diagnoses.

Receptive language disorder was diagnosed in many of the children with behavior or interactive disorders. In both studies, the severity of

TABLE 5.5. Change in Symptoms after Treatment with Theraplay

Symptoms	MCS (N = 291 toddler and preschool children with dual diagnoses)				CLS (N = 60 toddler and preschool children with dual diagnoses)				CGN (N = 30)	
	N	M_{t_1} (SD_{t_1})	M_{t_6} (SD_{t_6})	p	N	M_{t_1} (SD_{t_1})	M_{t_6} (SD_{t_6})	p	N	M_{t_1} (SD_{t_1})
Symptoms of attention, activity, and social behavior disorders										
Attention deficit	218	3.20 (0.8)	2.04 (0.8)	< .0001	50	3.04 (0.7)	2.22 (0.9)	< .0001	3	1.30 (0.5)
Attention deficit/ hyperactivity	105	3.17 (0.8)	1.84 (0.7)	< .0001	25	2.96 (0.8)	1.63 (0.8)	< .0001	2	1.27 (0.5)
Noncooperativeness	199	3.13 (0.8)	1.50 (0.7)	< .0001	45	3.00 (0.8)	1.66 (0.8)	< .0001	1	1.30 (0.5)
Oppositional defiance	161	3.15 (0.8)	1.39 (0.5)	< .0001	23	3.09 (0.7)	1.39 (0.5)	< .0001	1	1.10 (0.3)
Aggressiveness	69	2.93 (0.8)	1.26 (0.5)	< .0001	7	2.57 (0.8)	1.00 (0.0)	= .0023	0	1.00 (0.0)
Playing disorder	118	3.02 (0.8)	1.62 (0.8)	< .0001	20	3.05 (0.9)	1.79 (0.9)	< .0001	0	1.00 (0.0)
Symptoms of affective and anxiety disorders										
Shyness, bashfulness	149	3.04 (0.8)	1.36 (0.6)	< .0001	21	2.52 (0.7)	1.14 (0.4)	< .0001	3	1.23 (0.4)
Lack of self-confidence	111	3.11 (0.8)	1.39 (0.6)	< .0001	3	2.33 (0.6)	1.00 (0.0)	<.0001	0	1.00 (0.0)
Social anxiety	59	2.83 (0.8)	1.36 (0.6)	< .0001	3	3.00 (1.0)	1.00 (0.0)	n.s.	1	1.03 (0.2)
Performance anxiety	51	3.02 (0.8)	1.31 (0.5)	< .0001	2	2.00 (0.0)	1.00 (0.0)	< .0001	1	1.03 (0.2)
Selective mutism	38	3.11 (0.8)	1.71 (1.1)	< .0001	9	2.56 (0.7)	1.56 (1.1)	= .0152	0	1.00 (0.0)
Symptoms of language and pervasive developmental disorders										
Receptive language disorder	193	3.11 (0.8)	2.01 (0.8)	< .0001	52	3.13 (0.8)	2.25 (1.0)	< .0001	0	1.00 (0.0)
Autistic-like lack of social mutuality	56	2.98 (0.8)	1.88 (0.9)	< .0001	14	3.07 (0.8)	2.14 (1.0)	= .0009	0	1.00 (0.0)

Note. N, sample size; M_{t_1} (SD_{t_1}), mean (standard deviation) of the symptom's scale at the beginning of the therapy; $M_{t_6}(SD_{t_6})$, mean (standard deviation) of the reduced symptom's scale at the end of the therapy; p, statistical significance of the symptom's change. Other abbreviations as in Table 5.1.

receptive language disorders was high; in MCS, $N = 193$ of 291 children were identified as having receptive language disorder with a mean of M_{t_1} = 3.11 (SD = 0.8), and in CLS, N = 52 of 60 children were likewise identified with a mean of M_{t_1} = 3.13 (SD = 0.8) on the 4-point scale of CASCAP-D.

This coincidence of dual diagnoses of behavior disorders and language disorders is reported in the literature extensively (cf. Von Suchodoletz & Keiner, 1998) but without ranking the severity of the symptoms or giving data about the positive therapeutic change (see Table 5.5).

Reduction of Symptom Severity of Behavior Disorders after Treatment with Theraplay, and Clinical and Statistical Significance of Change

The positive change of the interactive behavior of clinically symptomatic children after being treated with Theraplay is clearly seen in Figures 5.1–5.3, showing the change of externalizing symptoms, and in Figures 5.4–5.6 showing the change of internalizing symptoms. Each of these figures demonstrates the therapeutically induced change of a symptom from the beginning (t_1) to the end (t_6) of the treatment with Theraplay and the lasting effect 2 years after the end of the therapy (t_7). The black triangle (▲) is the symbol for the clinically nonsymptomatic normal children of the CGN, in most cases showing no or very low degree of the relevant symptom, assessed at the beginning of the 16-week waiting period. This level is to be seen as a base line for comparison with the severity of the same symptom found in clinically symptomatic children of the MCS or CLS sample. This comparison demonstrates the high level of symptoms in the clinically disordered group of children before they were treated with Theraplay (t_1) and the degree of positive change at the end of the therapy (t_6). In addition, the curve of the CLS shows the lasting effect of the achieved therapeutic results 2 years after the end of the therapy (t_7). There was no relapse, and the achieved effect was stable.

The sample of the MCS was big enough to be subdivided into groups of children with initially severe, moderate, or mild symptoms. The squares with a straight line indicate the clinically symptomatic subsamples of the MCS and the resulting change. The black square (■) with an unbroken line (—) is the symbol for all children in the subsample with severe symptoms (CASCAP-D = 4). The gray square with an unbroken line marks all children with moderate symptoms (CASCAP-D = 3), and the white square (□) with an unbroken line indicates all children with mild symptoms (CASCAP-D = 2). The white diamond (◇) with a broken line (– – –) indicates the average of these three clinically symptomatic samples of the MCS, corresponding to the mean value (M_{t_1}) in Table 5.5. The black diamond (◆) with a broken line (– – –) indicates the average process of symptom change for all clinically symptomatic children from the CLS sample starting from the beginning of the therapy (t_1) to the end (t_6) and at a point 2 years after the end of the therapy (t_7). The course of the CLS curve 2 years after the end of treatment allows for evaluation of relapses or clinically relevant or statistically significant negative changes. Figures 5.1–5.3 demonstrate the therapeutic changes of the external symptoms after children were treated with Theraplay.

- *Noncooperative toddler and preschool children* (see Figure 5.1)
  MCS: $N = 199$ noncooperative children altogether (mean)
        $N = 78$ with severe noncooperative behavior
        $N = 69$ with moderate noncooperative behavior
        $N = 52$ with mild noncooperative behavior
  CLS: $N = 45$ noncooperative children altogether (mean)

- *Oppositional defiant toddler and preschool children* (see Figure 5.2)
  MCS: $N = 161$ oppositional defiant children altogether (mean)
        $N = 65$ with severe oppositional defiant behavior
        $N = 55$ with moderate oppositional defiant behavior
        $N = 41$ with mild moderate oppositional defiant
              behavior
  CLS: $N = 23$ oppositional defiant children altogether (mean)

- *Aggressive toddler and preschool children* (see Figure 5.3)
  MCS: $N = 69$ aggressive children altogether (mean)
        $N = 21$ with severe aggressiveness
        $N = 22$ with moderate aggression
        $N = 26$ with mild aggression
  CLS: $N = 7$ aggressive children altogether (mean)

Figures 5.4–5.6 demonstrate the therapeutically induced change of internal symptoms.

- *Shy, bashful toddler and preschool children* (see Figure 5.4)
  MCS: $N = 149$ shy children altogether (mean)
        $N = 51$ with severe shyness
        $N = 53$ with moderate shyness
        $N = 45$ with mild shyness
  CLS: $N = 21$ shy children altogether (mean)

- *Socially withdrawn toddler and preschool children* (see Figure 5.5)
  MCS: N = 103 socially withdrawn children altogether (mean)
  N = 26 with severe tendency for social withdrawal
  N = 38 with moderate tendency for social withdrawal
  N = 39 with mild tendency for social withdrawal
  CLS: N = 19 socially withdrawn children altogether (mean)

- *Socially anxious toddler and preschool children* (see Figure 5.6)
  MCS: N = 59 children with social anxiety altogether (mean)
  N = 15 with severe social anxiety
  N = 19 with moderate social anxiety
  N = 25 with mild social anxiety
  CLS: N = 3 children with social anxiety altogether (mean)

All of these symptoms typical of behavior disorders show a similar picture of change attributed to the Theraplay treatment. After treating the children with Theraplay, their symptoms marked as severe (■) in the beginning come near to milder degrees of the clinically nonsymptomatic children of the control group (▲). The effect of the treatment with Theraplay is a clinically significant reduction of the disordered symptoms of the interactive behavior of the children. Obviously, the effect of Theraplay is much greater if the symptom was originally marked as severe (■) than if it was originally only a moderate or mild notation (□). In other words, the more severe the relevant symptom originally identified, the more marked the change resulting from Theraplay treatment. These changes of the symptoms are clinically and statistically significant. Table 5.5 shows that even the mean of change of the symptoms is statistically highly significant ($M_{t_1} \rightarrow M_{t_6}$: $p < 0.0001$), with the exception of some of the very small subsamples of the CLS. There were only a few children in the sample of the CLS diagnosed with aggression, social anxiety, performance anxiety, or selective mutism; therefore, the evaluation of this data was omitted.

Figures 5.1–5.6 also give a first indication about the objectivity of the data to evaluate the effectiveness of Theraplay, indicating that the therapeutic method is independent of the diagnostic cohort, the type of therapeutic facility, and the therapist. The broken lines demonstrating the mean of the change of symptoms in both studies run widely parallel, in some cases even congruent, yielding research-based evidence of the degree of change of the symptoms as similar or the same in both independent studies and indicating the validity of Theraplay.

However, this example of the remarkable effectiveness of Theraplay to reduce the symptoms of the interactive behavior of clinically symptomatic

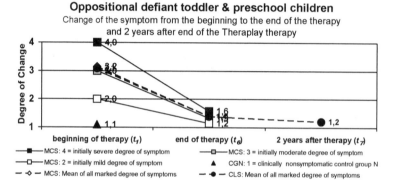

FIGURE 5.1. The effectiveness of Theraplay on noncooperative toddler and preschool children.

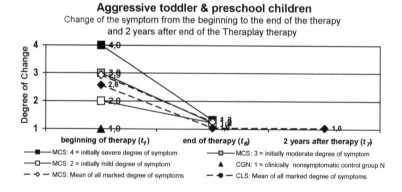

FIGURE 5.2. The effectiveness of Theraplay on oppositional defiant toddler and preschool children.

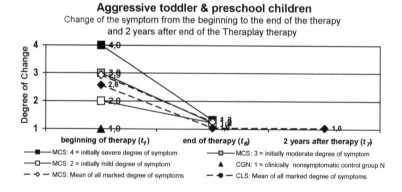

FIGURE 5.3. The effectiveness of Theraplay on aggressive toddler and preschool children.

124

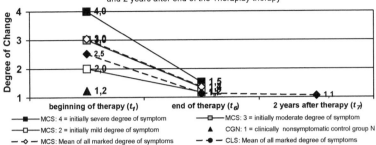

FIGURE 5.4. The effectiveness of Theraplay on shy, bashful toddler and pre-school children.

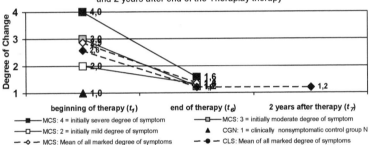

FIGURE 5.5. The effectiveness of Theraplay on socially withdrawn toddler and preschool children.

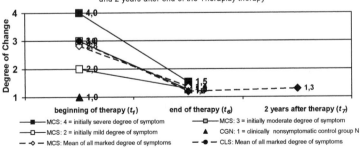

FIGURE 5.6. The effectiveness of Theraplay on socially anxious toddler and pre-school children.

toddler and preschool children to a level often coming near to that of clinically nonsymptomatic, normal children is not valid for all of the investigated symptoms. There are symptoms that are neuropsychologically influenced such as ADHD or the attention deficits of children with an autistic-like lack of social mutuality, typical also for children with early childhood autism or receptive language disorders, indicating a delayed development of language comprehension in toddler and preschool children. In these kinds of disorders, only children with originally mild symptoms improved to a degree similar to the interactive behavior of clinically nonsymptomatic children. Children demonstrating moderate or severe symptoms of this kind only improved to an ongoing level of mild or moderate symptoms when treated with Theraplay (see Figures 5.7–5.9), but even this reduction of the symptoms was clinically and statistically significant, with a very low probability of error $p < .0001$ to $p = .0009$ (see Table 5.5).

Figures 5.7–5.9 demonstrate the therapeutically conditioned change of such neuropsychologically influenced symptoms as attention-deficit/hyperactivity, autistic-like lack of social mutuality, or receptive language delay. In the following, the corresponding samples of Figures 5.7–5.9 are described.

- *Toddler and preschool children suffering from attention-deficit/hyperactivity* (see Figure 5.7)
  MCS: $N = 105$ inattentive, hyperactive children altogether (mean)
  >> $N = 41$ with severe attention-deficit/hyperactivity symptoms
  >> $N = 41$ with moderate attention-deficit/hyperactivity symptoms
  >> $N = 23$ with mild attention-deficit/hyperactivity symptoms
  CLS: $N = 25$ inattentive, hyperactive children altogether (mean)

- *Toddler and preschool children suffering from an autistic-like lack of social mutuality* (see Figure 5.8)
  MCS: $N = 44$ inattentive children with autistic-like lack of social mutuality (mean)
  >> $N = 15$ inattentive children with a severe lack of social mutuality
  >> $N = 16$ inattentive children with a moderate lack of social mutuality
  >> $N = 13$ inattentive children with a mild lack of social mutuality

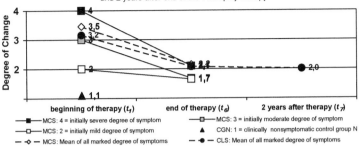

FIGURE 5.7. The effectiveness of Theraplay on inattentive toddler and preschool children suffering from attention-deficit/hyperactivity disorder (ADHD).

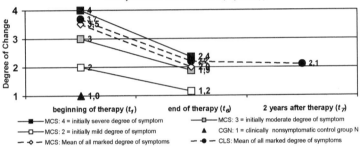

FIGURE 5.8. The effectiveness of Theraplay on toddler and preschool children suffering from an autistic-like lack of social mutuality.

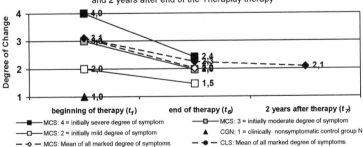

FIGURE 5.9. The effectiveness of Theraplay on receptive language-disordered toddler and preschool children.

127

CLS: N = 13 inattentive children with an autistic-like lack of
      social mutuality (mean)
          Out of these 13, 9 children were diagnosed with autism
          (Kanner syndrome).

- *Receptive language-disordered toddler and preschool children* (see Figure 5.9)
  MCS: N = 193 children with receptive language disorder
        altogether (mean)
            N = 73 with severe symptoms of receptive language
            disorders
            N = 68 with moderate symptoms of receptive language
            disorders
            N = 52 with mild symptoms of receptive language
            disorders
  CLS: N = 51 children with receptive language disorder
        altogether (mean)

Effect Size

Table 5.5 presents the statistically significant positive change in the symptoms. Another important way to demonstrate the effectiveness of Theraplay is to look at the size of the effect. There are several different ways to analyze the effect size (d). In this case, the following formula was used: $d = M_{t_6} - M_{t_1} / SD_{(t_1 + t_6)} / 2$. Jacobs (1999) claims that the result of this formula would come near the population's distribution of effect size (www.phil.uni-sb.de/jacobs/seminar/vpl/bedeutung.htm).

A small effect size of the reduction of a symptom caused by a treatment would be around d = 0.20, medium effect size value around d = 0.50, large effect size value around d = 0.80 (Bortz & Doering, 1995). In general, the effect sizes demonstrated by the MCS were very large (d > 1.00, see Table 5.6). Likewise, the effect size noted for the CLS in most of the symptoms was also very large ($d \geq 1.00$, see Table 5.6), apart from the effect size of attention-deficit with autistic-like lack of social mutuality (d = 0.91) and the effect size of receptive language disorder (d = 0.88), both of which still reflect a large effect. Like the statistical significance of the therapeutic change of the symptoms when treated with Theraplay, the large effect sizes described above confirm the effectiveness of Theraplay with toddlers and preschool children experiencing symptoms of interactive behavior disorders.

TABLE 5.6. Effect Size as an Indication of the Extent of the Symptom's Change after Treatment with Theraplay

Figure	Symptoms	MCS ($N = 291$ toddler and preschool children with dual diagnoses)				CLS ($N = 60$ toddler and preschool children with dual diagnoses)			
		N	M_{t_1} (SD_{t_1})	M_{t_6} (SD_{t_6})	d	N	M_{t_1} (SD_{t_1})	M_{t_6} (SD_{t_6})	d
	Effect size of the reduction of externalization behavior disorder symptoms								
5.1	Noncooperativeness	199	3.13	1.50	|2.51|	45	3.00	1.60	|1.91|
5.2	Oppositional defiance	161	3.15	1.39	|3.32|	23	3.09	1.39	|3.40|
5.3	Aggressiveness	69	2.93	1.26	|3.34|	7	2.57	1.00	|1.57|
	Effect size of the reduction of internalization behavior disorder symptoms								
5.4	Shyness, bashfulness	149	3.04	1.36	|2.71|	21	2.52	1.14	|3.83|
5.5	Socially withdrawn	103	2.87	1.36	|2.44|	19	2.58	1.21	|3.26|
5.6	Social anxiety	59	2.83	1.36	|2.53|	3	3.00	1.00	|2.00|
	Effect size of the reduction of neuropsychological conditioned behavior disorder symptoms								
5.7	Attention-deficit/ hyperactivity	105	3.17	1.84	|1.87|	25	2.96	1.63	|1.73|
5.8	Attention deficit with autistic-like lack of social mutuality	44	3.05	1.84	|1.49|	13	3.15	2.23	|0.91|
5.9	Receptive language disorder	193	3.11	2.01	|1.36|	52	3.13	2.25	|0.88|

Note. N, sample size; M_{t_1} (SD_{t_1}), mean (standard deviation) of the symptom's scale at the beginning of the therapy; M_{t_6} (SD_{t_6}), mean (standard deviation) of the symptom's reduced scale at the end of the therapy; d, effect size of the symptom's change (around $d = 0.20$, small; around $d = 0.50$, medium; around $d = 0.80$, large; $d > 1.00$, very large). Other abbreviations as in Table 5.1.

Duration of the Therapy: Average Number of Therapeutic Sessions

Generally, a therapeutic session treating a child with Theraplay takes 30 minutes, with additional time required to prepare the therapeutic plan prior to the interaction and to document the therapeutic process after each session. In the following, the duration of treatment is given as the average number of 30-minute sessions.

Theraplay claims to be a short-term play therapy, and this claim is confirmed by the results of both the MCS and CLS as independent studies (see Table 5.7).

The therapeutic aim has been to reduce the enduring and disturbing symptoms in the interactive behavior of disordered toddler and pre-school children between the ages of 2 years, 6 months and 6 years, 11 months. An average of 19–20 30-minute therapeutic sessions were neces-sary to achieve the goal for noncooperative, oppositional defiant, or aggressive behaviors, as noted in the externalizing behaviors of toddler and preschool children (see Table 5.7). The necessary number of sessions ranged from 9 to 30 sessions, due to mild, moderate, or severe degrees of their symptomatic presentation. Toddler and preschool children suffering from internalizing symptoms like shyness, tendency for social with-drawal, and social anxiety were also treated an average of 18–21 30-min-ute sessions to achieve the therapeutic aim of reducing the symptoms of these children to the degree that they become as open-minded, coura-geous, and approachable as clinically nonsymptomatic children of the

TABLE 5.7. Duration of Theraplay

Figure	Symptoms	Mean number of sessions: MCS (N = 291 toddler and preschool children with dual diagnoses)			Mean number of sessions: CLS (N = 60 toddler and preschool children with dual diagnoses)		
		N	M	SD	N	M	SD
	Effect size of the reduction of externalization behavior disorder symptoms						
5.1	Noncooperativeness	199	19.4	10.9	45	19.3	8.4
5.2	Oppositional defiance	161	19.2	10.4	23	18.2	6.5
5.3	Aggressiveness	69	19.8	10.6	7	15.9	5.8
	Effect size of the reduction of internalization behavior disorder symptoms						
5.4	Shyness, bashfulness	149	17.9	9.7	21	16.8	4.3
5.5	Socially withdrawn	103	20.5	11.3	19	20.7	7.9
5.6	Social anxiety	59	20.1	11.3	3	18.7	10.7
	Effect size of the reduction of neuropsychological conditioned behavior disorder symptoms						
5.7	Attention-deficit/hyperactivity	105	21.4	12.6	25	21.0	9.9
5.8	Attention deficit with autistic-like lack of social mutuality	44	26.0	13.0	13	26.0	8.9
5.9	Receptive language disorder	193	19.7	10.8	52	19.0	7.9

Note. N, sample size; *M*, mean number of 30-minute sessions needed to achieve the therapeutic aim (last-ing effect of symptom reduction after treatment with Theraplay); *SD*, standard deviation of the number of therapeutic sessions, also to be interpreted as the range between the shortest and longest number of ther-apeutic sessions. Other abbreviations as in Table 5.1.

same age and sex (see Table 5.7). The range also reached from 9 to 30 sessions, again based on the initial level of severity.

Toddler and preschool children with receptive language disorders also required an average of 19–20 therapeutic sessions with Theraplay to initiate verbal comprehension and to reduce the accompanying symptoms of behavior disorders (see Table 5.7). The number of sessions ranged from 8 to 32, each with a duration of 30 minutes of Theraplay.

Theraplay does not claim to heal children diagnosed with attention-deficit/hyperactivity disorders, but it may considerably reduce those symptoms that interfere with the interactive behavior of such children. After being treated with Theraplay, the children in these studies became much more calm, attentive, and interested; at the end of treatment they were still somewhat physically agitated and impulsive, but on a much lower level. Evidence indicates that an average of 21–22 30-minute sessions were needed to reduce the interfering symptoms so that a mutually satisfying interaction between the child and his or her caregiver became possible (see Table 5.7). The number of sessions required ranged from 8 sessions with children who were very easy to handle up to 34 sessions with children demonstrating a severe degree of attention-deficit/hyperactivity disorder.

To treat children with a comorbid disorder of attention-deficit and an autistic-like lack of social mutuality, more therapeutic sessions were necessary than with the previously reported cases of interactive behavior disorders. A lack of social mutuality is not only a symptom accompanying autism spectrum disorders; the lack of approachability for social interaction is also found in other diagnoses, but is pathognomic in children diagnosed with autism. Generally, it is well known that a long-term therapy is necessary to treat autistic children. To treat toddler and preschool children experiencing such complex symptoms, an average of 26 Theraplay sessions was needed (see Table 5.7) and, depending how severe the symptoms were, between 13 and 60 sessions. As noted, Theraplay cannot cure this disorder but makes the child much more approachable and amenable to interactions with his or her caregiver and others.

DISCUSSION OF THE RESULTS

The American Psychiatric Association (APA) has established criteria for evidence-based therapies. A coding system from A through G is used.

Based on these criteria, the CLS with an accumulated randomized sample of patients and control samples reached the code A- level, next to the first level. Code A- means a randomized clinical study of an intervention in which subjects are prospectively followed over time, there are treatment and control groups (e.g., a waiting-time control group), and subjects are randomly assigned to the two groups, but the approach is not double-blind as code A asks for. The other study, the MCS, may be placed between code A- and B. Code B, the third level of evidence, means a clinical trial by a prospective study in which an intervention is made and the results of that intervention are tracked longitudinally, but B does not meet the standards for a randomized clinical trial.

The convincing results of the CLS cannot be generalized, however, due to the unilateral specificity of the patient cohort, which may not be extrapolated to other populations of patients and therapeutic situations. The MCS does not fully meet the criteria for the third level of evidence (B), as it is a pre–post design without a control group. But the MCS is clearly aimed at analyzing different cohorts of patients under different therapeutic situations, treated by an increased number of Theraplay therapists. The point is that the results of the MCS are generalizable to a wider number of different populations of patients. On the basis of these criteria used to assess the practice-based evidence of these two studies, Theraplay may be seen as "presumably effective" on defined symptoms, especially on symptoms of externalizing or internalizing interactive behavior disorders. However, the results should be replicated by additional studies and extended to other populations of patients.

The results of these two studies show independently that Theraplay effectively reduced externalizing and internalizing symptoms of the disordered interactive behaviors of toddler and preschool children compared with the sample matched by age and sex. The clinical and statistical significance of the results is also proved by the statistical computation of the significant effect size of the reduced symptoms. Even neuropsychological syndromes such as ADHD, attention-deficit connected to an autistic-like lack of social mutuality as typically seen in autism spectrum disorders, and receptive language disorders have been effectively treated by Theraplay with statistically significant positive changes in the analyzed cohorts of patients.

The results of the controlled longitudinal study with a follow-up 2 years after the individual discharge from Theraplay treatment allow the conclusion that the effectiveness of Theraplay is lasting. There were neither relapses nor statistically significant changes of the symptoms; hence, the therapeutic results achieved with Theraplay were stable.

Looking at the results of research and counting the number of sessions, Theraplay is a real short-term play therapy. The average duration of therapy was 18–20 30-minute sessions, as measured by the number of therapeutic sessions needed to achieve a lasting reduction of symptoms of externalizing or internalizing behavior disorders. Depending on the mild, moderate, or severe degree of the symptoms, there were around ± 10–12 sessions needed. Additional sessions were typically necessary to reduce the symptoms of ADHD or of comorbid receptive language disorders. To reduce the symptoms of an autistic-like lack of social mutuality, there were on average 26 sessions needed to achieve the targeted result of the therapy. Having the necessary number of therapeutic sessions in mind, Theraplay can probably meet the claim to be an effective short-term play therapy for significantly reducing the symptoms as analyzed in these studies.

Finally, there were some deficiencies in these studies that should be avoided in future research. In both reported studies, the psychopathological diagnosis was assessed using CASCAP-D, the German version of the Clinical Assessment Scale for Child and Adolescent Psychopathology. Having in mind the need to standardize the research instruments for future intercultural studies in all countries where certified therapists treat patients with Theraplay, ideally there should be validated instruments to assess psychopathological and attachment disorders adapted to many different languages.

In the MCS, diagnosis and intervention were done by different clinicians, and in such a model, there will be inherent differences in clinical opinion. In future studies, careful attention should be paid to strictly separate diagnosis and intervention to control for variation and rule out any doubt about research results.

Future studies to evaluate the effectiveness of Theraplay should be carried out as prospective controlled studies with randomized samples of participants manifesting different symptoms and nonsymptomatic controls, both followed over time.

In spite of this criticism, the results of these two independent studies, financed by the researchers themselves, may contribute to the practice-based evidence evaluating the effectiveness of Theraplay.

NOTE

1. The term "Theraplay" is legally protected by Wz. 39518465 and The Theraplay Institute, Wilmette, Illinois.

REFERENCES

Achenbach, T. M. (1991). *Manual for the Child Behavior Checklist/4–18 and 1991 Profile.* Burlington, VT: University of Vermont, Department of Psychiatry.

Axline, V. (1947). *Play therapy: The inner dynamics of childhood.* Boston: Houghton-Mifflin. (German: *Spieltherapie im nicht-direktiven Verfahren.* Muenchen: Reinhardt, 1972)

Bortz, J., & Doering, N. (1995). *Forschungsmethoden und Evaluation.* 2. Auflage. Berlin: Springer.

Bowlby, J. (1988). *A secure base: Parent–child attachment and human development.* New York: Basic Books.

Bowlby, J. (1995). *Mutterliebe und kindliche Entwicklung.* Muenchen: Reinhardt.

Brisch, K. H. (2003). *Bindungsstörungen: Von der Bindungstheorie zur Therapie.* Stuttgart: Klett-Cotta.

Brody, V. (1978). Developmental play: A relationship-focused program for children. *Journal of Child Welfare, 57*(9), 591–599.

Doepfner, M., Berner, W., Flechtner, H., Lehmkuhl, G., & Steinhausen, H.-C. (1999). *Psychopathologisches Befund-System für Kinder und Jugendliche (CASCAP-D).* (English: *Clinical Assessment Scale for Child and Adolescent Psychopathology.*) Goettingen: Hogrefe Verlag für Psychologie.

Doepfner, M., Berner, W., Schwitzgebel, P., & Lehmkuhl, G. (1994). Dimensionen psychischer Störungen bei Kindern und Jugendlichen auf der Basis klinischer Beurteilungen. [Dimensions of psychological determined disorders of children and adolescents on base of clinical assessments]. *Zeitschrift für Kinder- und Jugenpsychiatrie, 22,* 299–317.

Field, T. (2001). *Touch.* Cambridge, MA: MIT Press.

Goetze, H. (2002). *Handbuch der personenzentrierten Spieltherapie.* Goettingen: Hogrefe.

Goldberg, S. (2000). *Attachment and development.* London: Arnold.

Harlow, H. F., & Harlow, M. K. (1966). Learning to love. *American Scientist, 54,* 244–277.

Hughes, D. A. (1998). *Building the bonds of attachment: Awakening love in deeply troubled children.* Northvale, NJ: Aronson.

Jacobs, B. [2005/07/27]. *Die Effektstärke (oder Effektgrösse).*[htm. last update 1999/10/22] www.phil.uni-sb.de/jacobs/seminar/vpl/bedeutung/bedeut.htm. alt.

Jernberg, A. M. (1979). *Theraplay: A new treatment using structured play for children and their families.* San Francisco: Jossey-Bass. (German: *Theraplay—Eine direktive Spieltherapie.* Trans. U. Franke. Stuttgart: Gustav Fischer, 1987)

Jernberg, A. M., & Booth, P. B. (1999). *Theraplay—Helping parents and children build better relationships through attachment-based play* (2nd ed.). San Francisco: Jossey-Bass.

Landreth, G. I. (2002). *Play therapy: The art of the relationship* (2nd ed.). New York: Brunner-Routledge.

Lowenfeld, V. (1969). Die "Welt"-Technik in der Kinder-Psychotherapie. In G.

Biermann (Hrsg.), *Handbuch der Kinderpsychotherapie* (pp. 442–451). Muenchen: Reinhardt.

Montagu, A. (1986). *Touching: The human significance of the skin.* New York: Harper & Row. (German: *Körperkontakt.* 5. Auflage. Stuttgart: Klett-Cotta, 1988)

Moustakas, C. E. (1953). *Children in play therapy.* New York: McGraw-Hill.

Moustakas, C. E. (1973). *The child's discovery of himself.* Northvale, NJ: Aronson.

Munns, E. (2003). Theraplay: Attachment-enhancing play therapy. In C. E. Schaefer (Ed.), *Foundations of play therapy* (pp. 156–174). Hoboken, NJ: Wiley.

Oaklander, V. (1978). *Windows to our children.* Moab, UT: Real People Press. (German: *Gestalttherapie mit Kindern und Jugendlichen.* Stuttgart: Klett, 1981)

Ritterfeld, U., & Franke, U. (1994). *Die Heidelberger Marschak-Interaktionsmethode. Zur Beurteilung der dyadischen Interaktion mit Vorschulkindern.* Stuttgart: Gustav Fischer.

Rutter, M. (1994). *Clinical implications of attachment concepts: Retrospect and prospect.* Paper presented at the International Conference on Attachment and Psychopathology, Toronto, Ontario, Canada.

Schore, A. N. (1994). *Affect regulation and the origin of the self. The neurobiology of emotional development.* Hillsdale, NJ: Erlbaum.

Schore, A. N. (2003). *Affect dysregulation and disorders of the self.* New York: Norton.

Siegel, D. J. (1999). *The developing mind: How relationships and the brain interact to shape who we are.* New York: Guilford Press.

Siegel, D. J., & Hartzell, M. (2003). *Parenting from the inside out.* New York: Tacher-Putnam.

Stern, D. (1974). The goal and structure of mother–infant play. *Journal of the American Academy of Child Psychiatry, 13,* 402–421.

Stern, D. (1986). *The interpersonal world of the infant.* New York: Basic Books. (German: [1992]: *Die Lebenserfahrung des Säuglings.* Stuttgart: Klett-Cotta)

Stern, D. (1995). *The motherhood constellation: A unified view of parent–child psychotherapy.* New York: Basic Books.

van IJzendoorn, M., & Sagi, A. (1999). Cross-cultural patterns of attachment. In J. Cassidy & P. Shaver (Eds.), *Handbook of attachment* (pp. 713–734). New York: Guilford Press.

Von Suchodoletz, W., & Keiner, T. (1998). Psychiatrische Aspekte bei sprachgestörten Kindern. *Pädiatrische Praxie, 54,* 395–402.

Waters, E., Weinfield, N., & Hamilton, C. (2000). The stability of attachment security from infancy to adolescence and early childhood: General discussion. *Child Development, 71*(3), 703–706.

Winnicott, D. W. (1958). *Collected papers: Through paediatrics to psychoanalysis.* London: Tavistock.

Ziegenhain, U., & Jacobsen, T. (1999). Assessing children's representational attachment models: Links to mother–child attachment quality in infancy and childhood. *Journal of Genetic Psychology, 160*(1), 22–30.

CHAPTER 6

Evidence-Based Play Therapy

DEE C. RAY

The U.S. Surgeon General's 2000 report on mental health described the shortage of appropriate services for children as a major health crisis and estimated that less than half of children in need receive any treatment (U.S. Public Health Service, 2000). Mental illness is now the leading cause of disability for all persons 5 years of age and older (U.S. Public Health Service, 2000). Evidence exists that untreated mental illness and behavioral problems in children follow the trajectory of continued behavioral problems at home and in school (Ackerman, Brown, & Izard, 2003; Keiley, Bates, Dodge, & Pettit, 2000). The president's New Freedom Commission on Mental Health (2003) recommended the promotion of screening, assessing, and providing services for the mental health of young children, in addition to the improving and expanding of school mental health. The commission also proposed the need for empirically based mental health interventions for children and adults. Public and private entities have emphasized the need for researchers and clinicians to demonstrate evidence of treatment effect prior to the dissemination of funding and/or support.

Play therapy has been used as a treatment of choice for young children since the early 1900s. Generally acknowledged as the originators of play therapy, Anna Freud (1928) and Melanie Klein (1932) used play as a substitute for verbalized free association in their efforts to apply analytical techniques to their work with children. Virginia Axline's (1947) use of play to apply nondirective therapeutic principles in her work with children popularized play therapy in the psychotherapy field, heavily influenced by Carl Rogers's (1942) person-centered theory. Her work and writings in the late 1940s and 1950s, including her accounting of play therapy with *Dibs* (1964), increased the knowledge and availability of play therapy. Axline (1949) was among the first to attempt to study the effects of play therapy and extend credibility to the intervention. Although by current standards, Axline's research does not address the rigor of research needed in the psychotherapy field to demonstrate efficacy of an intervention, she set the course for developing protocol and measuring effects of the play therapy approach. Founded in 1982, the Association for Play Therapy (APT) formed to develop and promote play therapy as a separate and distinct psychotherapy modality for treatment. APT currently serves more than 4,500 members identified as play therapy professionals.

META-ANALYTIC SUPPORT FOR PLAY THERAPY

As in most psychotherapy research, play therapy studies are limited by small sample sizes, which lead to a lack of generalizability of results (Ray, Bratton, Rhine, & Jones, 2001). In order to attain generalizable results, sample sizes would be daunting to the typical play therapy researcher. Chambless and Hollon (1998) suggest that treatment groups would need 50 clients per condition in order to reach sufficient statistical power in testing equivalency of groups. Because the necessity of large sample sizes hinders research practicality, psychotherapy has relied on meta-analytic reviews of research to address the effectiveness of interventions. Meta-analytic methodology combines the results from individual studies to produce an overall effect size, thereby determining the efficacy of the model intervention.

LeBlanc and Ritchie (1999) published the initial results of their meta-analysis of play therapy outcomes summarizing the results of 42 controlled studies, with an effect size of .66 standard deviations (SD). The researchers further detailed their study in a later publication, citing that benefits of play therapy appear to increase with the inclusion of parents and optimal treatment duration (LeBlanc & Ritchie, 2001). Using Cohen's (1988) guidelines for interpretation, an effect size (ES) of .66 denotes a moderate treatment effect, similar to effect sizes found in other child psychotherapy meta-analyses (Casey & Berman, 1985, ES = .71; Weisz, Weiss, Han, Granger, & Morton, 1995, ES = .71).

Ray et al. (2001), further detailed in Bratton, Ray, Rhine, and Jones (2005), conducted the largest meta-analysis on play therapy outcome research. This meta-analysis included the review of 180 documents dated

1942 to 2000 that appeared to measure the effectiveness of play therapy. Based on stringent criteria for inclusion, designating use of a controlled research design, sufficient data for computing effect size, and the identification by the author of a labeled "play therapy" intervention, 93 studies were included in the final calculation of effect size. The overall effect size was calculated at .80 SD, interpreted as a large effect, indicating that children receiving play therapy interventions performed .80 SD above children who did not receive play therapy. LeBlanc and Ritchie (2001) and Bratton et al. (2005) both included filial therapy research in their definitions of play therapy. Filial therapy is a parental intervention based on child-centered play therapy from which parents are taught basic child-centered therapy skills to facilitate weekly play sessions with their children.

Bratton et al. (2005) coded specific characteristics of play therapy that affected or had no effect on play therapy outcome. Effect sizes for humanistic (ES = .92) and nonhumanistic play therapy (ES = .71) interventions were considered to be effective regardless of theoretical approach. However, the effect size reported for humanistic approach was in the large effect category, while nonhumanistic was in the moderate category. This difference in effect may be attributed to a larger number of calculated humanistic studies (N = 73) compared to nonhumanistic studies (N = 12). When play therapy was delivered by a parent (ES = 1.15), the effect size was much larger than when delivered by a mental health professional (ES = .72), indicating the importance of involving parents in treatment to increase success of outcome. This finding was similar to the conclusions of LeBlanc and Ritchie (2001), who reported parent involvement as a predictor of play therapy outcome. Treatment duration was also a factor in the success of play therapy. Optimal treatment effects were obtained in 35–40 sessions, although many studies with fewer than 14 sessions also produced medium and large effect sizes. Age and sex were not found to be significant factors from which to predict the effects of play therapy. Play therapy appeared to be equally effective across age and sex. An effect size was not calculated for ethnicity due to the lack of specificity in the reporting of ethnicity in individual studies. In addressing presenting problems, the researchers encountered difficulty distinguishing specific diagnoses and symptoms due to the variation of the studies. However, 24 studies were calculated as investigating internalizing problems with an effect size of .81. Seventeen studies were calculated as examining the effects of play therapy on externalizing problems with an effect size of .78. Sixteen studies addressed a combination of internalizing and externalizing problems with an effect size of .93. These results indicated

that play therapy had a moderate to large beneficial effect for internalizing, externalizing, and combined problem types.

INDIVIDUAL STUDY SUPPORT FOR PLAY THERAPY

The field of play therapy has a history of more than 60 years of continuous research. Discussion of contemporary play therapy necessitates the
exploration of this research in the field. Play therapy most likely has the
longest history of research of any psychological intervention. In the earliest research I found, Dulsky (1942) attempted to study the relationship
between intellect and emotional problems. He inadvertently established
the effect of nondirective play therapy, which was to significantly improve social and emotional adjustments, yet no improvement was shown
on intellect. Dulsky's study is a typical example of historical play therapy
research. Although the research demonstrated a positive effect, neither a
control or comparison group nor randomization was utilized, and neither
a detailed description of participants nor a detailed description of treatment was published. Since Dulsky's 1942 study, an approximate count of
play therapy research, excluding filial therapy research, includes 103
studies, of which 71 were published in professional journals and 32 were
nonpublished, remaining in dissertation form. The majority of play therapy studies demonstrate some positive effect of play therapy on the participants. Over the last 15 years, since 1990, 36 research studies (27 published) on the impact of play therapy have been conducted. These most
recent studies have demonstrated the positive impact of play therapy on
general behavioral problems (Raman & Kapur, 1999; Shashi, Kapur, &
Subbakrishna, 1999), externalizing behavioral problems (Flahive, 2005;
Garza & Bratton, 2005; Karcher & Lewis, 2002; Kot, Landreth, &
Giordano, 1998; Schumann, 2004), internalizing problems (Packman &
Bratton, 2003), self-efficacy (Fall, Balvanz, Johnson, & Nelson, 1999), self-
concept (Kot et al., 1998; Post, 1999), anxiety (Baggerly, 2004; Shen, 2002),
depression (Baggerly, 2004), speech problems (Danger & Landreth, 2005),
and diabetes treatment compliance (Jones & Landreth, 2002).

The following section is a review of the play therapy research conducted over the last 15 years. The following criteria were applied when
selecting seven studies that exemplify current research methods and
reporting: (1) research published in a professional journal, (2) research
published since 1990, (3) research published in English, (4) use of a control group or comparison group, (5) sample size of 20 or more, (6) treatment described in detail or manualized, and (7) statistical methods and

results described in detail. Filial therapy research studies were not included in this review due to filial therapy's established power as a stand-alone intervention evidenced in Bratton et al. (2005) and more specifically in VanFleet, Ryan, and Smith (2005).

Play Therapy with Children Identified as Lacking in Coping Mechanisms

Fall et al. (1999) randomly selected children listed by teachers at three different schools as lacking in coping mechanisms that facilitate learning behaviors. Subjects were stratified by classroom teacher and grade level and randomly assigned to the control ($N = 31$) or experimental group ($N = 31$). There were 31 girls and 31 boys in the study. Age distribution was listed in the published article, ranging from 5 years to 9 years. The experimental group participated in six half-hour weekly child-centered play therapy sessions. All counselors were trained in research and child-centered protocol. The control group received no intervention. In a pretest–posttest design, all students were measured on three scales, including a classroom observation, Self-Efficacy Scale for Children (S-ES) and the Conners Teacher Rating Scale (CTRS). The classroom observation was conducted by research assistants trained to conduct a time sampling for off-task behaviors for 20 minutes with an established interrater reliability of 95%. Although both groups were found to increase favorable classroom behaviors through the CTRS and observation following treatment, they found that self-efficacy was significantly increased for those children participating in play therapy as measured by the S-ES.

Play Therapy with Hispanic Children

Participants for this study by Garza and Bratton (2005) were Hispanic children between the ages of 5 and 11 years old who were identified by teachers from three schools as experiencing behavioral problems. They were further screened with the Behavior Assessment System for Children (BASC) and scored in the at-risk or clinically significant range on any of the behavioral subscales. Twenty-nine students were identified and assigned to the either the child-centered play therapy intervention ($N = 15$) or the curriculum-based small group counseling group ($N = 14$). There were 17 boys and 12 girls who participated in the study. All participants were identified as Hispanic. Further distribution of age and grade breakdown is detailed in the published article. The child-centered play therapy

(CCPT) experimental treatment and Kids Connection curriculum comparison treatment were detailed in an accompanying manual to the study. Session summaries and videotapes were utilized to ensure treatment integrity. Both groups received 30 minutes of the assigned intervention once per week for 15 weeks. Using a pretest–posttest design, dependent variables were scores on the posttreatment BASC-parent report and BASC-teacher report. Results demonstrated that children receiving play therapy showed statistically significant decreases in externalizing behavior problems, specifically conduct problems, and moderate improvements in internalizing behavior problems, specifically anxiety. Effect sizes for several of the dependent measure scores indicated a moderate to large effect of play therapy, showing clinical significance in addition to statistical significance. Teacher BASC results demonstrated no statistical significance between the two groups.

Play Therapy with Children Diagnosed with Insulin-Dependent Diabetes

This study by Jones and Landreth (2002) sought to determine the effectiveness of play therapy with children diagnosed with insulin-dependent diabetes mellitus. Researchers recruited study participants from a summer camp for children with diabetes. Thirty children were selected for the study based on age (between 7 and 11 years) and other protocol criteria. There were 17 boys and 13 girls in the study. Ages and ethnicities are further detailed in the published study. The children were randomly assigned to the experimental or control group on the first day of camp. Children in the experimental group participated in 12 sessions of CCPT over the course of the 3-week camp. The control group received no additional intervention other than the summer camp. A pretest–posttest design was applied using the Revised Children's Manifest Anxiety Scale (RCMAS), Filial Problems Checklist (FPC), and Diabetes Adaptation Scale child form (DAS) as dependent measures. A 3-month posttest was also administered to participants through mail. Play therapists were trained in advanced play therapy and in issues related to diabetes. According to data analysis, both groups improved anxiety scores with no statistically significant difference in scores between groups. The experimental group showed greater improvement on the FPC than the control group but did not reach statistical significance. The experimental group showed a statistically significant increase in diabetes adaptation as indicated on the DAS.

Play Therapy with Child Witnesses of Domestic Violence

This study by Kot et al. (1998) employed a naturalistic design to accommodate the needs of residents of domestic violence shelters. During a 6-month period, CCPT was facilitated with all children between the ages of 4 and 10 years residing in the domestic shelter and whose parents agreed to be part of the study. Complete data was collected on 22 children in the experimental group. Following the collection of data on the experimental group, data was collected on 11 children who met the same conditions of the experimental group but entered the shelter following the end of residence of experimental group members. The experimental group received 12 45-minute sessions of individual CCPT in a period of 12 days to 3 weeks. Play therapists completed an advanced course in play therapy. The control group participated in regular shelter programs for the same length of time as the experimental group but received no play therapy. Pretest–posttest measures included Joseph Preschool and Primary Self-Concept Scale (JSCS), Child Behavior Checklist (CBCL), and Children's Play Session Behavior Rating Scale (CPSBRS). Raters blindly rated pre- and postintervention play therapy sessions according to the CPSBRS. Interrater reliability was .93 at posttesting. Following a treatment of play therapy, children in the experimental group scored significantly higher than children in the control group on self-concept as measured by the JSCS. Mothers of the children in the experimental group reported that their children exhibited significantly fewer externalizing behavior problems as measured by the CBCL and fewer total behavior problems than the mothers of children in the control group. Children in the experimental group scored significantly higher than children in the control group in physical proximity and play themes as measured by the CPSBRS.

Play Therapy with Learning-Disabled Preadolescents

Packman and Bratton (2003) recruited fourth- and fifth-grade volunteer students attending a private school specializing in the education of children with learning differences. Volunteer students were identified by parents or teachers as exhibiting behavioral difficulties. Thirty participants between the ages of 10 and 12 were randomly assigned to the treatment group ($N = 15$) or control group ($N = 15$). Breakdown of sex, ethnicity, and grade is detailed in the published article. The treatment group was further divided into groups of three and participated in a group play therapy intervention 1 hour per week for 12 weeks. The intervention was based on humanistic play therapy guidelines and is further outlined in the published article. The control group received no intervention. A pretest–posttest design was used with the Behavior Assessment System for Children—Parent Rating Form (BASC-PRF) and the Child Behavior Checklist—Parent Report Form (CBCL-PRF) serving as dependent variables. Children who participated in the play therapy intervention demonstrated statistically significant improvement in scores on the BASC-PRF on overall composite scores and internalizing problems over children in the control group. Although statistical significance was not achieved on the CBCL-PRF, effect sizes were in the large treatment effect category on total and internalizing problems. Externalizing problem scores also yielded a moderate effect on both the BASC-PRF and CBCL-PRF, although not a statistically significant one.

Play Therapy with At-Risk Students

This study by Post (1999) examined the effects of a play therapy program on children identified as at risk specifically through poverty designation, achieving below grade level, special education identification, and mobility in home environment. All at-risk students in the identified school were recruited to participate in the study. Seventy-seven students were assigned to the experimental group, and 91 were assigned to the control group. Further details on age, sex, ethnicity, and family background are included in the published study. Children in the experimental group participated in CCPT, which was facilitated by graduate students trained in an introductory play therapy course. Children in the experimental group received from 1 to 24 play therapy sessions once per week with a mean number of 4 sessions. The control group received no intervention. Dependent variables included the Coopersmith Self-Esteem Inventory (SEI), the Intellectual Achievement Responsibility Scale—Revised (IAR), and the State–Trait Anxiety Inventory for Children (STAIC). Pretest and posttest scores on the dependent variables were analyzed to determine the effect of play therapy over time. Although there was no difference between groups on anxiety, a statistically significant difference was found between groups on self-esteem and locus of control. Further analysis revealed that children participating in play therapy did not increase self-esteem and locus of control over time but maintained the pretest level. However, children in the control group not receiving play therapy suffered from a statistically significant loss in self-esteem and locus of control. The author concluded that play therapy might be needed to prevent at-risk children from developing lower self-esteem and from reducing their sense of responsibility for their academic progress.

Short-Term Play Therapy
with Chinese Earthquake Victims

This study by Shen (2002) investigated the impact of play therapy in an elementary school with Chinese children in Taiwan following an earthquake registering 7.3 on the Richter scale and resulting in the loss of many lives. The researcher recruited child participants from a rural elementary school located in an area of Taiwan that experienced the earthquake and more than 1,000 aftershocks in the subsequent months. Thirty students were identified as being at high risk for maladjustment using the Children's Mental Health Checklist (CMHC). The students, ranging from ages 8 to 12, were randomly and equally assigned to an experimental group and a control group. Breakdown of grade and sex is provided in the published study. The experimental group was further divided into play groups of three children per group. Each experimental small group received 10 40-minute group play therapy sessions during a 4-week span, meeting two to three times per week. Group play therapy was facilitated by a school counselor trained in CCPT. The control group received no intervention. Dependent measures included CMHC, FPC, RCMAS, and Multiscore Depression Inventory for Children (MDI-C). Results of the RCMAS demonstrated a significant decrease in anxiety, as well as a large treatment effect, for children participating in the experimental group as compared to the control group. Suicide risk as measured by the MDI-C was also found to be significantly less in the experimental group as compared to the control group.

Historical Play Therapy Studies

The use of these exemplary play therapy research studies by no means devalues the significant contribution that many other historical play therapy studies have made to the field. A rich history of play therapy efficacy has been established in the areas of hospitalized children with symptoms of anxiety (Cassell, 1965; Clatworthy, 1981; Johnson & Stockdale, 1975; Rae, Worchel, Upchurch, Sanner, & Daniel, 1989), self-concept (Crow, 1990; Gould, 1980; House, 1970; Perez, 1987), social adjustment (Cox, 1953; Oualline, 1976; Pelham, 1972; Thombs & Muro, 1973), and behavioral difficulties (Brandt, 2001; Gaulden, 1975; Hannah, 1986; Quayle, 1991). Detailed accounts of these studies can be found in the compilation of play therapy research summarized in Bratton and Ray (2000).

However, contemporary focus on research design and protocol rigor requires play therapy researchers to address cited flaws in the historical play therapy research. Ray et al. (2001) pointed to flaws regarding lack of experimental methods, reported statistics, descriptions of treatment, specificity of participants' descriptions, and ill-defined presenting problems as problematic. In the seven exemplary studies detailed in the previous description, historical flaws have been corrected and addressed. Contemporary play therapy researchers are detailing their designs, interventions, protocols, and statistical methods in order to maintain the highest research standards.

EFFECTIVENESS AND EFFICACY

As a result of external and internal pressure to present evidence of psychotherapy treatment, the American Psychological Association (APA) Division 12 Task Force on Promotion and Dissemination of Psychological Procedures issued the first major list of empirically supported treatments in 1995 (Chorpita, 2003). The purpose of defining and identifying empirically supported treatments was to find the most effective treatments for specific mental health problems and to help practitioners in their selection of client treatment (Steele & Roberts, 2003). The most articulated controversy regarding the identification of evidence-based treatments or empirically supported treatments, however, is the possible distinction between clinical trials and real-world interventions: efficacy versus effectiveness (Chorpita, 2003; Nathan, Stuart, & Dolan, 2003; Steele & Roberts, 2003). Nathan et al. (2003) described efficacy research as the focus on measurable effects of specific interventions, whereas effectiveness research focuses on whether treatments are feasible and have beneficial effects in real-world settings. Efficacy studies are well defined, with meticulous controls on inclusion and exclusion and strict adherence to research protocol. Due to the delivery of treatment in a realistic setting, effectiveness studies are plagued with research difficulties such as lack of specific diagnoses and lack of adherence to treatment protocol due to the clinical needs of clients. Some support exists for the lack of impact that efficacy studies have on practitioner settings.

Although Division 12's listing of empirically supported treatments was met with controversy over criteria and qualifications, as well as over the perceived need for such a list, other entities have followed suit. APA Division 53 further defined the criteria for evidence-based approaches and published the website "Evidence-Based Treatment for Children and Adolescents" (Society of Clinical Child and Adolescent Psychology and Network on Youth Mental Health, n.d.). Division 53 defines two categories of evidence-based approaches, which include "Best Support (well-established treatments)" and "Promising (probably efficacious treatments)." Criteria for Best Support include (1) at least two good between-group design experiments demonstrating efficacy in either demonstrating superiority to a placebo or another treatment or equivalent to an already established treatment in experiments with adequate statistical power, *or* (2) a large series of single-case design experiments ($N \geq 9$) demonstrating efficacy using good experimental designs and compared to another treatment, *and* (3) experiments must be conducted with treatment manuals, (4) characteristics of the client samples must be clearly specified, *and* (5) effects must have been demonstrated by at least two different investigators or teams of investigators. Criteria for Promising include (1) two experiments showing the treatment is statistically significantly superior to a waiting list control group, *or* (2) one between-group design experiment with clear specification of group, use of manuals, and demonstration of efficacy either through superiority to placebo or another treatment or equivalent to an already established treatment in experiments with adequate statistical power, *or* (3) a small series of single-case design experiments ($N \geq 3$) with clear specification of group, use of manuals, good experimental designs, and comparison of the intervention to a placebo or another treatment. Currently, this website lists four major types of disorders, including anxiety disorders, depression, attention-deficit/hyperactivity disorder, and conduct/oppositional problems. Several of the listed disorders identify no Best Support or Promising treatments, indicating the need for additional research on these and other diagnoses. It should be noted that currently no play therapy approaches are considered by Division 53 as Best Support or Promising.

Effectiveness of Play Therapy

Speaking to the issue of effectiveness, the strength of play therapy research appears to be in the history of and continued ability to conduct successful play therapy studies in natural real-world settings of schools, hospitals, clinics, and shelters. The New Freedom Commission on Mental Health (2003) recommended the expansion of preventive, proactive care in natural settings. Of the 103 research studies reviewed for this chapter, 41 were conducted in elementary schools. Five of the seven highlighted exemplary studies were conducted in a school environment with students during the school day. Although conducting research in the school setting presents the researcher with difficulties in controlling research groups and facilitating treatment as dictated by a protocol, it offers the practitioner a practical method for replicating treatment if it is discovered that treatment was effective. Owens and Murphy (2004) cited that when efficacy studies are conducted by professional researchers, results are often not generalizable because of low caseloads, high levels of supervision, and rigid inclusion and exclusion criteria. As evidenced by the play therapy research, researchers have attempted to provide services to a large number of children, including criteria such as, for example, "children who are identified by parents and/or teachers as exhibiting behavioral problems." This broader inclusion pattern allows the researcher to serve children who are experiencing problems but possibly not identified with a specific diagnosis or not exhibiting only criteria tied to a specific diagnosis. Although this inclusionary pattern dilutes the strength of an efficacy study, it increases the strength of an effectiveness study. For example, in a school setting, students, especially young students, often do not present with specific diagnosable disorders. They typically present with problems and related symptoms that can be associated with developmental issues, familial difficulties, interpersonal challenges, comorbid diagnoses, learning disabilities, and a variety of other associated causes. Treatment provided in school-setting studies can be replicated and provided by a full-time counselor, psychologist, or social worker in the public school setting.

In addition to the natural setting of school, several studies cited with children in hospital settings were conducted with children receiving other hospital services who might benefit from a play therapy treatment provided by hospital staff to reduce their anxiety. Shelters are perhaps the most difficult settings in which to conduct research, yet Kot et al. (1998) and Tyndall-Lind, Landreth, and Giordano (2001) directed research within the highly mobile environment of a domestic violence shelter, while Baggerly (2004) managed to conduct a quasi-experimental design in the mostly transient environment of a homeless shelter. Brandt (2001) demonstrated the impact of play therapy on children who received services from a mental health clinic that served clients of low income and education level.

Additional strengths of play therapy research include the ability to demonstrate effectiveness with younger age groups and diverse populations. Typically, child intervention research has focused on treatment for older children. Among studies highlighted as efficacy studies for the treatment of child depression, the youngest children were in third grade (Kaslow & Thompson, 1998). In a review of studies of conduct disorder in children, Brestan and Eyberg (1998) stated the mean age of children in the 82 reviewed studies was close to 10 years old (9.89 years). Other meta-analytic reviews of child therapy research outcomes cited similar mean ages, including Weisz et al.'s (1995) review of 150 studies, with a mean age of 10.5 years, and Kazdin, Bass, Ayers, and Rodgers's (1990) review of 105 studies with a mean age of 10.2 years. Play therapy research has, however, established play therapy as an appropriate intervention for younger children. LeBlanc and Ritchie's (2001) review of 42 play therapy studies and Ray et al.'s (2001) review of 93 play therapy studies cited mean ages of 7.9 years and 7.0 years, respectively. Because of the developmental language of play, many of the play therapy research studies investigated the impact of play therapy on children as young as 2 and 3 years old (Cassell, 1965; George, Braun, & Walker, 1982; Kot et al., 1998; Saucier, 1986; Shmukler & Naveh, 1984–1985; Trostle, 1988).

Diversity intervention also continues to be a focus of play therapy research. Play therapy researchers have sought to investigate play not only as a developmental intervention, but also as a universal language for children. Garza and Bratton (2005) demonstrated the positive effects of play therapy on problem behaviors for a sample of all Hispanic children, mostly identified as Mexican American. Shen (2002) confirmed the impact of play therapy in ameliorating symptoms of anxiety and suicide risk with Taiwanese child survivors of an earthquake. Trostle (1988) found that after 10 sessions of nondirective group play therapy, bilingual Puerto Rican children showed significant improvement in self-control and higher developmental level play behaviors when compared to their control group peers. When Post (1999) measured the effect of play therapy with 168 children, 82% of whom were African American, she found that a mean of four nondirective play therapy sessions helped them to maintain a stable level of self-esteem and internal locus of control. Although a large number of play therapy studies have failed to report ethnicity backgrounds for their participants, these few studies offer promising results for play therapy's impact on children of multicultural backgrounds.

Research in play therapy has shown effectiveness in natural settings, with younger children, and with diverse groups of children. Understanding play therapy as a distinct intervention that can be used in a generalized real-world setting with a younger population of varying backgrounds offers the intervention as a viable option for clinicians and practitioners. There are few other interventions that can boast a lengthy history of research with consistent positive results across a variety of populations and presenting problems. Certainly, for younger children, play therapy is unique in its capacity to offer mental health assistance for children who are suffering from a lack of services and interventions.

Efficacy of Play Therapy

Play therapy has demonstrated effectiveness in its ability to intervene with real-world children with real-world problems through a lengthy history of individual research and through a thorough analysis of the research (Bratton et al., 2005; LeBlanc & Ritchie, 2001). The meta-analyses have also helped the intervention of play therapy move toward the goal of efficacy. Chambless and Hollon (1998) provided a comprehensive description of efficacy to demonstrate that treatment benefits are due to the effects of the treatment and not to chance or confounding factors such as passage of time, effects of psychological assessment, or presence of different types of clients in the various treatment conditions. They further identified the need for randomization of the sample to a comparison condition, replication of the study by an independent team of investigators, and use of sound methodology. Sound methodology includes, but is not limited to, specificity in sample population description, selection of instruments that measure the specific focus of the population, followup methods, assessment of clinical significance, use of treatment manuals, monitoring of treatment protocol, and credible data analysis. Efficacy can be established through group design methods or single-case experiments.

Chorpita (2003) offered a broader interpretation of evidence-based research methods that includes four types of methods. Efficacy research links treatment with outcome, transportability examines the effectiveness of treatment for real-world settings, dissemination addresses the extent to which treatment can be implemented in real-world settings without researcher support, and system evaluation demonstrates efficacy when the system to be evaluated and the research team are completely independent. Through this continuum, there is a growing link between research and practice, evidentiary of effective treatments. Chambless and Hollon (1998) appeared to describe perfect research in which all conditions can be controlled and examined. The real-world application of play therapy research does not fit this criterion, but play therapy researchers can attempt to address issues noted by the narrow definitions of efficacy in order to strengthen the efficacy base of play therapy. Significant progress has been made in the areas of randomization of sample, addition of comparison groups, and use of credible data analysis and reporting. This progress needs to be maintained and enhanced. Yet, through this review, there appeared to exist three main criteria in which play therapy research has not aligned itself with the psychotherapy research on efficacy: manualization of treatment, specificity of population, and replication of studies. Several suggestions for improving clinical research in play therapy are proposed below.

Manualization of Treatment

The development and adherence to a treatment manual is a common theme in efficacy literature (Brestan & Eyberg, 1998; Chambless & Hollon, 1998; Nathan et al., 2003). Historically, play therapy has not adopted the use of manuals in specification of research protocol. Although play therapy researchers may identify a theoretical base such as a cognitive-behavioral or child-centered approach to play therapy, detailed descriptions are rarely provided. Play therapy is littered with recurring problems identifying treatment. For example, throughout research studies, child-centered play therapy is referred to as nondirective play therapy, play therapy according to Axline (1947), play therapy according to Landreth (2002), relationship play therapy, and self-directive play therapy, just to name a few. In the most recent research, Garza and Bratton (2005) took a step forward by identifying the use of a manual for a child-centered play therapy intervention. Possibly, play therapists have hesitated in using manuals because of the need to respond to each client as needed, but manuals are not required to be step-by-step outlines of sessions. In order to accommodate treatment, manuals can describe "broad principles and phases of treatment with examples of interventions consistent with these notions" (Chambless & Hollon, 1998, p. 11). This type of manual allows the play therapy researcher to define treatment according to theoretical principles and offer specific interventions to describe those principles, but it also allows for freedom in meeting the needs of the client through the principles outlined in the manual.

Adequate use of a treatment manual includes assurance that the treatment protocol is being followed. Adherence to treatment is a critical piece of conducting solid research, and it has been shown that without monitoring, researchers will drift from manualized treatments (Nathan et al., 2003). Monitoring of treatment goes beyond the general supervision and training of treatment providers in a given study. Steele and Roberts (2003) provided an example of treatment integrity measurement in suggesting randomized observation of recorded sessions by multiple observers. The use of trained observers who establish an acceptable level of inter-rater reliability to observe random sessions ensures that research protocol is being followed and is indeed responsible for outcome changes.

Specificity in Sample Population Description

As recently as a decade ago, researchers failed to include simple descriptive characteristics of the sample population. Play therapy research has greatly improved in the reporting of sex, age, ethnicity, and other distinguishing characteristics, yet improvement has not been made in the area of distinguishing presenting problems and symptoms. Using outcome measures such as the CBCL (Achenbach & Rescorla, 2001) or the BASC (Reynolds & Kamphaus, 1992), play therapy researchers continue to approach research with a broad net, attempting to serve all children with all behavioral problems. Although limiting to the number who can participate in research and the number of children who are served, identifying specific problems and examining only those problems will help build efficacy research in play therapy. This can be accomplished through the identification of DSM-IV diagnoses in children, then measuring the impact of play therapy on those diagnoses. Even though this approach sounds simple, it represents a unique problem for play therapists who provide services to young children, many of whom cannot be designated one specific diagnosis.

Hence, it is recommended that play therapy researchers attempt to study the effects of play therapy on grouped behaviors, such as hyperactivity, depressive problems, and anxiety problems. For example, instead of measuring problematic behavior of children according to the total problems score on the CBCL, a researcher could simply identify children who score borderline or clinically significant on the subscale of attention problems or aggressive problems. The researcher would proceed to measure the impact of a play therapy intervention on that specific scale. The hopeful outcome would be that instead of a general statement from some historical play therapy research studies in which it can be stated, "play therapy had a positive impact on problem behaviors of children," this new type of research would yield a statement such as "the specified play therapy intervention demonstrated a decrease in aggressive behaviors for children identified with clinically significant aggressive behaviors." Creating specificity in play therapy research helps the field to acknowledge how effective play therapy is with specific presenting problems.

Replication of Play Therapy Studies

As highlighted earlier, play therapy has a rich and lengthy history of research on various populations, across various presenting problems, in various settings, with various treatments. The downfall of such variation is the lack of replication in play therapy studies. Replication of research involves repeating studies on the use of a specific protocol with a specific presenting population in a specific setting. Valid replication also requires that similar studies be conducted by researchers independent of each other (Chambless & Hollon, 1998). Independent researchers are entities that are not working from the same resources or within the same unit. For example, a replicated study conducted by Professor Smith at XYZ University of a study that was conducted by Professor Jones at the same XYZ University would hold little weight as being independent research. However, if separate universities or entities, such as clinics or schools, conduct similar studies in different locations but with the same protocol and same type of setting, it *is* considered independent research. Manualization and specification are required in order for a study to be considered worthy of replication. Without these adherences to proper research protocol, there is no need to replicate a study. At this juncture, replication with loose research definitions and parameters is not particularly beneficial to the play therapy research.

Although play therapy does not have to meet these stringent requirements to be considered promising, best support treatments are marked by their manualization, specification of sample, and replication of results. As play therapy research continues to grow in its ability to present evidence of efficacy, focus must be placed on best efforts so that time, energy, and resources are not utilized in vain. The field of psychotherapy has pressured the field of play therapy to prove its worth. Anecdotal outcomes and historically valid research methods no longer meet the criteria being placed before the play therapy community to demonstrate efficacy. As play therapy researchers have shown, they will meet new standards by changing specific methods of conducting and reporting research, thereby addressing efficacy with a new evaluative audience.

CONCLUSION

Play therapy has an extensive history of research that demonstrates the practicality of using play therapy interventions with children across ages and issues. Play therapy clinicians, whose numbers have grown significantly in the last decade, base their therapeutic practice on known benefits that play therapy provides to young clients. Play therapy has been demonstrated to improve the self-concepts of children, decrease anxious behaviors, lessen externalizing and internalizing problem behaviors, and increase social adjustment. Play therapy delivered in the group or individual format appears to be equally effective in helping children deal with mental health issues and behavioral problems. An overall summarization of play therapy research over 60 years provides evidence that play therapy has a large beneficial treatment effect over comparison or nontreatment groups. Specific research studies are cited and reviewed in this chapter to reveal the overall impact of play therapy interventions.

The current trend among public and private organizations to move toward support of mental health treatments that have demonstrated efficacy has encouraged such entities to set standards for evidence-based practice. Play therapy research has responded to this trend by applying further rigor to field research. The strength of play therapy research lies in its application to real-world settings that validate play therapy as a usable model in working with real clients. In order for play therapy to be considered a well-established treatment, play therapy researchers must improve specific ways of implementing and reporting research designs. This chapter proposes several methods for addressing efficacy-based issues in play therapy research.

REFERENCES

Achenbach, T. M., & Rescorla, L. A. (2001). *Manual for the ASEBA school-age forms and profiles*. Burlington, VT: University of Vermont, Research Center for Children, Youth, and Families.

Ackerman, B., Brown, E., & Izard, C. (2003). Continuity and change in levels of externalizing behavior in school of children from economically disadvantaged families. *Child Development, 74*, 694–709.

Axline, V. (1947). *Play therapy*. New York: Ballantine.

Axline, V. (1949). Mental deficiency: Symptom or disease? *Journal of Consulting Psychology, 13*, 313–327.

Axline, V. (1964). *Dibs: In search of self*. New York: Ballantine.

Baggerly, J. (2004). The effects of child-centered group play therapy on self-concept, depression, and anxiety of children who are homeless. *International Journal of Play Therapy, 13*, 31–51.

Brandt, M. (2001). An investigation of the efficacy of play therapy with young children. (Doctoral dissertation, University of North Texas, 2001). *Dissertation Abstracts International, 61*, 2603.

Bratton, S., & Ray, D. (2000). What the research shows about play therapy. *International Journal of Play Therapy, 9*, 47–88.

Bratton, S., Ray, D., Rhine, T., & Jones, L. (2005). The efficacy of play therapy with children: A meta-analytic review of treatment outcomes. *Professional Psychology: Research and Practice, 36*, 376–390.

Brestan, E., & Eyberg, S. (1998). Effective psychosocial treatments of conduct-disordered children and adolescents: 29 years, 82 studies, and 5,272 kids. *Journal of Clinical Child Psychology, 27,* 180–189.

Casey, R., & Berman, J. (1985). The outcome of psychotherapy with children. *Psychological Bulletin, 98,* 388–400.

Cassell, S. (1965). Effect of brief puppet therapy upon the emotional responses of children undergoing cardiac catheterization. *Journal of Consulting Psychology, 29,* 1–8.

Chambless, D., & Hollon, S. (1998). Defining empirically supported therapies. *Journal of Consulting and Clinical Psychology, 66,* 7–18.

Chorpita, B. (2003). The frontier of evidence-based practice. In A. Kazdin & J. Weisz (Eds.), *Evidence-based psychotherapies for children and adolescents* (pp. 42–59). New York: Guilford Press.

Clatworthy, S. (1981). Therapeutic play: Effects on hospitalized children. *Journal of Association for Care of Children's Health, 9,* 108–113.

Cohen, J. (1988). *Statistical power analysis for the behavioral sciences* (2nd ed.). Hillside, NJ: Erlbaum.

Cox, F. (1953). Sociometric status and individual adjustment before and after play therapy. *Journal of Abnormal Social Psychology, 48,* 354–356.

Crow, J. (1990). Play therapy with low achievers in reading (Doctoral dissertation, University of North Texas, 1989). *Dissertation Abstracts International, 50,* 2789.

Danger, S., & Landreth, G. (2005). Child-centered group play therapy with children with speech difficulties. *International Journal of Play Therapy, 14,* 81–102.

Dulsky, S. (1942). Affect and intellect: An experimental study. *The Journal of General Psychology, 27,* 199–220.

Fall, M., Balvanz, J., Johnson, L., & Nelson, L. (1999). A play therapy intervention and its relationship to self-efficacy and learning behaviors. *Professional School Counseling, 2* (3), 194–204.

Flahive, M. (2005). *Group sandtray therapy at school with preadolescents identified with behavioral difficulties.* Unpublished doctoral dissertation, University of North Texas.

Freud, A. (1928). *Introduction to the technique of child analysis* (trans. L. P. Clark). New York: Nervous and Mental Disease Publishing.

Garza, Y., & Bratton, S. (2005). School-based child centered play therapy with Hispanic children: Outcomes and cultural considerations. *International Journal of Play Therapy, 14*(1), 51–80.

Gaulden, G. (1975). Developmental-play group counseling with early primary grade students exhibiting behavioral problems (Doctoral dissertation, North Texas State University, 1975). *Dissertation Abstracts International, 36,* 2628.

George, N., Braun, B., & Walker, J. (1982). A prevention and early intervention mental health program for disadvantaged preschool children. *The American Journal of Occupational Therapy, 36,* 99–106.

Gould, M. (1980). The effect of short-term intervention play therapy on the self-concept of selected elementary pupils (Doctoral dissertation, Florida Institute of Technology, 1980). *Dissertation Abstracts International, 41,* 1090.

Hannah, G. (1986). An investigation of play therapy: Process and outcome using interrupted time-series analysis (Doctoral dissertation, University of Northern Colorado, 1986). *Dissertation Abstracts International, 47,* 2615.

House, R. (1970). The effects of nondirective group play therapy upon the sociometric status and self-concept of selected second grade children (Doctoral dissertation, Oregon State University, 1970). *Dissertation Abstracts International, 31,* 2684.

Johnson, P., & Stockdale, D. (1975). Effects of puppet therapy on Palmar sweating of hospitalized children. *The Johns Hopkins Medical Journal, 137,* 1–5.

Jones, E., & Landreth, G. (2002). The efficacy of intensive individual play therapy for chronically ill children. *International Journal of Play Therapy, 11,* 117–140.

Karcher, M., & Lewis, S. (2002). Pair counseling: The effects of a dyadic developmental play therapy on interpersonal understanding and externalizing behaviors. *International Journal of Play Therapy, 11,* 19–42.

Kaslow, N., & Thompson, M. (1998). Applying the criteria for empirically supported treatments to studies of psychosocial interventions for child and adolescent depression. *Journal of Clinical Child Psychology, 27,* 146–155.

Kazdin, A., Bass, D., Ayers, W., & Rodgers, A. (1990). Empirical and clinical focus of child and adolescent psychotherapy research. *Journal of Consulting and Clinical Psychology, 58,* 729–740.

Keiley, M., Bates, J., Dodge, K., & Pettit, G. (2000). A cross-domain growth analysis: Externalizing and internalizing behaviors during 8 years of childhood. *Journal of Abnormal Child Psychology, 28,* 161–179.

Klein, M. (1932). *The psychoanalysis of children.* London: Hogarth.

Kot, S., Landreth, G., & Giordano, M. (1998). Intensive child-centered play therapy with child witnesses of domestic violence. *International Journal of Play Therapy, 7,* 17–36.

Landreth, G. (2002). *Play therapy: The art of the relationship* (2nd ed.). New York: Brunner-Routledge.

LeBlanc, M., & Ritchie, M. (1999). Predictors of play therapy outcomes. *International Journal of Play Therapy, 8,* 19–34.

LeBlanc, M., & Ritchie, M. (2001). A meta-analysis of play therapy outcomes. *Counseling Psychology Quarterly, 14,* 149–163.

Nathan, P., Stuart, S., & Dolan, S. (2003). Research on psychotherapy efficacy and effectiveness: Between Scylla and Charybdis? In A. Kazdin (Ed.), *Methodological issues and strategies in clinical research* (3rd ed., pp. 505–546). Washington, DC: American Psychological Association.

New Freedom Commission on Mental Health. (2003). *Achieving the promise: Transforming mental health care in America. Final Report.* DHHS Pub. No. SMA-03-3832. Rockville, MD: Department of Health and Human Services.

Oualline, B. (1976). Behavioral outcomes of short-term non-directive play therapy with preschool deaf children (Doctoral dissertation, North Texas State University, 1975). *Dissertation Abstracts International, 36,* 7870.

Owens, J., & Murphy, C. (2004). Effectiveness research in the context of school-based mental health. *Clinical Child and Family Psychology Review, 7,* 195–209.

Packman, J., & Bratton, S. (2003). A school-based group play/activity therapy intervention with learning disabled preadolescents exhibiting behavior problems. *International Journal of Play Therapy, 12*, 7–29.

Pelham, L. (1972). Self-directive play therapy with socially immature kindergarten students (Doctoral dissertation, University of Northern Colorado, 1971). *Dissertation Abstracts International, 32*, 3798.

Perez, C. (1987). A comparison of group play therapy and individual play therapy for sexually abused children (Doctoral dissertation, University of Northern Colorado, 1987). *Dissertation Abstracts International, 48*, 3079.

Post, P. (1999). Impact of child-centered play therapy on the self-esteem, locus of control, and anxiety of at-risk 4th-, 5th-, and 6th-grade students. *International Journal of Play Therapy, 8*, 1–18.

Quayle, R. (1991). The primary mental health project as a school-based approach for prevention of adjustment problems: An evaluation (Doctoral dissertation, Pennsylvania State University, 1991). *Dissertation Abstracts International, 52*, 1268.

Rae, W., Worchel, F., Upchurch, J., Sanner, J., & Daniel, C. (1989). The psychosocial impact of play on hospitalized children. *Journal of Pediatric Psychology, 14*, 617–627.

Raman, V., & Kapur, M. (1999). A study of play therapy in children with emotional disorders. *NIMHANS Journal, 17*, 93–98.

Ray, D., Bratton, S., Rhine, T., & Jones, L. (2001). The effectiveness of play therapy: Responding to the critics. *International Journal of Play Therapy, 10*, 85–108.

Reynolds, C., & Kamphaus, R. (1992). *Behavior assessment scale for children*. Circle Pines, MN: American Guidance Service.

Rogers, C. (1942). *Counseling and psychotherapy*. Boston: Houghton Mifflin.

Saucier, B. (1986). An intervention: The effects of play therapy on developmental achievement levels of abused children (Doctoral dissertation, Texas Woman's University, 1986). *Dissertation Abstracts International, 48*, 1007.

Schumann, B. (2004). *Effects of child-centered play therapy and curriculum-based small group guidance on the behaviors of children referred for aggression in an elementary school setting*. Unpublished doctoral dissertation, University of North Texas.

Shashi, K., Kapur, M., & Subbakrishna, D. (1999). Evaluation of play therapy in emotionally disturbed children. *NIMHANS Journal, 17*, 99–111.

Shen, Y. (2002). Short-term group play therapy with Chinese earthquake victims: Effects on anxiety, depression, and adjustment. *International Journal of Play Therapy, 11*, 43–63.

Shmukler, D., & Naveh, I. (1984–1985). Structured vs. unstructured play training with economically disadvantaged preschoolers. *Imagination, Cognition and Personality, 4*, 293–304.

Society of Clinical Child and Adolescent Psychology and Network on Youth Mental Health. (n.d.). *Evidence-based treatment for children and adolescents*. Retrieved July 15, 2005, from www.wjh.harvard.edu/%7Enock/Div53/EST/index.htm.

Steele, R., & Roberts, M. (2003). Therapy and interventions research with children and adolescents. In M. Roberts & S. Ilardi (Eds.), *Handbook of research methods in clinical psychology* (pp. 307–326). Malden, MA: Blackwell.

Thombs, M., & Muro, J. (1973). Group counseling and the sociometric status of second-grade children. *Elementary School Guidance and Counseling, 7,* 194–197.

Trostle, S. (1988). The effects of child-centered group play sessions on social-emotional growth of three- to six-year old bilingual Puerto Rican children. *Journal of Research in Childhood Education, 3,* 93–106.

Tyndall-Lind, A., Landreth, G., & Giordano, M. (2001). Intensive group play therapy with child witnesses of domestic violence. *International Journal of Play Therapy, 10,* 53–83.

U.S. Public Health Service. (2000). *Report of the Surgeon General's conference on children's mental health: A national action agenda.* Washington, DC: Author.

VanFleet, R., Ryan, S., & Smith, S. (2005). Filial therapy: A critical review. In L. Reddy, T. Files-Hall, & C. Schaefer (Eds.), *Empirically based play interventions for children* (pp. 241–264). Washington, DC: American Psychological Association.

Weisz, J., Weiss, B., Han, S., Granger, D., & Morton, T. (1995). Effects of psychotherapy with children and adolescents revisited: A meta-analysis of treatment outcomes studies. *Psychological Bulletin, 117,* 450–468.

PART III

APPLICATIONS

CHAPTER 7

"I'm Rich"

Play Therapy with Children Who Are Homeless

JENNIFER BAGGERLY

"I'm rich!" exclaims a child during her play therapy session at a homeless shelter. She throws play money in the air and watches it fall to the ground, as quickly as her world fell when her family was evicted from their home. Numerous toys in the playroom and a caring play therapist are her solace from the harsh reality of homelessness. By playing "I'm rich," she gains in fantasy what she longs for in reality.

This play behavior could be enacted by more than 1 million children who are homeless in the United States in a given year (Institute for Children and Poverty [ICP], 2001; National Coalition for the Homeless [NCH], 2002b). According to the Stewart B. McKinney Act, 42 U.S.C. § 11301, et seq. (1994), families and children are homeless if they lack a fixed, regular, and adequate nighttime residence and if they have a primary nighttime residence that is a shelter or place not ordinarily designed for residence, such as a car, abandoned building, or public park (NCH, 2004). The threat of homelessness affects another 13 million children who live below the poverty line in the United States. The number of children who are homeless continues to increase. The fastest growing segment of the homeless population is families with children, who represent 40% of people who are homeless (NCH, 2004). Since 1 in 5 adults who are homeless was homeless as a child, the cycle of homelessness appears to be accelerating (NCH 2004).

The purpose of this chapter is to help play therapists develop needed attitudes, knowledge, and skills to work with the increasing number of children who are homeless. First, the causes and impact of homelessness are described to increase play therapists' empathy. Second, the rationale for and research on play therapy with children who are homeless are discussed. Third, perspectives and procedures for implementing child-centered play therapy with children who are homeless are presented. Fourth, conjoint interventions such as classroom guidance lessons and teacher consultation are described. Finally, a case study that illustrates play therapy and other interventions is presented.

CAUSES OF HOMELESSNESS

The causes of homelessness are numerous. Poverty and lack of affordable housing are leading causes (NCH, 2002c). Although more than 26% of parents who are homeless are employed, the low wages they earn result in a crisis of not being able to afford medical care, food, and housing (ICP, 2001). A one- or two-bedroom apartment at fair market rent requires more than minimum wage: "In the median state, a minimum-wage worker would have to work 89 hours each week to afford a two-bedroom apartment at 30% of his or her income, which is the federal definition of affordable housing" (NCH, 2002c, ¶ 7). The number of people needing but unable to afford low-cost housing grew by 1 million in the 1990s (NCH, 2002c).

Decline in public assistance also contributes to homelessness. The myth that welfare provides relief from poverty must be dispelled. NCH (2002c) states that "The median Temporary Assistance to Needy Families (TANF) benefit for a family of three is approximately one-third of the poverty level" (¶ 11). A study by ICP (2001) found that 20–50% of families who lost their TANF benefits became homeless.

Lack of affordable health care can also financially devastate a family that struggles to pay bills and then has a medical crisis (NCH, 2002c). Loss of time from work along with insurmountable medical bills can result in homelessness. One single mother of a 10-year-old boy reported she became homeless because she had to quit her job to get Medicaid so she could receive treatment for lupus (personal communication, October 2000).

Domestic violence is another contributor to homelessness, as many women who choose to leave a violent relationship do not have the financial means to pay for housing. A study of 777 homeless parents found that 22% of them left their last place of residence because of domestic violence (NCH, 2002c). Many women who leave their state due to domestic violence reside at homeless shelters because domestic violence shelters typically serve only county or state residents.

Mental illness and addiction are also cited as causes of homelessness (NCH, 2002c). Of the single adult population, approximately 20–25% suffers from mental illness. The lack of appropriate treatment leaves people with mental illness or addiction in a vulnerable position of not having the wherewithal to maintain housing for their families.

Overall, "homelessness results from a complex set of circumstances, which require people to choose between food, shelter, and other basic needs" (NCH, 2002c, ¶ 34). Understanding these causes of homelessness may increase play therapists' empathy for families who are homeless and may also help them recognize children's play reenactment of events leading to homelessness.

IMPACT OF HOMELESSNESS ON CHILDREN

Behavioral and Social

Behaviorally, children who are homeless tend to exhibit more externalizing problems, such as delinquent and aggressive behavior, than their peers from a normative sample (Buckner, Bassuk, Weinreb, & Brooks, 1999). Koblinsky, Gordon, and Anderson (2000) also found that preschool children who were homeless had more behavioral problems than children who were not homeless. Prevalence of aggression in children who are homeless may be due to exposure to violence in homeless environments and in their families (Anooshian, 2005). Socially, children living in a homeless shelter are hindered in their development of social skills due to the shame of their homelessness and frequent family moves (Buckner et al., 1999; Walsh & Buckley, 1994). Children who were homeless were found to have less social support and fewer coping behaviors than children who were either never homeless or previously homeless (Menke, 2000).

Emotional and Psychological

Emotionally, children who are homeless tend to experience more depression and anxiety than children who are housed (Buckner et al., 1999). Approximately 47% of children who were homeless were found to have clinically significant internalizing problems, such as depression and anxiety, compared to only 21% of children who were housed (Buckner et al., 1999). Menke and Wagner (1997) also found depression and anxiety were significantly higher in children who were homeless compared to children who were never homeless. Other researchers (Homeless Children, 1999) found that 20% of children who were homeless had severe emotional difficulties that warranted clinical intervention, although these children seldom received intervention. Many children who are homeless have witnessed domestic violence. Approximately 80% of mothers who are homeless, compared to 66% of mothers who are housed, stated they experienced domestic violence (Buckner et al., 1999).

Academic

Academic achievement problems also have been reported for children who are homeless (Masten, Sesma, Si-Asar, Lawrence, Miliotis, & Dionne, 1997). Rubin, Erickson, Agustin, Cleary, Allen, and Cohen (1996) found elementary schoolchildren who were homeless performed significantly worse on academic tests than children who were not homeless. Biggar (2002) found that lifetime history of homelessness negatively predicted students' academic performance as measured by GPA. Other research indicates that children who are homeless were diagnosed with learning disabilities at double the rate of children who are not homeless (Homeless Children, 1999).

RATIONALE FOR PLAY THERAPY

Due to these intense social, emotional, behavioral, academic, and familial problems, many children who are homeless need mental health interventions (Buckner & Bassuk, 1997). The McKinney Act mandates that state and local education agencies provide resources to children who are homeless to increase their school success (NCH, 2002a). Therefore, it is incumbent upon school, community mental health, and homeless shelter counselors to ensure that children who are homeless receive developmentally appropriate mental health interventions to promote their academic, personal, and social success.

Play therapy is the most developmentally appropriate mental health intervention with children because it utilizes their natural language of play during the therapeutic process (Landreth, 2002). Piaget (1962) stated that play bridged the gap between children's concrete experience and abstract thought, which helps children organize and master their experiences. During play therapy, children who are homeless use play to master troubling experiences such as lack of money and eviction from their home (Baggerly, 2003).

The effectiveness of play therapy in resolving children's emotional and behavioral problems was shown in Ray, Bratton, Rhine, and Jones's (2001) meta-analysis of 94 play therapy studies, which revealed a large effect size of $d = .80$. Other research indicating that play therapy is an evidence-based practice has been identified by Reddy, Files-Hall, and Schaefer (2005). In addition, Baggerly's (2004) research involving 42 homeless children showed significant improvements in their self-esteem, anxiety, and depression after receiving child-centered play therapy. Preliminary research findings from Nana's Children Mental Health Founzdation indicate that children who were homeless and received child-centered play therapy showed significant improvement in The Boxall Profile's (Bennathan & Boxall, 1998) Developmental Strands of Internalization of Controls and Diagnostic Strands of Self-Limiting Features and Unsupported Development when compared to control group children (Baggerly, Jenkins, & Drewes, 2005). These researchers also found that more children who received at least 15 sessions of play therapy, compared to those who did not, achieved their reading goals on AIMSweb Reading-Curriculum-Based Measurement (Shin & Shin, 2002). Hence, research is growing to establish play therapy as a developmentally appropriate evidence-based treatment for children who are homeless.

PERSPECTIVE AND PROCEDURES
OF CHILD-CENTERED PLAY THERAPY

Perspective

Prior to working with children who are homeless, play therapists need a clear perspective of therapeutic core conditions to meet homeless children's intense psychological need for safety (Baggerly, 2003). One theoretical approach that emphasizes a safe relationship is child-centered play therapy.

> Play therapy is a dynamic interpersonal *relationship* [italics added] between a child and a therapist trained in play therapy procedures who provides selected play materials and facilitates the development of a *safe relationship* [italics added] for the child to fully express and explore self (feelings, thoughts, experiences, and behaviors) through play, the child's natural medium of communication, for optimal growth and development. (Landreth, 2002, p. 16)

This safe, therapeutic relationship between play therapist and children who are homeless is based on therapeutic core conditions, that is, unconditional positive regard, empathy, and genuineness (Landreth, 2002; Rogers, 1951). To effectively convey these core conditions to children who are homeless, play therapists should pursue several strategies of personal preparation. To offer unconditional positive regard, play therapists should convey to children who are homeless that every person is worthy of respect, regardless of his or her economic status. Play therapists are advised to engage in frequent self-reflection to address feelings of guilt over their own economic well-being. Otherwise, play therapists' guilt may lead to disdain and a blame the victim attitude, thereby diminishing warmth and acceptance.

Genuineness, or openness to feelings and attitudes that flow through the play therapist, is enhanced when play therapists "listen to self and accept without fear their own complexity of feelings and experiences" (Rogers, 1951, p. 53). When working with children who are homeless, play therapists should monitor their own feelings and experiences related to their racial, cultural, and socioeconomic identity developmental level (Sue & Sue, 1999). Since most play therapists are white and middle class (Ryan, 2002), it is imperative for them to progress through the White Racial Identity Development stages of resistance, introspection, and integrative awareness (Sue & Sue, 1999). This progression can be accomplished by implementing strategies such as self-exploration, development of friendships with diverse people, and commitment to community change (Sue & Sue, 1999). Genuineness is also strengthened when play therapists reevaluate their personal basis for hope, such as financial gain or faith and healthy relationships. If play therapists' sense of hope is based on money, then their genuineness will communicate hopelessness to children who are poor and homeless; however, if their hope is based on faith and healthy relationships, then their genuineness will communicate hopefulness since faith and healthy relationships are available regardless of financial status.

Empathy is conveyed when play therapists "sense the feelings and personal meanings which clients experience in each moment and communicate that understanding to clients" (Rogers & Stevens, 1967, p. 54). To develop empathy for children who are homeless, play therapists are advised to ponder two questions: "What does it mean to be middle class?" and "What is it like to live in poverty?" The difference between being middle class and living in poverty includes (1) an intense daily struggle for survival, such as choosing between medicine for a sick family member and a meal for other family members (NCH, 2002c), and (2) a mistrust of those in the helping professionals who may appear judgmental and condescending (Sue & Sue, 1999). When play therapists honestly face the harsh reality of poverty and accept their social responsibility of mitigating its effects on children, they will begin to understand the struggle of homelessness and empathize with children who are homeless.

In addition to these core conditions, a safe therapeutic relationship with children who are homeless is facilitated through a nondirective approach in play therapy. When play therapists allow children to lead the play session, children will unfold their stories of homelessness and other experiences and will use play as their narrative to communicate their greatest concerns, which may or may not be homelessness (Walsh & Buckley, 1994). For example, some children's most pressing concern could be their parents' divorce or witnessing gang violence, rather than homelessness. Giving children freedom to resolve their trauma in their time frame in a safe, therapeutic environment will empower them to gain a sense of mastery and resolution and strengthen them to cope with other experiences (Gil, 1991).

Play Therapy Procedures and Maslow's Hierarchy of Needs

The therapeutic approach discussed above and play therapy procedures for children who are homeless are most appropriately implemented in light of Maslow's hierarchy of needs: physiological survival, safety, love and belonging, self-esteem, and self-actualization (Daniels, 1992; Maslow, 1968). The physiological survival need of children who are homeless is met by providing snacks, such as fruit, crackers, and juice, as well as a comfortable place to rest. Many children will arrive at the playroom hungry and physically exhausted and will not be able to engage in meaningful play until these needs are met.

Safety

The safety need of children who are homeless is met by creating a safe, private therapeutic setting within the playroom (Walsh & Buckley, 1994). Providing play therapy in a quiet setting at the homeless shelter or school adds to children's sense of safety. Confidentiality should be explained to children in a concrete manner, such as "this is a confidential or private time for you. If you want to tell others what you did or said, you can, but I will not unless you or someone else is being hurt a lot." Personal space and privacy could be emphasized by posting a privacy sign on the door.

A safe, therapeutic environment is also created by providing children with carefully selected toys in the following categories; (1) real-life items such as a bendable doll family, a cardboard box top with rooms indicated by strips of tape, a baby bottle, plastic dishes, a small car, a small plane, and a telephone, (2) aggressive release items such as handcuffs, a dart gun, a rubber knife, toy soldiers, and an inflatable plastic punching toy, and (3) creative expressive items such as Play-Doh, a small plain mask, paper, crayons, and blunt scissors (Landreth, 2002). Given the limited budgets of homeless shelters and schools, the least expensive way to obtain these toys is through garage sales, thrift stores, dollar stores, or in a play therapy totebag (available at www.playtherapy-toys.com). If funding is available, Landreth's (2002) more extensive list of therapeutic toys is preferable.

Since more than 60% of homeless children are African American or Hispanic (NCH, 2002b), ethnic dolls, artwork, and play food items should be added to the playroom (Glover, 2001). In addition, play therapists are advised to seek understanding of children's cultural backgrounds, beliefs, and values through discussions with parents, reading ethnic literature, and participating in ethnic community events. However, play therapists should respect the uniqueness of each child by avoiding stereotypes and overculturalization, or attributing characteristics to ethnicity rather than poverty (Glover, 2001; Sue & Sue, 1999).

Safety within play sessions is also established when play therapists appropriately and consistently set therapeutic limits to protect people and toys (Landreth, 2002). Therapeutic limit setting through a three step A-C-T process of acknowledging children's feelings or intentions, communicating limits, and targeting an alternative provides a caring and consistent structure for children to regulate their own behavior. For example:

> RITCHIE: Give me that money. I need it. (*Grabs money from Andy and runs to the other side of the room.*)
>
> ANDY: I'll get you. (*Loads dart gun and aims at Ritchie.*)
>
> PLAY THERAPIST: Andy, I know you are mad at Ritchie for taking your money, but people are not for shooting. You can choose to pretend the Bobo is Andy and shoot the Bobo or tell him you're mad.

Love and Belonging

The need for love and belonging in children who are homeless is met by consistently implementing Axline's eight basic principles of

1) developing a warm, friendly relationship, 2) accepting children exactly as they are, 3) establishing a feeling of permissiveness, 4) reflecting children's feelings, 5) maintaining a deep respect for children's problem-solving ability, 6) allowing the child to lead the session, 7) being patient with the process, and 8) only setting limits as needed. (Axline, 1969, pp. 73–74)

Through these principles, play therapists communicate an attitude of love and create an atmosphere of belonging that reaffirm children's inherent value as important people in society.

When children participate in group play therapy (Sweeney & Homeyer, 1999), they experience a sense of belonging with other children who are homeless and gain the added therapeutic benefit of universality (Yalom, 1995). These benefits are observed in the following dialogue between 6-year-old Mark and Darron who both reside at a homeless shelter.

MARK: I'm going to work so I can have money to pay the rent.

DARRON: Yeah, me too. I don't want to get kicked out of my house.

MARK: I'm going to be a banker to make lots of money for my family.

DARRON: I'm going to be a doctor.

PLAY THERAPIST: You're both excited to make money and keep your family safe.

In this group interaction, the boys validated each other's fear of losing their home and encouraged each other in finding solutions.

Self-Esteem

The need for self-esteem in children who are homeless is met as play therapists return responsibility to children, encourage them through a difficult process, and give them credit for succeeding on their own (Landreth, 2002). For example, consider the following dialogue between 6-year-old Mark and his play therapist.

MARK: I can't get these [bowling pins] to stand up. (*Grimaces.*)

PLAY THERAPIST: You're frustrated, but you're still trying. (*Reflects feeling; encourages.*)

MARK: You do it.

PLAY THERAPIST: Mark, I know you're frustrated, but that's something you can keep on trying.

MARK: Well, I got this row up. (*Continues working.*) I got them all up. (*Smiles.*)

PLAY THERAPIST: You're proud you did it on your own!

Through such interactions, children who are homeless learn mastery of situations that seem hopeless and develop the self-esteem to overcome future challenges.

Self-Actualization

Children's highest need, as identified by Maslow, is "a basic human drive toward growth, completeness, and fulfillment" (Corsini & Wedding, 2000, p. 469). The self-actualization of children who are homeless is facilitated through consistent implementation of play therapy procedures such as following their lead, avoiding judgmental statements, reflecting feelings and content, facilitating decision making, enhancing self-esteem, setting therapeutic limits, and enlarging the meaning of children's play to increase insight (Landreth, 2002).

Glimpses of an 8-year-old boy's self-actualization process are seen in the following transcript.

ANDY: I have handcuffs, a cop's badge, a cop's license, and a cop's ID. I have everything I need to be a cop.

PLAY THERAPIST: You have everything you need to be an important person.

ANDY: Now, you can't arrest me.

PLAY THERAPIST: You're safe.

ANDY: I'm going to put on my battery charger. Going turbo. Zoom. (*Twirls around and then stands with hands on his hips.*)

PLAY THERAPIST: Now you're powerful!

ANDY: Now that I'm turbo. I may look the same, same clothes. But I'm different. I'm super strong. You can't mess with me. Pow! (*Punches down Bobo doll.*)

PLAY THERAPIST: You're different now. You feel strong and protective.

Through his play, Andy was in the process of changing his self-concept from feeling unimportant and powerless, a common feeling of homeless children, to becoming important and powerful. In the safe, supportive, permissive, and therapeutic environment of play therapy, Andy empowered himself, rather than relying on someone else. As he incorporates these positive experiences into his self-concept, he will see himself as possessing positive power and a bright future, which will lead him toward self-actualization.

Play Themes and Facilitative Responses. The growth and development of children who are homeless is greatly enhanced as play therapists implement the procedure of enlarging the meaning of children's play. Using toys for their words and play as their language (Landreth, 2002), children symbolically reenact troubling experiences to resolve conflicts and compensate for unsatisfied needs (Piaget, 1962). To expedite this process, play therapists should enlarge the meaning of children's play by identifying common play themes, linking these themes to children's experiences, and verbally reflecting this understanding of feelings, beliefs, and desires to children, thereby increasing children's awareness and insight.

This procedure is illustrated by the following therapeutic reflections to prevalent play themes of children who are homeless. Two unique play themes of children who are homeless appear to be eviction and "I'm rich" (Baggerly, 2003). However, children who are homeless also display common play themes such as power and control, aggression, and nurturing (Benedict et al., 1995; Holmberg, Benedict, & Hynan, 1998).

Eviction. Homeless children frequently reenact the experience of being evicted from their home during their play. Feelings of helplessness, anger, confusion, and loss become evident as children use the toys to relive their eviction. This theme is illustrated in the play of 7-year-old Tyronne who lived in a homeless shelter and was referred for play therapy by his mother due to frequent anger outbursts and low self-esteem.

During Tyronne's first sessions, he created disorganized and chaotic battles between toy soldiers and animal families, frequently throwing all the toys together. Therapeutic responses of reflecting his feelings and play content included "the soldiers and animals are so angry that they are fighting" and "they are confused about what to do." During the 10th session, Tyronne's story became more organized, with the following distinct scene. He carefully set up the furniture and a family of people in the playhouse. He pretended the people were going about their daily routine of cooking, eating, and sleeping, when suddenly the soldiers entered the house, knocked over furniture, and threw the people out. The animals helped the people by checking to see if they were safe and bringing the family back together. Then the animals tried to fight the soldiers to regain the house, but the soldiers prevailed. The meaning of Tyronne's play was enlarged by first recognizing the play theme of eviction and then linking it to his experience through reflections such as "The family is scared that the soldiers are kicking them out of the house. You know what that's like" and "The animals are helping the people just like you are helped here."

The progression of Tyronne's play themes from disorganized aggression to specific reenactment of eviction reflects identifiable stages of therapeutic progress, from general hostility to specific symbolization (Hendricks, 1971; Moustakas, 1955). In his play, Tyronne appeared to be reliving the fear and frustration of his family's eviction, the perceived hostility of the landlord's (soldiers') actions, the nurturing he received from the homeless shelter staff (animals), and the reality of not being able to return home. Providing therapeutic responses along with core conditions helped Tyronne (1) become aware of repressed emotions and beliefs that were clamoring for his attention, (2) reprocess intrusive memories of the traumatic event, (3) gain a sense of mastery and control over overwhelming experiences, (4) integrate these experiences into his self-structure, and (5) become a more organized whole, thereby moving from maladjusted incongruence to adjusted congruence (Landreth & Sweeney, 1997; Rogers, 1951).

"I'm Rich." Another common play theme of children who are homeless is called "I'm rich." In it, children count play money or toss it up in the air and exclaim "I'm rich!" Children who are homeless appear to have an intense awareness of their family's lack of money. For example, one 10-year-old girl stated, "I didn't get to have a birthday party, and I only got one present because we didn't have a house or money." Children who are homeless introject into their self-structure their parents' statements such as "If we just had enough money for rent, we'd be OK," or "If we only won the lottery, we wouldn't have to worry." In an attempt to gain in fantasy what they do not have in reality, children use the play money to pretend they are rich. Therapeutic responses to enlarge the meaning for the "I'm rich" play theme include "You feel happy and powerful with all that money" and "You really wish you had lots of money so you could have your own home."

Children who are homeless often reveal inaccurate perceptions about money. Some children believe money can only be obtained in an unconventional manner. For example, some children toss money up in the air as if it magically falls from the sky, rather than obtaining it from working. Other children pretend to sell drugs to get money so that they can buy sodas and fast food. In addition, some children who are homeless seem to believe that money is more reliable and valuable than relationships. For example, during play, some children pretended to trick or kill a friend to steal his or her money. Their valuing money over relationships may reflect their experience of an unreliable parent or relative who left them without basic necessities. Play therapists should communicate this understanding through empathic, nonjudgmental therapeutic responses such as "You were so hungry you decided to steal the money" or "You know one way to get money fast; perhaps you've seen that before." Play therapists can also address this complex issue by consulting with parents, teachers, and community leaders about family dynamics, money management, career planning, and social justice.

Power and Control

Children who are homeless have even less power and control over themselves and their circumstances than children who have a home. When children live at homeless shelters, they have little control over when, what, and where they will eat, when they will go to bed, and where they can play. Since children at shelters usually reside in one dorm-type room with their parent(s) and siblings, they have limited privacy and space. In addition, prior to becoming homeless, many children experienced a lack of power and control within communities where drugs, prostitution, and crime were rampant.

Consequently, a play theme of power and control is common among children who are homeless. Therapeutic responses to enlarge the meaning help children gain a sense of power and control, as illustrated in the following scenario.

TRAY: I'm a secret agent for the president.

DAVID: I'm a bodyguard for the princess.

PLAY THERAPIST: You're both someone real important!

TRAY: I'll shoot the bad guys! They can't get me!

DAVID: Me, too. I'll get them first!

PLAY THERAPIST: You're both powerful and in control now!

TRAY: Yeah, we're in charge!

Through such play, children who are homeless assert their sense of power and develop their identities as powerful people. Thus, even when their current experience at the shelter limits their power, children will find hope for the future in their strengthened sense of self.

Children's empowerment can be facilitated further by encouraging parents and teachers to offer children as many choices as possible, such as, "Do you want to go outside before or after doing your homework?"

Aggression: Abuser/Victim/Protector

Since many children who are homeless have witnessed domestic and community violence (NCH, 2002c), aggression is a common play theme. Children frequently reenact violent scenes by playing the role of the abuser, victim, or protector. Although this play can be emotionally overwhelming, it is crucial that play therapists maintain a nonanxious presence in order to create a sense of safety for children. As play therapists reflect children's feelings, motives, and physiological responses, such as rapid heart rate and clenched muscles, children begin to associate physiological responses with feelings and learn to self-regulate. Consider the following scenario:

MARTY: Don't be messin' with my wife. (*Punches and jumps on top of bop bag.*)

PLAY THERAPIST: You're protecting your wife! You're angry. Your muscles are tight. (*Punches bop bag for several minutes.*)

MARTY: I'm letting you have money to buy a house. But when I see you, you owe me. (*Stands over bop bag and jumps on it.*)

PLAY THERAPIST: You're helping him out, but you're tough and in control.

MARTY: (*Picks up money.*) This money is for my family. You think I'm going to get kicked out of my house? No way! (*Kicks and punches bop bag.*)

PLAY THERAPIST: You're mad! You don't want to get kicked out of your house. You want to provide for your family.

Through such therapeutic responses, children will learn to differentiate the feelings of aggression (anger and rage) from the motives of aggression (protection and safety). As children become aware of their motives, they can begin to explore alternative, nonviolent strategies to create safety and protection.

Nurturing. Nurturing is another common play theme for children who are homeless. Since the basic needs of food and a safe comfortable bed have not been available for children who are homeless, they often symbolically meet this need through play activities such as feeding baby dolls, cooking meals, making beds, and doctoring each other. Consider the following scenario:

MARY: I'm giving the baby her oatmeal.

PLAY THERAPIST: You're making sure she has enough to eat.

MARY: Here's a blanket so she won't get cold while she sleeps.

PLAY THERAPIST: You know it's important to keep her warm.

MARY: Time for her checkup from the doctor.

PLAY THERAPIST: You're making sure she's well. You like taking care of the baby.

Through such play, children who are homeless satisfy their own desire for care, experience the power and pleasure of positive caregiving, and affirm themselves as nurturing people, thereby integrating nurturing values into their self-structure.

Occasionally, children will reenact failed nurturance by activities such as pretending to spank a crying baby rather than comforting it (Benedict et al., 1995). When they project feelings of distress and helplessness through this play, therapeutic responses such as "the baby is scared and sad when she doesn't get what she needs" will increase children's awareness of their feelings and affirm that their needs are legitimate. Thus, rather than introjecting the experience of failed nurturance as an indication of lack of worth, they will begin to accept their need for nurturing as an indication of their self-worth.

CONJOINT INTERVENTIONS: ASCA NATIONAL MODEL

In addition to play therapy, it is recommended that play therapists facilitate several other interventions to meet the needs of children who are homeless. In terms of the American School Counseling Association's (ASCA) national model (ASCA, 2002), children who are homeless will benefit from (1) guidance curriculum in social skills training, (2) individual student planning via assessment instruments, (3) responsive services through play therapy as described above and parent consultation, and (4) program and system support through teacher consultation (Baggerly & Borkowski, 2004). These four components of the ASCA national model will be illustrated through a case description of a 7-year-old African American girl who was homeless (Baggerly & Borkowski, 2004).

Case Description

Regina (alias) was a 7-year-old African American female who resided with her mother and 10-year-old brother in one dormitory-like room at a homeless shelter in a southeastern U.S. metropolitan city. After several months in the shelter, Regina's mother married, and her new stepfather moved into the room with the family. Regina's mother reported a family history of homelessness and poverty, frequent moves, past domestic violence, and a lack of recent contact with the children's biological father.

Regina was enrolled in the first grade in a general education K–2 classroom at the on-site charter school in the homeless shelter where they resided. Her mother and the school cumulative folder provided only a small amount of useful family and academic background information. Regina's mother said her daughter had no known academic deficiencies but did have social and behavioral problems. Her teachers reported Regina's academic performance in the classroom was on grade level, despite learning gaps in basic achievement skills (e.g., reading, writing, and math).

According to her teachers and mother, Regina's problem behaviors at home and school included excessive dependency and attention seeking from adults (e.g., repeatedly asking "Do you love me?" and constantly approaching and interrupting), peer difficulties (e.g., making and keeping friends), low frustration tolerance (e.g., raising her voice and talking out of turn), stealing, lying, and denying responsibility for her actions. In addition, her teachers reported a history of somatic complaints, poor self-concept, impulsivity, depressed mood, distractibility, oversensitivity, anxiety, and irritability. Regina's strengths included friendliness, helpfulness, attractive appearance, and an active energy level.

Education/Prevention

The first component of the ASCA national model, education/prevention, was conducted through large-group classroom guidance. Specifically, a weekly social skills training program entitled "Stop and Think" (Knoff, 1999) was implemented in Regina's class. The major components of the Stop and Think model are (1) discussion of social skills, (2) modeling, (3) role playing, (4) performance feedback, and (5) transfer of training via application in the everyday environment (Knoff, 1999). During weekly large-group guidance lessons, a part-time school psychology graduate assistant presented the following Stop and Think steps (Knoff, 1999): (1)

identify a problem and verbalize "stop and think," (2) activate decision making by asking "What are my choices?" (3) evaluate options and ask "Do I want to make a good choice or a bad choice?" (4) select an option and state, "Just do it," and (5) conduct self-evaluation and encourage self by saying "good job." The teachers reviewed these steps on a daily basis with Regina and other students in her classroom.

In addition, the school psychologist encouraged teachers to implement a classroomwide behavior management system that entailed a token economy using a behavior-monitoring chart with written stars as a secondary reinforcer (Cooper, Herron, & Heward, 1987). If Regina met her individualized behavior goals of being honest rather than lying, asking to borrow items rather than stealing, cooperating with teachers by raising her hand or waiting her turn rather than interrupting, and completing her assigned tasks, then she was rewarded with a star on her behavior-monitoring form at the end of each day. At the end of the week, if she earned five stars, she received a primary reinforcer of a grab bag toy or school supplies. In addition, teachers were encouraged to give her frequent praise and to reward her with extra stars for positive behavior.

Individual Student Planning

The second component of the ASCA national model, individual student planning, was conducted through assessment. In order to assess Regina's behavioral and emotional progress, the following three assessment instruments were administered. These instruments were selected based on prevalent use in other studies of children who are homeless (Buckner et al., 1999) and based on availability, which was limited by the homeless shelter's budget. The Child Behavior Checklist Parent Report Form (CBCL-PRF), developed by Achenbach (1994), is a 113-item scale on which parents rate their child's behavior. Results are described in two domains, internalizing and externalizing behavior, and nine subscales. The Child Anxiety Scale (CAS), developed by Gillis (1980), is a 20-item questionnaire specifically designed to measure anxiety in children ages 5 to 12. The Joseph Preschool and Primary Self-Concept Scale (JSCS), developed by Joseph (1979), is a 15-item test that measures the self-concept of children ages 3 to 9. Scores are based on the child's identification with either a negative or positive picture of a child doing different activities. The child's self-concept is rated on a global index scale of 0 (low) to 30 (high) and is categorized as high risk negative, poor, watch list, moderate positive, or high positive.

Responsive/Intervention Services

The third component of the ASCA national model, responsive/intervention services, was conducted through group play therapy. Group work with children who are homeless was recommended by several researchers (Daniels, D'Andrea, Omizo, & Pier, 1999; Davey & Neff, 2001; Hunter, 1993; Nabors, Proescher, & DeSilva, 2001; Strawser, Markos, Yamaguchi, & Higgins, 2000). Group play therapy offers the extra benefit of helping children assume responsibility in interpersonal relationships (Landreth, 2002).

I am a licensed mental health counselor supervisor and a registered play therapist supervisor. I provided 10 weekly sessions of child-centered group play therapy to Regina and Twanda (alias), another female student in her class. Basic child-centered play therapy principles of following the child's lead, avoiding judgmental statements, creating a safe, accepting atmosphere, reflecting feelings, facilitating decision making, enhancing self-esteem, and setting therapeutic limits were followed (Landreth, 2002). Sessions were conducted in a private room with play therapy totebag toys such as a doll family, plastic dishes, handcuffs, toy soldiers, an inflatable plastic punching toy, Play-Doh, paper, and crayons (Landreth, 2002).

Another responsive service provided was parent consultation, based on recommendations by Nabors et al. (2001). Through parent consultation, I provided Regina's parents with positive feedback about her, such as "Regina responds well when limits are set in a friendly but firm way and when she is given choices." In addition, parents were encouraged to use a more effective, democratic parenting style of encouragement and problem solving within flexible limits rather than an authoritarian parenting style of harsh commands and corporal punishment (Steinberg, Lamborn, Darling, Mounts, & Dornbusch, 1994). Unfortunately, Regina's mother and stepfather were distracted by meeting more basic needs and, thus, did not choose to implement a more positive approach to parenting at that time.

Program and System Support

Since teacher training in mental health prevention activities was suggested by Nabors et al. (2001), consultation was provided to Regina's teachers, who were encouraged to consistently implement the behavior management system for Regina and were provided with alternative understanding of her behavior, such as "She is motivated by a desire to please peers and adults." As a result of these ASCA interventions, Regina's behavior improved according to verbal reports from her mother and teachers, her anxiety decreased as measured by the CAS and her self-concept improved as measured by the JSCS (Baggerly, 2004).

Case Study Results of Play Therapy and Conjoint Interventions

After implementation of these interventions during the 12 weeks that Regina attended the charter school and the family resided at the homeless shelter, the following results were noted in Regina's assessment scores and behavior (Baggerly & Borkowski, 2004). Regina's preassessment on the CBCL-PRF revealed a total t score of 74, which indicated clinical significance of behavior problems. Her internalizing score ($t = 66$) and externalizing score ($t = 74$) were also in the clinically significant range as they are 1.5 standard deviations above the norm. Specifically, her anxious/depressed subscale score ($t = 69$) was in the borderline clinical range while thought problems ($t = 73$), attention problems ($t = 78$), delinquent behavior ($t = 71$), and aggressive behavior ($t = 76$) subscale scores were in the clinically significant range. On this preassessment, specific concerns reported by Regina's mother included "not understanding that she have to stay in her seat [sic]," "always writing notes because she knows she be wrong [sic]," "hides her food as if someone going to take it [sic]," "wants to grow up to fast [sic]," and "wants to be the boss." In order to determine the integrity of the mother's responses, we reviewed individual items on the protocol and found no pattern of extreme ratings nor scores skewed in either direction.

Although Regina's mother was asked to complete the post-assessment CBCL-PRF, she did not comply, as she stated that she was pre-occupied with moving out of the homeless shelter. However, she did give a verbal report that Regina's behavior improved in that she demonstrated less dependency, lying, and stealing in the last few weeks of treatment. Since the post–CBCL-PRF was not completed, the validity of Regina's behavior change is questionable.

Anxiety

Results measured by CAS indicated a decrease in Regina's anxiety. Regina's preassessment standard sten score of 10 on the CAS placed her in the 99th percentile for a child of her age, indicating that she experienced more anxiety than 99% of the normative group. Her post-assessment standard sten score of 8 on the CAS placed her in the 91st percentile. Although Regina's posttest sten score of 8 still indicates a significant departure from the norm, her anxiety score was a full standard deviation lower than her pretest score.

Self-Concept

Results measured by JSCS indicate an increase in Regina's self-concept. Her JSCS pretest global self-concept score was 4, which is in the "high risk negative" category, while her posttest global self-concept score was 22, which borders on the "poor" category. Specific questions reveal improvement in Regina's self-concept. For the question, "One of these girls is a bad girl, and the other girl is a good girl. Which one are you?" Regina answered, "I'm a bad girl" in the pretest but answered, "I'm a good girl" in the posttest. For the question, "One of these girls is smiling, and the other girl is crying. Which one do you do the most?" Regina answered "Cry" in the pretest but "Smile" in the posttest.

Behavior

Based on reports from Regina's teachers and review of behavior-monitoring charts by the school's psychology graduate assistant, Regina demonstrated substantial improvement in her classroom behavior by the end of treatment. Unfortunately, due to personnel changes within school staff, behavior-monitoring charts were misplaced at the end of the school year, and, thus, specific data is not available to indicate when and at what rate Regina's behaviors changed. However, teachers verbally reported that Regina's lying, stealing, and interrupting had decreased and that she completed more of her weekly assignments by the end of treatment. Teachers also verbally reported that several days before Regina and her family were to move out of the shelter and away from the school, her behavior regressed to stealing and lying once a day.

Observations of Regina's behavior during group play therapy sessions suggest that Regina understood and integrated the concepts of the behavior-management system. For example, during session 7, she played teacher and said, "Don't do that. Sit down. Good. You earned a star." She appeared to associate good behavior with the reward of earning a star on the behavior-monitoring chart. Regina also began to integrate social skills such as "stop and think" into her daily routine. For example, during one play session, while trying to make a decision, she verbalized, "Stop and think. What are my choices? Do I want to make a good choice or a bad choice? Just do it. Good job!" and demonstrated the accompanying hand signs for each step. She also frequently stated, "I'm supposed to make good choices."

In addition, Regina demonstrated more collaboration with Twanda during the last few play sessions. For example, instead of insisting that she be the boss, she was more likely to yield to Twanda's suggestions for play. In the classroom, Regina's teachers and the school's psychology graduate assistant anecdotally observed Regina exhibiting less attention-getting and dependent behavior. They observed Regina demonstrating more appropriate social skills to gain attention, such as volunteering in role plays and increasing her participation in peer activities.

Group Play Therapy Behavior and Themes

Variations in Regina's play therapy themes throughout the 10 sessions were observed by using the Benedict Play Theme Analysis System (Benedict et al., 1995). During the first four play sessions, Regina's play themes predominantly entailed nurturing themes, such as feeding the baby doll, and dependency themes, such as repeatedly asking "How do you do this?" Beginning at session 6, Regina began displaying mastery themes, such as adding menu prices on her own and stating "let me do it," and positive power themes, such as playing an encouraging teacher. In addition, observations of Regina's play revealed a shift toward positive self-perception throughout the sessions. For example, in group play therapy session 3, Regina wrote, "I'm sorry for doing bad," while in session 6, she wrote, "I'm being a good star." During the last session, Regina maintained play themes of mastery and positive power but also displayed conflict related to moving out of the shelter.

Parent and Teacher Response

Before program interventions began, Regina's parents and teachers expressed frustration and exasperation with her dependency, lying, and stealing. Both her parents and teachers attempted to address her behavior with an authoritarian discipline approach of harsh words and punishment. Although neither her parents nor teachers consistently implement a more positive, democratic approach to discipline, both parents and teachers verbally indicated satisfaction with the group play therapy and social skills training and decreases in their own frustration. They also reported decreases in Regina's dependency, lying, and stealing toward the end of treatment.

CONCLUSION

Play therapy and conjoint interventions as described above provide many benefits for children like Regina who are homeless. Play therapy helps fulfill their needs for physiological survival, psychological safety, love and belonging, self-esteem, and self-actualization. Play therapy also mitigates the mental health impact of homelessness on children by providing a therapeutic environment where children can reenact and resolve traumatic experiences and develop skills and confidence to face future challenges.

To facilitate the growth and development of children who are homeless, play therapists need a perspective on the prevalence, causes, and impact of homelessness. In addition, they need to prepare themselves personally to offer unconditional positive regard, genuineness, and empathy through ongoing self-reflection. Play therapists should also implement procedures of a nondirective approach and therapeutic responses including enlarging the meaning of common play themes. As play therapists fulfill their social responsibility by providing play therapy to children who are homeless, they will empower them and help them break the cycle of homelessness.

ACKNOWLEDGMENTS

Sections from Baggerly (2003). Copyright 2003 by the Association for Play Therapy. Reprinted by permission; sections from Baggerly and Borkowski (2004). Copyright 2004 by the American School Counselor Association. Reprinted by permission.

REFERENCES

Achenbach, T. M. (1994). *Child Behavior Checklist*. Burlington, VT: Child Behavior Checklist, University Medical Education Associates.

American School Counseling Association. (2002). *The ASCA national model: A framework for school counseling programs*. Herndon, VA: Author.

Anooshian, L. J. (2005). Violence and aggression in the lives of homeless children: A review. *Aggression and Violent Behavior, 10*(2), 129–152.

Axline, V. M. (1969). *Play therapy*. New York: Ballantine Books.

Baggerly, J. N. (2003). Play therapy with homeless children: Perspectives and procedures. *International Journal of Play Therapy, 12*(2), 87–106.

Baggerly, J. N. (2004). The effects of child-centered group play therapy on self-concept, depression, and anxiety of children who are homeless. *International Journal of Play Therapy, 13*(2), 31–51.

Baggerly, J. N., & Borkowski, T. (2004). Applying the ASCA national model to elementary school students who are homeless: A case study. *Professional School Counseling, 8*(2), 116–123.

Baggerly, J. N., Jenkins, W., & Drewes, A. (2005, October). *The effects of play therapy on academics, development, and mental health of homeless children.* Paper presented at the annual meeting of the Association for Play Therapy, Nashville, TN.

Benedict, H. E., Chavez, D., Holmberg, J., McClain, J., McGee, W., Narcavage, C. J., et al. (1995). *Benedict play therapy theme codes.* Unpublished manuscript, Baylor University, Waco, TX.

Bennathan, M., & Boxall, M. (1998). *The Boxall Profile: A guide to effective intervention in the education of pupils with emotional and behavioural difficulties.* London: Association of Workers for Children with Emotional and Behavioural Difficulties.

Biggar, H. A. (2002). Homeless children's self-report of experiences and the role of age, history of homelessness, and current residence in academic performance. *Dissertation Abstracts International, 63*(1-B), 563.

Buckner, J. C., & Bassuk, E. L. (1997). Mental disorders and service utilization among youths from homeless and low-income housed families. *Journal of the American Academy of Child and Adolescent Psychiatry, 36* (7), 890–900.

Buckner, J. C., Bassuk, E. L., Weinreb, L. F., & Brooks, M. G. (1999). Homelessness and its relation to the mental health and behavior of low income school-age children. *Developmental Psychology, 35*(1), 246–257.

Cooper, J., Herron, T., & Heward, W. (1987). *Applied behavior analysis.* Upper Saddle River, NJ: Prentice-Hall.

Corsini, R. J., & Wedding, D. (Eds.). (2000). *Current psychotherapies* (6th ed.). Itasca, IL: Peacock.

Daniels, J. (1992). Empowering homeless children through school counseling. *Elementary School Guidance and Counseling, 27*, 104–112.

Daniels, J., D'Andrea, M., Omizo, M., & Pier, P. (1999). Group work with homeless youngsters and their mothers. *Journal for Specialists in Group Work, 24*, 164–185.

Davey, T. L., & Neff, J. A. (2001). A shelter-based stress-reduction group intervention targeting self-esteem, social competence, and behavior problems among homeless children. *Journal of Social Distress and the Homeless, 10*(3), 279–291.

Gil, E. (1991). *The healing power of play. Working with abused children.* New York: Guilford Press.

Gillis, J. S. (1980). *Child anxiety manual.* Champaign, IL: Institute for Personality and Ability Testing, Inc.

Glover, G. (2001). Cultural considerations in play therapy. In G. L. Landreth (Ed.), *Innovations in play therapy: Issues, process, and special populations* (pp. 31–41). Philadelphia: Taylor & Francis.

Hendricks, S. (1971). A descriptive analysis of the process of client-centered play therapy (Doctoral dissertation, North Texas State University, 1971). *Dissertation Abstracts International, 32*, 3689A.

Holmberg, J. R., Benedict, H. E., & Hynan, L. S. (1998). Gender differences in children's play therapy themes: Comparisons of children with a history of attachment disturbance or exposure to violence. *International Journal of Play Therapy, 7*(2), 67–92.

Homeless Children (1999, November). *America, 181*(15), 3.

Hunter, L. B. (1993). Sibling play therapy with homeless children: An opportunity in the crisis. *Child Welfare, 72*(1), 65–75.

Institute for Children and Poverty. (2001). *A shelter is not a home—or is it?* New York: Author. Retrieved December 19, 2002, from www.homesforthehomeless.com/facts.html

Joseph, J. (1979). *Joseph preschool and primary self-concept screening test.* Chicago: Stoelting.

Knoff, H. (1999). *The stop and think teachers manual: Early to middle elementary school edition.* Unpublished document, University of South Florida, Tampa.

Koblinsky, S. A., Gordon, A. L., & Anderson, E. A. (2000). Changes in the social skills and behavior problems of homeless and housed children during the preschool year. *Early Education and Development, 11*(3), 321–338.

Landreth, G. L. (2002). *Play therapy: The art of the relationship.* (2nd ed.). New York: Brunner-Routledge.

Landreth, G. L., & Sweeney, D. S. (1997). Child-centered play therapy. In K. J. O'Connor & L. M. Braverman (Eds.), *Play therapy: Theory and practice* (pp. 17–45). New York: Wiley.

Maslow, A. H. (1968). *Toward a psychology of being* (2nd ed.). Princeton, NJ: Van Nostrand.

Masten, A. S., Sesma, A., Si-Asar, R., Lawrence, C., Miliotis, D., & Dionne, J. A. (1997). Educational risks for children experiencing homelessness. *Journal of School Psychology, 35,* 27–46.

Menke, E. M. (2000). Comparison of the stressors and coping behaviors of homeless, previously homeless, and never homeless poor children. *Issues in Mental Health Nursing, 21*(7), 691–710.

Menke, E. M., & Wagner, J. D. (1997). A comparative study of homeless, previously homeless, and never homeless school-aged children's health. *Issues in Comprehensive Pediatric Nursing, 20*(3), 153–173.

Moustakas, C. (1955). Emotional adjustment and the play therapy process. *Journal of Genetic Psychology, 86,* 79–99.

Nabors, L., Proescher, E., & DeSilva, M. (2001). School based mental health prevention activities for homeless and at-risk youth. *Child and Youth Care Forum, 30*(1), 3–18.

National Coalition for the Homeless. (2002a). *Education of homeless children and youth. NCH Fact Sheet #10.* Washington, DC: Author. Retrieved December 19, 2002, from www.nationalhomeless.org/facts.html

National Coalition for the Homeless. (2002b). *How many people experience homelessness. NCH Fact Sheet #2.* Washington, DC: Author. Retrieved July 26, 2005, from www.nationalhomeless.org/facts.html

National Coalition for the Homeless. (2002c). *Why are people homeless. NCH Fact*

Sheet #1. Washington, DC: Author. Retrieved December 19, 2002, from www.nationalhomeless.org/facts.html

National Coalition for the Homeless. (2004). *Who is homeless. NCH Fact Sheet #3*. Washington, DC: Author. Retrieved July 26, 2005, from www.nationalhomeless. org/facts.html

Piaget, J. (1962). *Play, dreams, and imitation in childhood*. New York: Norton.

Ray, D., Bratton, S., Rhine, T., & Jones, L. (2001). The effectiveness of play therapy: Responding to the critics. *International Journal of Play Therapy, 10*(1), 85–108.

Reddy, L. A., Files-Hall, T. M., & Schaefer, C. E. (2005). *Empirically based play interventions for children*. Washington, DC: American Psychological Association.

Rogers, C. (1951). *Client-centered therapy, Its current practice, implications, and theory*. Boston: Houghton-Mifflin.

Rogers, C., & Stevens, B. (1967). *Person to person: The problem of being human*. Lafayette, CA: Real People Press.

Rubin, D. H., Erickson, C. J., Agustin, M. S., Cleary, S. D., Allen, J. K., & Cohen, P. (1996). Cognitive and academic functioning of homeless children compared with housed children. *Pediatrics, 97*, 289–294.

Ryan, S. (2002). *Who are we? Findings from the Association for Play Therapy membership survey*. Paper presented at the 19th Annual Association for Play Therapy International Conference, St. Louis, MO.

Shin, M. R., & Shin, M. M. (2002). *AIMSweb Training Workbook: Administration and scoring of Reading Curriculum-Based Measurement (R-CBM) for use in general outcome measurement*. Eden Prairie, MN: Edformation, Inc.

Steinberg, L., Lamborn, S. D., Darling, N., Mounts, N. S., & Dornbusch, S. M. (1994). Over-time changes in adjustment and competence among adolescents from authoritative, authoritarian, indulgent, and neglectful families. *Child Development, 65*, 754–770.

Stewart B. McKinney Act, 42 U.S.C. § 11301 et seq. (1994).

Strawser, S., Markos, P. A., Yamaguchi, B. J., & Higgins, K. (2000). A new challenge for school counselors: Children who are homeless. *Professional School Counseling, 3*(3), 162–171.

Sue, D., & Sue, D. (1999). *Counseling the culturally different: Theory and practice* (3rd ed.). New York: Wiley.

Sweeney, D. S., & Homeyer, L. E. (Eds.). (1999). *Group play therapy: How to do it, how it works, whom it's best for*. San Francisco: Jossey-Bass.

Torquati, J. C., & Gamble, W. C. (2001). Social resources and psychosocial adaptation of homeless school-aged children. *Journal of Social Distress and the Homeless, 10*(4), 305–321.

Walsh, M. E., & Buckley, M. A. (1994). Children's experiences of homelessness: Implications for school counselors. *Elementary School Guidance and Counseling, 29*(1), 4–15.

Yalom, I. D. (1995). *The theory and practice of group psychotherapy* (3rd ed.). New York: Basic Books.

Treatment of Sexually Abused Children

MARY MARGARET KELLY
HOPE C. ODENWALT

The harmful consequences of child sexual abuse have been copiously detailed in decades of empirical studies and case descriptions. Yet no consistent set of symptoms has been found that uniquely characterizes sexually abused children (Green, 1993; Kendall-Tackett, Williams, & Finkelhor, 1993; Saywitz, Mannarino, Berliner, & Cohen, 2000). Some consistency exists with regard to demographic characteristics of sexual abuse victims and perpetrators. Girls are at significantly greater risk for sexual abuse than boys, and perpetrators are frequently family members or close family friends (Berliner & Elliott, 1996; Briere & Elliot, 2003). Still, there is no typical victim of child sexual abuse. Instead, the substantial descriptive literature reveals a remarkably wide array of possible aftereffects.

The inability to predict how a given child may react to sexual abuse presents a challenge to the clinician charged with that child's treatment. At the same time, the considerable variability in the clinical presentations of sexual abuse victims is not at all surprising. It is understandable that children's responses are so extremely unpredictable given that sexual abuse is an experience, not a diagnostic category, and can be significantly modified by contextual factors, such as the extent of the abuse, family functioning, the relationship with the abuser, and developmental differences in the way the child processes the abuse (Heflin & Deblinger, 2003; O'Donohue, Fannetti, & Elliott, 1998).

SEQUELAE OF CHILD SEXUAL ABUSE

While no specific child sexual abuse syndrome has been identified, child victims are at significant risk for a number of psychological problems. Symptoms associated with internalization such as anxiety and fear are frequently the earliest problems presented by sexually abused children (Kendall-Tackett et al., 1993; McClellan, Adams, Douglas, McCurry, & Storck, 1995). Other commonly observed internalizing symptoms include depression (Wozencraft, Wagner, & Pelligrin, 1991), negative self-perceptions (Cohen, Deblinger, Maedel, & Stauffer, 1999), somatic complaints (Livingston, 1987), sleep difficulties (Wells, McCann, Adams, Voris, & Ensign, 1995), and suicidality (McClellan et al., 1995). Externalizing behaviors can be prominent in the clinical presentation of the sexually abused child as well. The most widely studied single correlate of child sexual abuse is problematic sexual behavior on the part of the child (Friedrich et al., 1992). Child sexual abuse is also associated with aggression and oppositionalism (Kendall-Tackett et al., 1993), poor peer interaction (Einbender & Friedrich, 1989), substance abuse (Heflin & Deblinger, 2003), and school performance problems (Wells et al., 1995).

Significant numbers of sexually abused children meet the criteria for DSM psychiatric diagnoses, notably posttraumatic stress disorder (Collin-Vezina & Hebert, 2005; Deblinger, McLeer, Atkins, Ralphe, & Foa, 1989; Wolf & Birt, 1995) as well as dissociative disorders (Collin-Vezina & Hebert, 2005; Gil, 2002). At the other end of the continuum is an especially puzzling subgroup of sexually abused children who present no discernable psychological difficulties. Estimates of asymptomatic child victims range from 21–49% of the total population of sexually abused children. These youngsters may have particularly high levels of support, or they may belong to a group of sexual abuse survivors whose symptom manifestation is delayed. Adjustment levels of these children generally worsen over time (Kendall-Tackett et al., 1993).

It is also possible that the phenomenon of the asymptomatic sexual abuse victim is a function of empirical methodology. Perhaps these children suffer with painful but subtle symptoms that are not easily identifiable by the standardized measures employed in empirical investigations (Saywitz et al., 2000). Simon-Roper (1996) includes internal sequelae as well as observable symptoms in her description of the impact of victimization. She states that while much effort has gone toward documenting the behavioral level of victims' responses, covert injuries exist within child sexual abuse survivors, and these internal injuries are more resistant to change.

Leahy, Pretty, and Tenenbaum (2003) consider the sequelae of child sexual abuse to be multilayered. They warn that correlational data linking overtly measurable symptomology with child sexual abuse should not be the sole research tool if one is to achieve a thorough understanding of victimization effects. Burgess's (1987) concept of trauma encapsulation provides clarity about the nature of sometimes elusive child sexual abuse sequelae. "Trauma encapsulation" refers to the child's propensity to hold memories and feelings associated with the overwhelming trauma of sexual abuse in a cognitively unprocessed state. To the extent that the child victim's self-awareness is limited by the encapsulation process, "objective" self-report measures may be of questionable value as criterion variables in correlational research. The very psychological processes (e.g., avoidance, dissociation) that drive symptoms out of awareness are likely to contribute to subsequent psychological problems, such as dysregulation and cognitive problems (Strand, 1999).

In addition to its immediate impact, long-term correlates of child sexual abuse have been well-documented. A considerable body of research points to child sexual abuse as a major risk factor for adjustment problems in adulthood (Briere & Elliot, 2003; Neuman, Houskamp, Pollock, & Briere, 1996; Polusny & Follette, 1995; Saywitz et al., 2000). Briere (1992) identified seven categories of longstanding dysfunction likely to be found in child sexual abuse survivors: symptoms of posttraumatic stress and dissociation, cognitive distortions, impaired self-reference and -relatedness, avoidance, and altered emotionality. Additionally, anxiety, depression, interpersonal trust issues, and patterns of revictimization are frequently identified long-term sequelae of child sexual abuse (Hansen, Hecht, & Futa, 1998).

Several studies have revealed associations between self-destructive behavior and experiences of childhood sexual abuse. A history of child sexual abuse has been correlated with suicidal thoughts and suicide attempts in clinical as well as nonclinical community samples (Polusny & Follette, 1995). Relationships between child sexual abuse and self-mutilation have been reported in studies of several different clinical populations (Briere & Gil, 1998; van der Kolk, Perry, & Herman, 1991).

Empirical studies have consistently revealed significant associations between child sexual abuse and substance abuse in both clinical and community samples (Burgdorf, Chen, Walker, Porowski, & Herrell, 2004; Polusny & Follette, 1995). Herman, Perry, and van der Kolk (1989) found a significantly higher incidence of childhood sexual abuse in individuals diagnosed with borderline personality disorder as compared to other groups. Premature sexual behavior, including early pregnancy, has been consistently found to be associated with a history of sexual abuse (Brown, Cohen, Chen, Smailes, & Johnson, 2004). Male victims of child sexual abuse are at increased risk for confusion and concern about sexual identity as well as inappropriate attempts to assert masculinity (Durham, 2003; Watkins & Bentovim, 1992).

In a large-scale investigation of long-term sequelae of child sexual abuse, Teegan (1999) found 93% of adult female survivors continue to suffer from trauma-related symptoms. Additionally, he found that 79% of survivors experience dissociative symptoms. Furthermore, Teegan identified four primary predictors of long-term symptomology in sexual abuse survivors:

1. *Distorted self-concept*, which consists of low self-efficacy, unassertiveness, feelings of shame and helplessness, and distrust of others
2. *Avoidance of intimacy*, which is employed to control fears and shame
3. *Body awareness problems*, which refer to the inability to sense all or part of one's body as well as negative body-oriented attributions
4. *Adult coping strategies*, which consist of efforts at self-exploration and healing, such as reading relevant literature, involvement in psychotherapy, and social support. This final predictor would be expected to correlate negatively with long-term adjustment problems.

Clearly, while sexual abuse can have profound effects on children, the exact nature of those effects is quite unpredictable. Several conceptual models have been developed to account for the heterogeneity of children's responses to sexual abuse. Since understanding the impact of sexual abuse can inform strategies for intervention, these models can also serve as frameworks to organize clinicians' thinking about the likely treatment needs of sexually abused children.

Perhaps the most widely referenced model is that of Finkelhor and Browne (1985), who proposed that child sexual abuse consists of four traumatizing factors, each of which is experienced in varying degrees by sexually abused children. Their traumagenic model seeks to predict how each of the four sources of trauma impacts affective and cognitive aspects of the child victim's adaptation. The specific pattern of symptoms displayed in any given case is linked to the trauma sources that are most prominent in the child's situation. Finkelhor and Browne's trauma sources are (1) traumatic sexualization, (2) stigmatization, (3) powerlessness, and (4) betrayal.

Traumatic sexualization hinders healthy sexual adjustment because it results in the distortion of the victim's perceptions of sexuality. For example, sexuality may become linked with fear in the child's mind, or the child may come to consider sexual behavior as a valid means of pursuing nonsexual goals such as attention, status, or other privileges. Stigmatization results from unwarranted guilt experienced by the child for participating in the abuse and places the child at risk for diminished self-esteem and even for self-loathing. Durham (2003) has aptly described the result of stigmatization as an enduring "internalization of oppression" within the child (p. 22). Powerlessness ensues from repeatedly thwarted attempts on the part of the child to stop the abuse or enlist help from others to stop it. Finkelhor and Browne (1985) hypothesize that such a chronic pattern of frustration and helplessness can culminate in pervasive anxiety or dissociative symptoms. Betrayal stems from the breach of trust suffered by a child who is abused by the very figure responsible for providing stability, support, and safety. Finkelhor and Browne predict that enduring trust and interpersonal anger issues are likely results of the betrayal factor.

Friedrich (1994) developed a model that depicts the trauma of child sexual abuse as disruptive to development in three major domains: attachment, self-regulation, and self-esteem. For each of these areas of impact, he describes expected patterns of symptomatic behavior and corresponding intervention strategies. For example, the inner working models that shape sexually abused children's expectancies for interpersonal relationships are likely to be heavily influenced by the inconsistency and fear that characterize relationships with abusive attachment figures. Such interpersonal histories point to the need for therapists to anticipate trust issues and boundary problems in the therapy relationship.

Sexual abuse is also likely to interfere with the ability to self-regulate because the victim's efforts to understand the abuse are typically invalidated by the abuser, leaving the child with no consistent, dependable way of thinking about the connections among experiences, thoughts, and feelings. As a result, the abused child's ability to enlist cognitive strategies to recognize and manage emotions is compromised, as is the child's capacity for self-soothing in the face of overstimulating emotional arousal. Friedrich recommends psychoeducational interventions to reduce dysregulation and build coping strategies. The experience of sexual abuse is likely to affect the child victim's self-image, resulting in symptoms such as somatic concerns, depleted self-esteem, and an inability to observe or reflect on oneself. Relevant treatment priorities include increasing self-efficacy and accuracy of self-perception.

PRELIMINARY TREATMENT CONSIDERATIONS

Before beginning treatment, therapists must first attend to a number of practical aspects of the abuse situation. The success of treatment depends largely on the effective management of these critically important matters. Chief among these preliminary considerations are the child's safety and maximizing the involvement of the family and community resources.

The most immediate priority for the therapist is the establishment of safety. The child must feel safe in the most concrete sense; the abuse must be discontinued. Reflecting on her work with sexually abused children, Elianna Gil (1991, p. 59) states, "probably the greatest lesson I have learned from abused children and adults is that everything they do after they have been abused is designed to keep themselves feeling safe." Friedrich (1994) also considers safety to be an essential precondition to therapy with sexually abused children. Clearly it would be unreasonable and decidedly unempathetic to expect a child to turn her attention to engagement in the psychotherapy process if she is not safe from continued victimization at home (Ambridge, 2001). In the task of establishing safety, Friedrich includes providing support for the child through further losses and separation that may ensue following the disclosure of the abuse. This support is particularly helpful for children whose offender has entered the corrections system or has abandoned the family, as well as children who have been removed from their families.

To be complete, the treatment plan must include strategies for creating a safe environment in the therapy office. Both Gil (1991) and Green (1988) have described aspects of the treatment process that can contribute to an atmosphere of safety, including emphasizing trust in the therapy relationship and establishing healthy boundaries in the session. Teegan (1999) recommends a careful, nonjudgmental approach for building therapeutic safety. Herman (1992) described an initial safety and stabilization stage in the treatment of sexually abused children.

Inclusion of prevention training is a widely recognized treatment component that addresses safety issues as well as many other needs of sexually abused children (O'Donohue & Elliott, 1992). In addition to teaching children concrete skills to equip them to cope with future threats and prevent revictimization, prevention training can build self-awareness and -assertion skills and develop a sense of personal boundaries in the child, all characteristics of healthy self-esteem. An emphasis on prevention may be particularly relevant for child victims who present sexual behavior problems. Gray and Prithers (1993) propose the use of a prevention team comprising caregivers and other adults in the child's life who collaborate to prevent a recurrence of problematic sexual behavior on the part of the child.

In addition to addressing safety needs, potentially influential situational factors create a demand for contextual pretreatment planning, including evaluations of the child's family as well as the broader societal milieu. The treatment plan must include identification of family and community supports that can be accessed by the therapist for the purpose of ameliorating the effects of the abuse (Cicchetti & Toth, 1995b; Ross & O'Carroll, 2004). Friedrich (1994, p. 799) refers to this pretherapy obligation as the duty of the therapist to "know all the players."

Knowledge of the child's family situation is essential. Child sexual abuse does not occur in isolation. Whether the abuse takes place outside the family or is intrafamilial, it impacts each family member. Family factors influence the course of sexually abused children's development so profoundly that the majority of long-term sequelae are more closely determined by family functioning than by the abuse itself (Alexander, 1992).

Several aspects of family life have been shown to shape the child victim's adjustment, including family cohesion and control (Cohen & Mannarino, 1996; Friedrich, Beilke, & Urquiza, 1987). O'Donohue et al. (1998) sort family influences on the child's adjustment along a timeline including preabuse factors such as the child's attachment history, abuse characteristics such as duration and relationship with the abuser, and postabuse influences such as family members' responses to the disclosure. The symptoms manifested by the sexually abused child may in large part be a product of longstanding family dysfunction, chronically pathological patterns of relatedness among family members, or the crises that arise in the family following the disclosure (Green, 1993).

Most influential among family characteristics is the nature of abuse victims' relationships with nonoffending parents (Conte & Schuerman, 1987; Hansen et al., 1998; Nelson-Gardell, 2001). Peters (1988) found maternal warmth to be a stronger predictor of the child victim's adjustment than abuse-related variables. Eisenhower (2002) found that perceived parental support was significantly associated with long-term resilience in both African American and European American victims, confirming two decades of research that consistently points to postdisclosure parental support as a key contributor to recovery of sexually abused children (Kendall-Tackett et al., 1993). The protective value of abuse victims' relationships with nonoffending parents may be related to the impact of parental support on children's cognitive processing of abuse. The presence of a warm, supportive parent discourages the development within the child of negative appraisals of self and others (Spaccarelli & Kim, 1995).

Closely related to parental support is the issue of the nonoffending parent's level of distress. The weighty tasks that face nonoffending parents following disclosure (e.g., protecting the child from further abuse, dealing with law enforcement agencies) are indeed awesome and demand significant resourcefulness at the very time that parents are likely to feel most vulnerable (Ambridge, 2001).

Cohen and Mannarino (1996) found parental emotional reactions to the child's sexual abuse to be strongly related to behavioral and emotional symptoms in the victim. Specifically, they found parental stress to be the single most significant predictor of treatment outcome for preschool victims of sexual abuse. Parental depression and distress correlated significantly with both internalizing and externalizing symptoms in children. Parental depression was associated with sexual behavior problems in child victims as well. Clearly, parental stress levels and emotional availability significantly affect children's postabuse adjustment, including their potential to benefit from therapy (Friedrich, 1994; Heflin & Deblinger, 2003).

One mechanism that might explain the impact of parents' emotional state on their children's postdisclosure adjustment is modeling (Bandura, 1977). Young victims of abuse are likely to look to nonoffending parents for an emotional blueprint they can emulate in their attempts to cope with the abuse. Children are unable to learn adaptive coping strategies from parents whose coping is marginal or ineffective. In contrast, lower levels of parental distress and dysfunction are likely to increase parents' emotional availability as positive models for their children. In a study of parent distress and coping following sexual abuse disclosure, Davies (1995) found that most nonoffending parents experience multiple types of emotional distress, including anger, depression, and symptoms of posttraumatic stress. Parents also reported that they needed support in order to deal with the family crisis of sexual abuse, particularly immediately after the disclosure.

In another study that sheds light on the relationship between parent stress and recovery of the child victim, Bolen and Lamb (2004) found that children whose guardians believed their reports that abuse occurred were more emotionally supported than children whose nonoffending parents were ambivalent about their reports of abuse. Remarkably, parental belief that the abuse occurred was a better predictor of subsequent emotional support than parental provision for the child's continued safety. Furthermore, parents' distress levels were consistently and closely associated with ambivalent feelings toward their abused children.

It is noteworthy that parent well-being and support have emerged as significant ameliorative factors in investigations of cognitive-behavioral interventions for sexually abused children. While cognitive-behavioral research is primarily focused on internal cognitive factors that influence adjustment, the impact of parent stress level and emotional availability has been documented in this body of literature as a major determinant of children's adjustment and response to treatment (Deblinger, Stauffer, & Steer, 2001).

Clearly, when nonoffending parents are supported and child victims are validated and cared for, their adjustment is more successful. Parental support of the victimized child counteracts the effects of the manipulation and secrecy that are so central to abusive relationships. Treatment preparations would be incomplete without plans to enhance nonoffending parents' capacity to affirm and support their sexually abused children (Durham, 2003; Gil, 2002).

APPROACHES TO TREATMENT: THE NEED FOR THERAPIST FLEXIBILITY

Given the heterogeneity of symptoms presented by sexually abused children as well as the myriad family and social circumstances affecting their adjustment, treatment planning should be individualized to meet each child's unique needs. Perhaps in response to the complexity of clinical presentations in this population, the treatment outcome literature has increasingly reflected a trend toward combining techniques from a variety of theoretical traditions to address the varied problems presented by sexually abused children.

Rasmussen's (2001) integrative approach to treating sexually abused children with sexual behavior problems includes multiple components: supportive encouragement of expression of feelings associated with the abuse, behavioral skill building, and modification of cognitive distortions stemming from the abuse. Faust (2000) has proposed an intervention for sexually abused children that integrates family systems theory and cognitive therapy techniques. Mannarino and Cohen (2000) described a multimodal approach that includes cognitive interventions combined with behavioral strategies, psychoeducational experiences, and a humanistic component to create a safe therapeutic alliance that allows the child to work on problems of interpersonal trust. Mannarino and Cohen include humanistic interventions for nonoffending parents as well. They report that the parents of sexual abuse victims readily acknowledge their need for support, and they are generally more receptive to therapeutic support than the child victims. Silberg's (2004) integrated developmental model incorporates techniques derived from both attachment and family systems theories with cognitive-behavioral interventions to address the need for complex treatment of the multiple problems presented by sexually abused children. Bacon (2001) integrates attachment theory, family systems approaches, and traditional play therapy as well as a cognitive perspective in her description of the healing process for sexually abused children.

In addition to integrative treatment models and outcome studies, attempts have been made to identify commonalities across different theoretical approaches to the treatment of abused children. Both Lyness (1993) and Schaefer (1994), for example, offer conceptualizations of play therapy as consisting, in part, of a classical conditioning process, a cornerstone of many behavioral interventions. They propose that as the child gradually reapproaches traumatic material in the play, the troubling stimuli associated with the trauma are repeatedly paired with the comforting stimuli inherent in the play process, resulting in a diminution of painful responses to the trauma, and a reduction of discomfort from facing traumatic memories. Indeed, classical conditioning may be operating in the play therapy process and may be a significant contributor to the symptom relief children experience in play therapy.

Clearly, clinicians improve their chances of success if they are prepared to utilize a variety of techniques derived from different theoretical traditions. Additionally, flexibility and openness enhance the clinician's approach to defining goals. The effective therapist finds a balance between aggressively focused approaches, which target an overly narrow range of the child's presenting problems, and, at the other extreme, an excessively passive, unfocused orientation. Dufour and Chamberland (2004) urge clinicians to resist an overfocused approach to treatment of sexually abused children because there are typically so many problem areas in these children's lives. Directing therapeutic efforts exclusively at one target reduces the child's chances for recovery.

While an excessively narrow focus is likely to be problematic, a preponderance of evidence points to the superiority of relatively directive, goal-focused approaches in clinical work with sexually abused children (Gil, 2002). Smith and Bentovim (1994) advise that therapy with sexually abused children should be directive and supportive since silence on the part of the therapist may be reminiscent of the silence that often characterizes children's abuse histories. Consequently, nondirective approaches may inadvertently promote avoidance in sexually abused children. Additionally, sexually abused children are likely to be particularly reluctant to deal with the trauma that brings them to therapy. The material is likely to be humiliating, or the child may dissociate in the therapy room. Since the child typically has little or no basis upon which to expect a safe, trustworthy relationship with adults, he or she may fear talking about any aspect of the abuse. Friedrich (1994) recommends that the child be directly encouraged to address the abuse either in words or through play. He points out that, in contrast to sexually abusive relationships where children are discouraged from talking about feelings, the therapy relationship must distinguish itself by encouraging awareness and openness of communication.

ESSENTIAL ELEMENTS OF TREATMENT

Reviews of the sexual abuse treatment literature are encouraging as they indicate generally positive effects for children in treatment (Finkelhor & Berliner, 1995; Saywitz et al., 2000). Additionally, some consensus exists about key characteristics of the treatment process that enhance effectiveness. Several core therapeutic experiences have been consistently identified as promoting healing in sexually abused children. These experiences include the following therapeutic opportunities:

- the opportunity to be involved in a safe, affirming relationship with a trustworthy therapist
- the opportunity to reevaluate and revise self-perceptions and perceptions of others that have been damaged and distorted by the abuse experience
- the opportunity to revisit the abuse psychologically, gradually confronting troubling memories in order to master emotionally the trauma of the abuse

The Therapeutic Relationship

The therapeutic relationship has long been considered a major change agent in psychotherapy. Its significance is central to the treatment of sexually abused children because these children carry into therapy psychologically bruising interpersonal histories along with the products of their abuse histories: distorted perceptions of themselves and the interactional world. Sexual abuse is inherently interactive, and so the opportunity to be involved in a safe, supportive interpersonal relationship with a trustworthy adult is particularly healing (Gil, 1991).

Each therapeutic encounter is an opportunity for the child incrementally to build alternative perspectives of the interpersonal world and his or her role in it. Without such reparative interactions, the sexually abused child is vulnerable to repeated reliving of the anguish of past abusive relationships in which he or she was emotionally exploited to meet the needs of the abuser (Chop, 2003). The relationship with the attuned therapist provides the child with a new, more optimistic model of the interpersonal world, including more realistically positive perceptions of others and expectations for relationships (Harris & Landreth, 2001). The therapist's personal emotional congruence is particularly important as a model of stability and genuineness in relationships. Additionally, the therapeutic relationship can provide an emotional anchor for the child during painful transitions and crises that frequently accompany disclosure of sexual abuse (Cicchetti & Toth, 1995a).

In addition to its direct benefits, a supportive relationship with the therapist is necessary in order for other healing experiences to take place in the therapy process (Schaefer, 1994). For example, one cannot reasonably expect a child to take on the arduous task of recalling and reevaluating abuse experiences and learning to cope with their aftermath unless he or she has first established that the therapy relationship is safe and secure. In order for the child to share his or her inner world, he or she must first trust the integrity of the therapist and the therapeutic relationship (Harris & Landreth, 2001). Additionally, the therapist must be a model of willingness to face difficult realities by consistently demonstrating the ability to deal directly with problem situations that occur in the therapy room. Belief in the therapist's competence instills hope in the child, which, in turn, gives the child a reason to commit him- or herself to the therapy process (Rasmussen, 2001).

As essential as the therapeutic alliance is to ensure effective treatment, the capacity of many sexually abused children to form such an alliance is limited. Prior to therapy, many of these children learned to associate intimacy with fear and hopelessness in the face of danger (Gil, 2002). For these children, to be close to an adult authority figure is to risk injury and degradation (Eltz, Shirk, & Sarlin, 1995). They arrive in the therapy room having learned to anticipate danger when they experience interpersonal closeness.

Certainly the therapy relationship is weighted with expectations for closeness. Faced with such expectations, the sexually abused child may attempt to flee the connection with the therapist through acting out or avoidance (Schaefer, 1994). Ideally, the therapist responds to the child's resistance by observing and describing the child's behavior, inquiring about how the child is experiencing the therapy relationship, naming the emotions associated with those experiences, encouraging discussion and normalization of the child's rationale for resisting, and gently but persistently asserting the immediate realities of the therapy relationship in contrast to the child's anxiety-laden expectations.

The therapist repeatedly orients the child's attention to the discrepancy between the child's inaccurate and disturbing interpersonal expectations and the immediate, here-and-now interpersonal realities in the therapy room. This interpersonal learning process is essential to establish a sufficiently safe environment for the sexual abuse victim to begin the process of surrendering his or her typically vulnerable and vigilant style of processing interpersonal relationships in favor of tentatively trusting the therapist and the therapeutic alliance and ultimately generalizing these healthy interpersonal perceptions to relationships outside of the therapy room (Gil, 1991, 2002).

While the child is making use of the therapeutic relationship in ways that enhance interpersonal competence, the relationship with the therapist is, at the same time, providing ongoing learning experiences that yield significant benefits for the child's self-image (Fall, 1994). A safe, supportive alliance between therapist and child can provide a corrective emotional experience for the abused child whose self-image has gradually become distorted to accommodate consistently punishing and disrespectful abusive experiences.

The corrective emotional experience (Alexander & French, 1946), a time-honored component of the psychoanalytic psychotherapy process, uses the interaction patterns between therapist and child to produce new learning for the child concerning his or her self-worth and self-presentation to others. It involves a gradual, incremental interpersonal learning experience that allows the child to discard old, distorted views of him- or herself and replace them with new, more accurate self-perceptions.

Friedrich (1994) has described how interaction cycles that take place in the relationship between therapists and sexually abused children can yield a corrective emotional experience. The opportunity for a corrective emotional experience begins when the child engages in problematic behavior in the therapy room. The specific nature of the behavior varies depending on each child's unique relationship history. Some behaviors that the therapist might encounter include reluctance to talk, oppositionalism, sexual behavior, or accusations aimed at the therapist (Durham, 2003). These behaviors are likely to be noteworthy for their irrelevance to the ongoing supportive, respectful relationship offered by the therapist. It is as if the child is acting out a script from his or her prior relationship with the abuser. His or her behavioral choices are more reflective of old relational contingencies than current relational realities. The impact of the abuse frequently can be clearly seen still influencing the child's behavioral options in the therapy room long after the abuse has been stopped (Durham, 2003).

In addition to their irrelevance, the sexually abused child's behaviors are likely to elicit extremely strong negative reactions from others who are engaged in relationships with him or her. In the case of the therapeutic relationship, progression toward a corrective emotional experience continues as the therapist becomes aware of his or her own uncomfortable feelings evoked by the child's interaction style. It is not at all surprising for the therapist to be struck by the amount of anger felt at the child or the sense that the therapist has lost control of the therapy process (Gil, 2002). These personal reactions on the part of the therapist signal the opportunity to achieve a corrective emotional experience by interrupting maladaptive interaction patterns in which the child's damaged self-image is reinforced by others' abusive and retaliatory responses to her self-defeating behavior.

In a corrective emotional experience, the child's behavior is not met with rejection, but with an invitation to join forces with the therapist in thinking about the child's behavior patterns, including their roots in past abuse, as well as examining their current effectiveness. The therapist's enduring commitment to encouraging more rewarding, increasingly effective methods of self-expression in the child provides a corrective emotional experience because the therapist's concern is incompatible with the child's lack of self-respect, the source of her self-defeating behavior. The experience of being taken seriously, respected, and valued in the therapist's eyes gives the sexually abused child at least a preliminary glimpse of his or her own fundamental worth.

The interpersonal reality testing that goes on in the corrective emotional experience overlaps in many respects with the cognitive-behavioral emphasis on the role of cognitive distortions in perpetuating symptomatic behavior in sexually abused children. The psychoanalytic technique of identifying and correcting distortions caused by primitive defenses is analogous to the more directive cognitive-behavioral strategies for remediating maladaptive perceptions and expectancies. Both traditions recognize the significance of the distorted self-image created by child sexual abuse (Green, 1992; King et al., 1999), and in both perspectives, enhancing the accuracy and adaptability of the child's perceptions is considered essential for successful recovery from sexual abuse.

The therapeutic relationship is described in spatial terms in many discussions of treatment of sexually abused children (Walker & Bolkovatz, 1988). The relationship between therapist and child is very frequently conceptualized as an emotional "place" or "space," recalling Winnicott's (1965) image of the very first powerfully influential attachment relationship, the holding environment, where the self of the infant is shaped through safe, predictable, and validating parenting. In fact, attachment theory provides a rich and highly relevant model to guide the therapist's thinking about the powerfully healing components in the therapeutic relationship with sexually abused children who must negotiate the unique developmental ordeal of having been attached to an adult figure who was a source of danger rather than safety and protection (Bacon, 2001; Bacon & Richardson, 2001; Holmes, 2000). Perhaps, then, the therapeutic relationship can be viewed as a safe reparative retreat that allows the child to restore fundamental trust and self-worth.

In summary, Herman (1992, p. 197) aptly characterizes the goal of the therapeutic relationship in these words: "if helplessness and isolation are the core experiences of psychological trauma, then empowerment and reconnection are the core experiences of recovery." The therapist is a relationship partner who encourages the development of the child's potential by providing validation that springs from empathy with the child. The child can learn to feel safely related to the therapist, and what flows from that experience of safety is a growing faith in the likelihood that future relationships will be supportive (Hazell, 2000). The therapeutic relationship provides the child with consistent experiential evidence that trust in others can be a reasonable approach to many relationships.

Self-Image and Self-Expression

Self-esteem is especially relevant in the treatment of sexually abused children because of the shame and stigmatization associated with their abuse experiences (Gil, 2002). Several factors may contribute to the sexually abused child's typically depleted self-image. Very young, cognitively egocentric victims may blame themselves for the abuse because of their level of cognitive development. In other cases, victims' self-blame may reflect the need to feel in control following a history of helplessness and vulnerability in abusive relationships. Blaming themselves for the abuse may be less painful than full awareness of just how powerless they have been (Marvasti, 1994). Often the abuser suggests and reinforces the notion that the victim is responsible for the abuse, a reflection of patent denial and cognitive distortion on the part of the abuse perpetrator. Child victims whose welfare depends on maintaining their relationship with their abusers may adopt an attribution of guilt in hope of preserving their precarious connection to the abuser, who is capable of frightening retaliation for lack of cooperation (Leahy et al., 2003; Simon-Roper, 1996).

While the child's acceptance of responsibility for the abuse may temporarily placate the abuser, the long-term psychological cost is considerable. The child's self-esteem is eroded, and her expectations for future relationships are contaminated with fear and suspiciousness. The lack of congruence between the actual circumstances of the abuse and the distorted ways she has learned to think about it is likely to lead the child to question her overall ability to accurately perceive and understand the world around her. Over time, the child's awareness of competing sources of information about her self-worth becomes restricted. She may automatically screen out positive feedback about herself because it is incompatible with the self-image that is most familiar (Simon-Roper, 1996).

Some sexually abused children develop a false self in an attempt to prevent the loss of insecure, abusive attachments. Their behavior reveals only what is approved of and expected. In the process, they may lose touch with the genuine defining features of their true identity (Palmer, Farrar, & Ghahary, 2002). The inner world of many of these children is silenced. They have so thoroughly lost touch with themselves that they are unable to experience their own affect. Vas Dias (2000) describes these abuse victims as existing with a self that is not fully alive.

Treatment for sexually abused children with problems in self-worth and self-development can take many forms. The presence of a therapist who witnesses and validates the child's painful life story is most useful in helping children gain awareness of their hidden inner selves. The therapist's eagerness to listen and learn about the child directs the child's attention toward the existence of his inner world and opens the door to eventual reflection on inner experiences. The genuine validation of the therapist also makes it possible for the child to revise his self-image so that he can begin experiencing himself as a worthwhile human being, welcome in the world of human relatedness (Vas Dias, 2000; Ambridge, 2001).

This aspect of therapy with sexually abused children is often described as helping the child to find his or her voice. It is empowering for children to learn how to assert feelings that could not be acknowledged during the abuse (Gil, 2002). However, the fear of consequences of speaking the truth about the abuse may linger in the child, inhibiting self-awareness and self-expression in the therapy room (Durham, 2003). Gil (1991) recommends that the therapist directly and supportively encourage self-expression. She details a variety of practical, directive play techniques to facilitate self-awareness and -expression in abused children. In some cases, the therapist may need to model how to play in order to guide a chronically silenced child toward self-expression. Directive behavioral rehearsal of assertion skills has been found to be useful in encouraging self-expression in sexually abused children as well (Heflin & Deblinger, 2003).

Self-reflection is a central treatment goal for sexually abused children. The capacity to think about one's inner world is a necessity for successful adjustment and resilience. Fonagy (1998) has eloquently detailed the origins of the reflective self in primary attachment relationships. The child gradually discovers him- or herself interpersonally in the caregiver's attuned responses to the child's inner needs and mental states. The capacity for self-reflection is understandably compromised in many sexually abused children for whom attachments center on meeting the needs of an abusive caregiver, excluding essential validation of the child's inner world (Fonagy & Target, 1997). Viewed from this perspective, the therapeutic relationship can be considered a corrective attachment relationship, providing the child with a new chance to discover and reflect on him- or herself in interactions with the therapist (Friedrich, 1994).

Self-reflection is a widely recognized objective in virtually all major child therapy traditions. Child therapists operating out of the psychoanalytic tradition aim for the development of an observing ego within the child. Accurate self-perception is a cornerstone of cognitive-behavioral therapy that offers a number of directive psychoeducational techniques applicable to self-perception and self-esteem problems in sexually abused children (Kendall, 1991; King et al., 1999). In the cognitive-behavioral perspective, the child's perception of her abuse and the meanings she ascribes to it are critical determinants of her beliefs about herself (Briere & Elliott, 1994).

It is important to include in the therapy process a reservoir of experiences that allow the child to see him- or herself as competent, effective, and able successfully to influence the world around her (Ambridge, 2001). Engaging the child in expressive activities such as art or storytelling can enhance the child's sense of personal efficacy. The therapist can also promote a sense of competence by setting attainable treatment goals for the child, providing skill building to attain those goals, and building in appropriate recognition for accomplishment of those goals (Gil, 2002).

Experiential opportunities that highlight personal effectiveness generally have a greater impact on children's attitudes than discussions aimed at insight about self-worth (Friedrich, 1994).

Mastery Experiences

The first systematic psychological observations of children's play, described by Sigmund Freud in 1920, serve as our earliest guidelines for understanding how children recover from traumas such as sexual abuse. Freud noted that children consistently reconstruct distinctly unpleasant experiences in their play. Traumatized children, in particular, appear to utilize play spontaneously to address emotionally overwhelming experiences.

In the century since Freud's initial observations, much has been learned about how play facilitates adjustment in traumatized children. The psychoanalytic view conceptualizes play as a typical childhood expression of repetition compulsion, the natural inclination to return energy and attention to unfinished, uncomfortable events or experiences that have not yet been satisfactorily resolved. While adults may revisit emotionally troubling issues in repetitive thought or conversation, the child's preferred medium for repetition for mastery is play (Gil, 1991).

Repetition for mastery takes place in play as the child begins to deal with large, overwhelming problems such as sexual abuse one component part at a time. Divided into manageable parts, traumas such as abuse are more easily faced. As the child repeatedly addresses each aspect of the trauma in his or her play, the tension associated with the overall experience is gradually diminished, moderating the impact of the abuse (Ginsberg, 1993). Play is restorative because it deintensifies stressful experiences (Del Po & Frick, 1988). Mastery is made even more attainable because the child's play activities involve symbolic metaphors of the abuse, allowing for initial distance from direct, potentially overwhelming reliving of the abuse (Wershba-Gershon, 1996). The symbolic nature of make-believe play shields the child from having to prematurely face overwhelmingly frightening memories that might engage defensive avoidance and stall the recovery process (Landreth, 2001).

Repetition for mastery is a gradual process of facing ever more directly the aspects of traumatizing experiences that must be acknowledged and accurately understood (Waelder, 1932). As the child gradually allows bits of overwhelming experiences into awareness, he can explore and practice ways of thinking about and coping with those experiences and develop solutions that are uniquely his own (Landreth, 2001).

Noteworthy overlap exists between the traditional psychodynamic notion of repetition for mastery in the child's play and Piaget's (1962) concept of assimilation, a fundamental process for cognitive adaptation to environmental demands. Assimilation in children's spontaneous play increases their ability to adapt to challenging developmental problems. By returning again and again in play to demanding situations that could potentially overwhelm their resources, children achieve understanding, resolution, and adjustment to those problem situations incrementally.

Repeated imaginal experiencing of abuse is a central component in the cognitive-behavioral treatment of sexually abused children (Heflin & Deblinger, 2003; King et al., 1999). In cognitive exposure techniques, the therapist directs the child's attention to thoughts and memories of the abuse. Repeated recollection of the abuse in the absence of frightening abuse experiences gradually reduces anxiety as a result of habituation (Deblinger, Lippmann, & Steer, 1996; Ross & O'Carroll, 2004). The consistencies between the psychodynamic tradition of repetition for mastery and the behavioral emphasis on repeated confrontation of the trauma present clinicians with the opportunity to creatively combine approaches to fostering mastery in sexually abused children. Knell and Ruma (2003), for example, developed a multimodal approach that combines features of play therapy and directive cognitive-behavioral techniques in an integrative model of treatment for sexually abused children.

Ideally, as the child gains mastery over difficult external circumstances such as abuse, she is at the same time, examining and investigating her internal world (Del Po & Frick, 1988). Facing and reworking the trauma allows for psychological integration to take place. Integration is an essential goal for many sexually abused children in whom traumatic experiences are walled off from awareness through unconscious protective mechanisms such as dissociation (Gil, 2002). Other fragmenting adaptations to the abuse may involve separating mental processes that normally belong together. For example, a sexually abused child may reexperience aspects of the trauma with affect completely split off from consciousness (Durham, 2003). In these cases, defensive barriers that were constructed to reduce the emotional impact of the abuse persist even when they are no longer effective, and, in fact, may become impediments to healthy adjustment.

Repetition in play is restorative because it provides multiple opportunities for the child, with the guidance of the therapist, to link together fragmented aspects of the personality, organize thoughts about the abuse, assign appropriate meaning to memories of the abuse, and coherently place these memories in the child's past so that he can use his psychological resources to move forward developmentally (Gil, 2002).

In order for the child's play to be healing, her recollections of abuse must not be mere intellectual exercises. She must emotionally confront the abuse before she can successfully recover from it. Revisiting the abuse must be accompanied by an appropriate release of affect (Oremland, 1993). Additionally, the emotions associated with the abuse must eventually be put into words (Gil, 1991). Continual replaying of abuse scenarios without any emotional component of the experience can significantly impede recovery rather than facilitating it (Terr, 1990). Therefore, an essential role of the therapist is to encourage the child to link traumatic memories with corresponding affect. Additionally, the therapist must help the child find words to express the affect associated with the trauma and verbalize the ways she copes with her trauma-related affect.

In order to lead to mastery, the child's play should involve a shift from a passive overall orientation, which frequently emanates from a history of victimization, to an active approach in the play. Moving from passive to active play allows the child to experience active agency in shaping his environment. In doing so, he can practice proactive behaviors and attitudes that counteract the helplessness of his abuse history (Lyness, 1993). Erik Erikson (1977) described a typical way that active mastery is achieved through play. He observed that children often create models of demanding situations in their play, accompanied by playful experimentation with coping strategies to address those situations. Thus, the play often involves active exploring of problem-solving options. The opportunity to explore and experiment with problem solving while remaining in control of the pace, process, and outcome of the play is particularly valuable to sexual abuse victims, who were not able to control critical aspects of their lives during their abuse (Landreth, 2001).

In sum, repeatedly revisiting the trauma of the abuse creates an increased sense of familiarity, predictability, and mastery over the abuse. All the while, the child is practicing new skills and coping strategies in her play. Each successive replaying of the abuse reduces the affective residue associated with it (Lyness, 1993; Oremland, 1993). The need for psychological defenses to protect the child from overwhelming tension is, in turn, gradually reduced (Landreth, 2001). Psychological resources that had been dedicated to driving the effects of the abuse out of awareness are diverted to more developmentally appropriate tasks (Marvasti, 1994). Repetition for mastery allows the child to take in difficult experiences, understand them, and make them part of herself and her history in a nonharmful way. In the process, the child changes, as does her perception of herself and the world around her (McMahon, 1992).

REFERENCES

Alexander, F., & French, T. (1946). *Psychoanalytic therapy: Principles and applications.* New York: Ronald Press.

Alexander, P. C. (1992). Application of attachment theory to the study of sexual abuse. *Journal of Consulting and Clinical Psychology, 60(2),* 185–195.

Ambridge, M. (2001). Monsters and angels: How can child victims achieve resolution? In S. Richardson & H. Bacon (Eds.), *Creative responses to child sexual abuse: Challenges and dilemmas* (pp. 167–182). London: Jessica Kingsley.

Bacon, H. (2001). Attachment, trauma and child sexual abuse. In S. Richardson & H. Bacon (Eds.), *Creative responses to child sexual abuse: Challenges and dilemmas* (pp. 44–59). London: Jessica Kingsley.

Bacon, H., & Richardson, S. (2001). Attachment theory and child abuse: An overview of the literature for practitioners. *Child Abuse Review, 10(6),* 377–397.

Bandura, A. (1977). *Social learning theory.* Englewood Cliffs, NJ: Prentice-Hall.

Berliner, L., & Elliott, D. M. (1996). Sexual abuse of children. In J. Briere, L. Berliner, J. A. Bulkley, C. Jenny, & T. Reid (Eds.), *The APSAC handbook on child maltreatment.* Thousand Oaks, CA: Sage.

Bolen, R. M., & Lamb, J. H. (2004). Ambivalence of nonoffending guardians after child sexual abuse disclosure. *Journal of Interpersonal Violence, 19(2),* 185–211.

Briere, J. (1992). *Child abuse trauma: Theory and treatment of the lasting effects.* Newbury Park, CA: Sage.

Briere, J., & Elliott, D. (1994). Immediate and long-term impacts of child sexual abuse. *The Future of Children: Sexual Abuse of Children, 4(2),* 54–69.

Briere, J., & Elliott, D. M. (2003). Prevalence and psychological sequelae of self-reported childhood physical and sexual abuse in a general population sample of men and women. *Child Abuse and Neglect, 27(10),* 1205–1222.

Briere, J., & Gil, E. (1998). Self-mutilation in clinical and general population samples: Prevalence, correlates, and functions. *American Journal of Orthopsychiatry, 68(4),* 609–620.

Brown, J., Cohen, P., Chen, H., Smailes, E., & Johnson, J. (2004). Sexual trajectories of abused and neglected youths. *Journal of Developmental and Behavioral Pediatrics, 25(2),* 77–82.

Burgdorf, K., Chen, X., Walker, T., Porowski, A., & Herrell, J. (2004). The prevalence and prognostic significance of sexual abuse in substance abuse treatment of women. *Addictive Disorders and Their Treatment, 3(1),* 1–13.

Burgess, A. (1987). Child molesting: Assessing impact in multiple victims. *Archives of Psychiatric Nursing, 1,* 33–39.

Chop, S. M. (2003). Relationship therapy with child victims of sexual abuse placed in residential care. *Child and Adolescent Social Work Journal, 20(4),* 297–301.

Cicchetti, D., & Toth, S. L. (1995a). Child maltreatment and attachment organization. In S. Goldberg, R. Muir, & J. Kerr (Eds.), *Attachment theory: Social, developmental, and clinical perspectives* (pp. 279–308). Hillsdale, NJ: Analytic Press.

Cicchetti, D., & Toth, S. L. (1995b). A developmental psychopathology perspective
on child abuse and neglect. *Journal of the American Academy of Child and Adolescent Psychiatry, 34*(5), 541–565.

Cohen, J. A., Deblinger, E., Maedel, A. B., & Stauffer, L. B. (1999). Examining sex-
related thoughts and feelings of sexually abused and nonabused children.
Journal of Interpersonal Violence, 14(7), 701–712.

Cohen, J. A., & Mannarino, A. P. (1996). Factors that mediate treatment outcome
of sexually abused preschool children. *Journal of the American Academy of
Child and Adolescent Psychiatry, 35*(10), 1402–1410.

Collin-Vezina, D., & Hebert, M. (2005). Comparing dissociation and PTSD in sexually abused, school-aged girls. *Journal of Nervous and Mental Disease, 193*(1),
47–52.

Conte, J. R., & Schuerman, J. R. (1987). Factors associated with an increased
impact of child sexual abuse. *Child Abuse and Neglect, 11*(2), 201–211.

Davies, M. G. (1995). Parental distress and ability to cope following disclosure of
extrafamilial sexual abuse. *Child Abuse and Neglect, 19*(4), 399–408.

Deblinger, E., Lippmann, J., & Steer, R. (1996). Sexually abused children suffering
posttraumatic stress symptoms. Initial treatment outcome findings. *Child
Maltreatment, 1,* 310–321.

Deblinger, E., McLeer, S. V., Atkins, M., Ralphe, D., & Foa, E. (1989). Posttraumatic stress in sexually abused, physically abused, and non-abused children. *Child Abuse and Neglect, 13*(3), 403–408.

Deblinger, E., Stauffer, L. B., & Steer, R. A. (2001). Comparative efficacies of supportive and cognitive-behavioral group therapies for young children who
have been sexually abused and their nonoffending mothers. *Child Maltreatment, 6*(4), 332–345.

Del Po, E., & Frick, S. (1988). Directed and nondirected play as therapeutic modalities. *Children's Health Care, 16*(4), 261–267.

Dufour, S., & Chamberland, C. (2004). The effectiveness of selected interventions
for previous maltreatment: enhancing the well-being of children who live at
home. *Child and Family Social Work, 9*(1), 39–56.

Durham, A. (2003). *Young men surviving child sexual abuse: Research stories and lessons for therapeutic practice.* New York: Wiley.

Einbender, A. J., & Friedrich, W. N. (1989). Psychological functioning and behavior of sexually abused girls. *Journal of Consulting and Clinical Psychology,
57*(1), 155–157.

Eisenhower, J. W. (2002). Family support and internalized beliefs as mediators of
the long-term effects of child sexual abuse in African American and European American women. *Dissertation Abstracts International Section A: Human-
ities and Social Sciences, 62*(12A), 4331.

Eltz, M. J., Shirk, S. R., & Sarlin, N. (1995). Alliance formation and treatment outcome among maltreated adolescents. *Child Abuse and Neglect, 19*(4), 419–431.

Erikson, E. (1977). *Toys and reasons*. New York: Norton.

Fall, M. (1994). Self-efficacy: An additional dimension in play therapy. *International Journal of Play Therapy, 3*(2), 21–32.

Faust, J. (2000). Integration of family and cognitive-behavioral therapy for treating sexually abused children. *Cognitive and Behavioral Practice, 7*(3), 361–368.

Finkelhor, D., & Berliner, L. (1995). Research on the treatment of sexually abused children: A review and recommendations. *Journal of the American Academy of Child and Adolescent Psychiatry, 34*(11), 1408–1423.

Finkelhor, D., & Browne, A. (1985). The traumatic impact of child sexual abuse: A conceptualization. *American Journal of Orthopsychiatry, 55*(4), 530–541.

Fonagy, P. (1998). An attachment theory approach to treatment of the difficult patient. *Bulletin of the Menninger Clinic, 62*(2), 147–163.

Fonagy, P., & Target, M. (1997). Attachment and reflective function: Their role in self-organization. *Development and Psychopathology, 9*(4), 679–700.

Freud, S. (1920). Beyond the pleasure principle. In *The standard edition of the complete psychological works of Sigmund Freud* (Vol. 18, 7–64). London: Hogarth Press.

Friedrich, W. N. (1994). Individual psychotherapy for child abuse victims. *Child and Adolescent Pediatric Clinics of North America, 3*(4), 797–812.

Friedrich, W. N., Beilke, R. L., & Urquiza, A. J. (1987). Children from sexually abusive families: A behavioral comparison. *Journal of Interpersonal Violence, 2*(4), 391–402.

Friedrich, W. N., Grambsch, P., Damon, L., Hewitt, S. K., Koverola, C., Lang, R. A., et al. (1992). Child sexual behavior inventory: Normative and clinical comparisons. *Psychological Assessment, 4*(3), 303–311.

Gil, E. (1991). *The healing power of play*. New York: Guilford Press.

Gil, E. (2002). Play therapy with abused children. In F. Kaslow (Ed.), *Comprehensive handbook of psychotherapy: Volume 3. Interpersonal/humanistic/existential* (pp. 61–82). New York: Wiley.

Ginsberg, B. G. (1993). Catharsis. In C. E. Schaefer (Ed.), *The therapeutic powers of play* (pp. 107–141). Northvale, NJ: Aronson.

Gray, A., & Prithers, W. D. (1993). Relapse prevention with sexually aggressive adolescents and children: Expanding treatment and supervision. In H. Barbaree, W. Marshall, & S. Hudson (Eds.), *The juvenile sexual offender* (pp. 289–319). New York: Guilford Press.

Green, A. H. (1988). The abused child and adolescent. In C. J. Kestenbaum & D. T. Williams (Eds.), *Handbook of clinical assessment of children and adolescents* (Vol. 2, pp. 842–863). New York: University Press.

Green, A. H. (1992). Applications of psychoanalytic theory in the treatment of the victim and the family. In W. O'Donohue & J. Geer (Eds.), *The sexual abuse of children* (Vol. 2, pp. 285–300). Hillsdale, NJ: Erlbaum.

Green, A. H. (1993). Child sexual abuse: Immediate and long-term effects and intervention. *Journal of the American Academy of Child and Adolescent Psychiatry, 32*(5), 890–902.

Hansen, D. J., Hecht, D. B., & Futa, K. T. (1998). Child sexual abuse. In V. B. Van

Hasselt & M. Hersen (Eds.), *Handbook of psychological treatment protocols for children and adolescents* (pp. 153–178). Mahwah, NJ: Erlbaum.

Harris, T. E., & Landreth, G. L. (2001). Essential personality characteristics of effective play therapists. In G. L. Landreth (Ed.), *Innovations in play therapy: Issues, process, and special populations* (pp. 23–29). New York: Brunner-Routledge.

Hazell, J. (2000). An object relations perspective on the development of the person. In U. McCluskey & C. A. Hooper (Eds.), *Psychodynamic perspectives on abuse: The cost of fear* (pp. 25–39). London: Jessica Kingsley.

Heflin, A. H., & Deblinger, E. (2003). Treatment of a sexually abused adolescent with posttraumatic stress disorder. In M. A. Reinecke, F. M. Dattilio, & A. Freeman (Eds.), *Cognitive therapy with children and adolescents: A casebook for clinical practice* (pp. 214–246). New York: Guilford Press.

Herman, J. L. (1992). *Trauma and recovery.* New York: Basic Books.

Herman, J. L., Perry, J. C., & van der Kolk, B. A. (1989). Childhood trauma in borderline personality disorder. *American Journal of Psychiatry, 146*(4), 490–495.

Holmes, J. (2000). Attachment theory and abuse: A developmental perspective. In U. McCluskey & C. A. Hooper (Eds.), *Psychodynamic perspectives on abuse: The cost of fear* (pp. 40–53). London: Jessica Kingsley.

Kendall, P. C. (1991). *Child and adolescent therapy.* New York: Guilford Press.

Kendall-Tackett, K. A., Williams, L. M., & Finkelhor, D. (1993). Impact of sexual abuse on children: A review and synthesis of recent empirical studies. *Psychological Bulletin, 113*(1), 164–180.

King, N. J., Tonge, B. J., Mullen, P., Myerson, N., Heyne, D., & Ollendick, T. H. (1999). Cognitive-behavioral treatment of sexually abused children: A review of research. *Behavioral and Cognitive Psychotherapy, 27*(4), 295–309.

Knell, S. M., & Ruma, C. D. (2003). Play therapy with a sexually abused child. In M. Reinecke & F. Dattilio (Eds.), *Cognitive therapy with children and adolescents* (pp. 338–368). New York: Guilford Press.

Landreth, G. (2001). Facilitative dimensions of play in the play therapy process. In G. L. Landreth (Ed.), *Innovations in play therapy: Issues, process, and special populations* (pp. 3–22). New York: Brunner-Routledge.

Leahy, T., Pretty, G., & Tenenbaum, G. (2003). Childhood sexual abuse narratives in clinically and nonclinically distressed adult survivors. *Professional Psychology: Research and Practice, 34*(6), 657–665.

Livingston, R. (1987). Sexually and physically abused children. *Journal of the American Academy of Child and Adolescent Psychiatry, 26*(3), 413–415.

Lyness, D. (1993). Mastery of childhood fears. In C. E. Schaefer (Ed.), *The therapeutic powers of play* (pp. 309–322). Northvale, NJ: Aronson.

Mannarino, A. P., & Cohen, J. A. (2000). Integrating cognitive-behavioral and humanistic approaches. *Cognitive and Behavioral Practice, 7*(3), 357–361.

Marvasti, J. A. (1994). Play diagnosis and play therapy with child victims of incest. In K. J. O'Connor & C. E. Schaefer (Eds.), *Handbook of play therapy, Vol. 2: Advances and innovations* (pp. 320–348). New York: Wiley.

McClellan, J., Adams, J., Douglas, D., McCurry, C., & Storck, M. (1995). Clinical characteristics related to severity of sexual abuse: A study of seriously mentally ill youth. *Child Abuse and Neglect, 19*(10), 1245–1254.

McMahon, L. (1992). *The handbook of play therapy.* New York: Tavistock/Routledge.

Nelson-Gardell, D. (2001). The voices of victims: Surviving child sexual abuse. *Child and Adolescent Social Work Journal, 18*(6), 401–416.

Neumann, D. A., Houskamp, B. M., Pollock, B. M., & Briere, J. (1996). The long-term sequelae of childhood sexual abuse in women: A meta-analytic review. *Child Maltreatment, 1*(1), 6–16.

O'Donohue, W. T., & Elliott, A. N. (1992). Treatment of the sexually abused child: A review. *Journal of Clinical Child Psychology, 21*(3), 218–228.

O'Donohue, W., Fanetti, M., & Elliott, A. (1998). Trauma in children. In V. M. Follette, J. I. Ruzek, & F. R. Abueg (Eds.), *Cognitive-behavioral therapies for trauma* (pp. 355–382). New York: Guilford Press.

Oremland, E. K. (1993). Abreaction. In C. E. Schaefer (Ed.), *The therapeutic powers of play* (pp. 143–165). Northvale, NJ: Aronson.

Palmer, L., Farrar, A. R., & Ghahary, N. (2002). A biopsychosocial approach to play therapy with maltreated children. In F. Kaslow (Ed.), *Comprehensive handbook of psychotherapy: Interpersonal/humanistic/existential* (pp. 109–130). New York: Wiley.

Peters, S. D. (1988). Child sexual abuse and later psychological problems. In G. E. Wyatt & G. J. Powell (Eds.), *Lasting effects of child sexual abuse* (pp. 101–117). Newbury Park, CA: Sage.

Piaget, J. (1962). *Play, dreams, and imitation in childhood.* New York: Norton.

Polusny, M. A., & Follette, V. M. (1995). Long-term correlates of child sexual abuse: Theory and review of the empirical literature. *Applied and Preventative Psychology, 4*(3), 143–166.

Rasmussen, L. (2001). Integrating cognitive-behavioral and expressive therapy interventions: Applying the trauma outcome process in treating children with sexually abusive behavior problems. *Journal of Child Sexual Abuse, 10*(4), 1–29.

Ross, G., & O'Carroll, P. (2004). Cognitive-behavioral psychotherapy in intervention in childhood sexual abuse: Identifying new directions from the literature. *Child Abuse Review, 13*(1), 51–64.

Saywitz, K. J., Mannarino, A. P., Berliner, L., & Cohen, J. A. (2000). Treatment for sexually abused children and adolescents. *American Psychologist, 55*(9), 1040–1056.

Schaefer, C. E. (1994). Play therapy for psychic trauma in children. In K. O'Connor & C. E. Schaefer (Eds.), *Handbook of play therapy, Vol. 2: Advances and innovations* (pp. 297–318). New York: Wiley.

Silberg, J. L. (2004). The treatment of dissociation in sexually abused children from a family/attachment perspective. *Psychotherapy: Theory, Research, Practice, Training, 41*(4), 487–495.

Simon-Roper, L. (1996). Victims' response cycle: A model for understanding the incestuous victim-offender relationship. *Journal of Child Sexual Abuse, 5*(2), 59–79.

Smith, M., & Bentovim, A. (1994). Sexual abuse. In M. Rutter, E. Taylor, & L. Hersov (Eds.), *Child and adolescent psychiatry* (pp. 230–251). Oxford, UK: Blackwell.

Spaccarelli, S., & Kim, S. (1995). Resilience criteria and factors associated with resilience in sexually abused girls. *Child Abuse and Neglect, 19*(9), 171–182.

Strand, V. C. (1999). The assessment and treatment of family sexual abuse. In N. B. Webb (Ed.), *Play therapy with children in crisis: Individual, group, and family treatment* (2nd ed., pp. 104–130). New York: Guilford Press.

Teegan, F. (1999). Childhood sexual abuse and long-term sequelae. In A. Maercker, M. Schutzwohl, & A. Solomon (Eds.), *Posttraumatic stress disorder: A lifespan developmental perspective* (pp. 97–112). Seattle: Hogrefe & Huber.

Terr, L. C. (1990). *Too scared to cry: Psychic trauma in childhood.* New York: Harper & Row.

van der Kolk, B. A., Perry, J. C., & Herman, J. L. (1991). Childhood origins of self-destructive behavior. *American Journal of Psychiatry, 148*(12), 1665–1671.

Vas Dias, S. (2000). Inner silence. In U. McCluskey & C. A. Hooper (Eds.), *Psychodynamic perspectives on abuse: The cost of fear* (pp. 159–171). London: Jessica Kingsley.

Waelder, R. (1932). The psychoanalytic theory of play. *Psychoanalytic Quarterly, 2,* 208–224.

Walker, L. E., & Bolkovatz, M. A. (1988). Play therapy with children who have experienced sexual assault. In L. Walher (Ed.), *Handbook on sexual abuse of children: Assessment and treatment issues* (pp. 249–269). New York: Springer.

Watkins, B., & Bentovim, A. (1992). The sexual abuse of male children and adolescents: A review of current research. *Journal of Child Psychology and Psychiatry, 33*(1), 197–248.

Wells, R. D., McCann, J., Adams, J., Voris, J., & Ensign, J. (1995). Emotional, behavioral, and physical symptoms reported by parents of sexually abused, nonabused, and allegedly abused prepubescent females. *Child Abuse and Neglect, 19*(2), 155–163.

Wershba-Gershon, P. (1996). Free symbolic play and assessment of the nature of child sexual abuse. *Journal of Child Sexual Abuse, 5*(2), 37–57.

Winnicott, D. W. (1965). *Maturational processes in the facilitating environment.* New York: International Universities Press.

Wolf, V., & Birt, J. (1995). The psychological sequelae of child sexual abuse. In T. H. Ollendick & R. J. Prinz (Eds.), *Advances in clinical child psychology* (pp. 233–263). New York: Plenum Press.

Wozencraft, T., Wagner, W., & Pelligrin, A. (1991). Depression and suicidal ideation in sexually abused children. *Child Abuse and Neglect, 15*(4), 505–511.

Play Therapy for Girls Displaying Social Aggression

MYRA M. LAWRENCE
KRISTIN CONDON
KATHRYN S. JACOBI
EMILY NICHOLSON

Social or relational aggression, the use of relationships and social influence to hurt others, often characterizes the interaction among school-age and teenage girls. Considered to be more typical of girls' than of boys' behavior, social aggression includes such behaviors as name-calling, gossiping, spreading rumors, isolating and excluding girls, and giving girls the "silent treatment" (Galen and Underwood, 1997). It is quite prevalent (72% of all girls report being victims of such aggression [Underwood, 2003]) and increases in frequency and intensity during the preteen and early teenage years. As they develop a better understanding of social situations and the importance of relationships, girls sometimes apply this knowledge to attack and destroy the valued relationships within their peer group (Wiseman, 2002; Simmons, 2002; Underwood, 2003).

Many researchers and clinicians interchangeably refer to social and relational aggression to identify these destructive interactions among girls. Others distinguish between indirect, covert social aggression, as when girls spread rumors, try to influence and shift alliances, or undermine another girl's social position; and direct, overt social aggression, as when girls engage in "openly maligning someone else to others with no pretense of benign intentions" (Underwood, 2003, p. 32). We will use the term social aggression to describe both indirect and direct behavior, as this term encompasses all types of aggression among girls and "best describes the function of these behaviors, namely, to do social harm" (Galen & Underwood, 1997, cited in Underwood, 2003, p. 23).

While some aims of socially aggressive behavior are instrumental in nature, intended to achieve a specific outcome such as increased status or importance within a desired group, socially aware girls know that they are expected to "be nice"—not harsh, aggressive, or obviously angry. Lyn Mikel Brown (2003) remarks on the need for girls to find their own voices to express a variety of emotions, observing that girls struggle with the cultural expectations directing acceptable feminine behavior. She describes girls as held within the grip of the prescribed "Good Girl Code of Ethics," where being soft-spoken, kind, and thoughtful to others is essential, where being "nice" becomes the power word, the power position. Operating within this code, girls often select subtle actions like eye rolling, hair tossing, or couching their language in a way that allows them to disavow or minimize the meaning of their words and actual motives. Siegel and Hartzell (2003) point out that these "nonverbal messages of eye contact, facial expression, tone of voice, gestures, body posture, and the timing and intensity of response are also extremely important elements of communication" (p. 10). Brown (2003) writes that girls learn "to hurt another person in such a way that it looks as though there has been no intention at all" (p. 16), but Wiseman (2002) shows that "girls' competition with and judgment of each other weakens their friendship and effectively isolates all of them" (p. 13).

In contrast to boys, who often engage in higher levels of obvious verbal and physical aggression (Thompson & Grace, 2001; Underwood, 2003), girls' negative peer interactions generally are minimized and dismissed because they are less overtly aggressive in nature. At school and at home, teachers and parents see and respond to obvious aggressive behaviors— hitting, shoving, or engaging in physical posturing and verbal threats— and overlook the often subtle ways in which girls communicate to one another that someone is no longer part of the group, no longer welcome at the lunch table, or no longer included in social plans, phone calls, or e-mails. The more covert behaviors in which girls often engage are rarely observed, rarely reported, and are easily minimized or denied by a perpetrating girl who is called on them at school or at home. Particularly with the advent of e-mail, instant messages, chat rooms, and websites, girls find that "whereas targets of physical aggression at least know who has attacked them, victims of social aggression may not know who the perpetrators are and often must cope with their victimization with the sense that everyone else is involved and working against them" (Underwood, 2003, p. 15). Only seemingly less destructive than the aggression and bullying behaviors considered typical in boys, social aggression is highly damaging to the emotional, academic, and social development of girls, often having a lifelong negative effect on adjustment. In contrast to more overt aggressive behaviors that are easier to recognize and discipline, social aggression may go unnoticed by everyone but the social group of girls involved. Yet, fear of social aggression, teasing, and bullying are reported to account for more absences from school than any other factor.

In incidents of social aggression girls assume certain roles, which we will define as follows: The Aggressor, popularly referred to as the Queen Bee, is the girl who initiates socially aggressive behavior and usually has one or more allies. The Ally or Sidekick is the girl who is closest to and models her behavior and mannerisms after the Queen Bee. Second in command, she enforces directives and presents a united front with the Queen Bee that creates a formidable force within the group. The Bystander is the girl or girls who observe what occurs and may be torn between groups without overtly affiliating with either side in a conflict. The Floater is the girl who moves from girl to girl or group to group, maintaining connections with all participants. And the Target or Victim is the girl singled out and placed under siege (Wiseman, 2002; Underwood, 2003). The girl who is targeted for social aggression often feels completely alone and without resources to alter her situation. The Aggressor often feels that she has omnipotent, unregulated power and influence. Bystanders who might want to intervene typically are paralyzed because they fear becoming the next target of the Aggressor and her Allies. Thus, some Bystanders will be drawn into roles that support the girl or girls in power, hoping to solidify their own safety and security, whereas other Bystanders will remain quiet, hoping to avoid any action that might turn the attention of the Aggressor toward them.

It is clear that each participant experiences uncertainty on this social terrain, and the players are well aware that the roles they assume are fluid and subject to change. All the players recognize that they are potential targets, for Aggressors may come home from school in tears over social interactions, and girls who are victimized sometimes turn and target other girls in their peer group. Those in power are eager to remain so to protect themselves from any incursions into their position of supposed safety; those who are victimized hope to vanish or vanquish, uncertain how best to proceed; and those girls who are Bystanders recognize that one cannot simply be an observer, as they risk identification as "with" or "against" the Victim or Aggressor, with all this portends.

From the earliest moments of infancy, our sense of self and others is developed within the crucible of meaningful relationships with others. When important relationships are betrayed, the effect is to undermine an individual's sense of self. Girls who directly or indirectly experience social aggression typically develop feelings of distress that result from an attack on their social connections and relatedness to their peer group, which is central to female development and relationships. Intended to get a girl "where it hurts," social aggression achieves not only the impact caused by a specific act—shunning, isolating a girl from social activities, spreading rumors, turning a best friend into a worst enemy, or exposing a girl's innermost secrets—all hallmarks of interpersonal violence, but also places the framework of a girl's social existence under siege, undermining the girders of support that friendships and relationships constitute for girls. Social aggression typically is manifested as an interactional process contrived to hurt or expel a girl from her essential social group and threatens to deconstruct that girl's entire social network. To complicate the situation further, social aggression is often easily denied by the Aggressors because of the way it is conveyed; a Victim can be told with apparent sincerity that she has misread a situation or incident or that she is overreacting to an unintentional slight, a small gesture or a few words that were never meant to hurt. This compounds the problem for the Victim, who may both hope and be led to believe that her perception is wrong. Because of her self-doubt, the destruction of security, trust, and connection with other girls is even more traumatic for the girl on the receiving end of socially aggressive behavior.

When girls experience trauma, they feel overwhelmed, and their usual protective mechanisms no longer provide them with a sense of security (Flashman, 2003). Social, psychological, and emotional difficulties accompany mild, moderate, and more severe forms of social aggression and require careful, informed intervention to restore a supportive network of relationships in which girls can thrive. In extreme cases, based both on the severity of the actions perpetrated and the emotional make-up of the girl who is targeted, a loss of trust and sense of alienation and disconnection can begin to pervade every relationship the girl subsequently engages in or avoids. What emerges as we look more closely at the dynamics of social aggression is that girls who are expelled from their position of security in relationships are then subjected to further trauma; they may be repeatedly treated as an object of isolation and exclusion, of rumor and betrayal, with no obvious path of escape. It is primarily because intimate relationships are grounded in shared histories, expectations, secrets, and vulnerabilities that girls can truly betray, reject, or humiliate another. The impact of this traumatic experience forces the girl to relive all earlier developmental struggles related to her autonomy, her sense of initiative and competence, her underlying sense of identity, her self-esteem, and her capacity for intimacy (Herman, 1992). It is these issues that surface in the therapy relationship and become the focus for play therapy intervention.

THE AIMS OF PLAY THERAPY

Girls victimized by social aggression might seem likely to do anything to free themselves from such entanglements, but this rarely happens. First, girls often feel that they have somehow brought this rejection and humiliation on themselves. This perception adds to their self-doubt, self-blame, and uncertainty about how to proceed. They do not know what they did to get into this predicament, and they have no idea how to get out—they only know that they are desperate to do so. Second, since these girls often come to mistrust their experience and judgment (e.g., the Aggressor says "I didn't really mean it," "We were only joking," or "You take things too seriously"), they cease to trust their own perspective. Third, such reassurances encourage girls to believe that what just happened was really only in their imaginations; they are desperate not to lose their social group and prefer minimizing or discounting their reactions to facing the painful possibility that their friends are no longer trustworthy and that they are no longer secure within their group. Finally, some girls who do make the effort to extricate themselves from being the identified Victim find that efforts to escape only serve to intensify the social connections that hold them, leaving them more stuck. Sometimes, a girl's attempts to ignore socially aggressive behavior or to respond with her own witty or cutting remarks, reactions often supported by well-meaning parents, teachers, and therapists, tend to increase the derision she faces.

The distress and trauma of social aggression, as described by Herman (1992) and Flashman (2003) disrupt a girl's sense of security, trust, connection with others, and ability to establish and trust the meaning of the painful experience as she understands it in the face of peer and adult pressure to dismiss it as unimportant. Therefore, any intervention in and treatment of social aggression must include in its approach an effort to restore functioning in these four basic domains and focus on

1. Establishing safety and helping girls create a sense of *security*
2. Creating an environment in which *trust* is established

3. Assisting girls as they *reconstruct the story* through describing their experiences in order to establish its true *meaning* and *significance* to each participant

4. Restoring the *connection* between the person traumatized and her peer community

It is of critical importance that the adults who implement programs targeting social aggression do not minimize its traumatic impact. Because the upsetting experience may be an aggregate of such discrete, covert communications as eye-rolling, not inviting a girl to a party, or creating instant-messaging rumors, it is easy for adults to perceive these events as somewhat inconsequential. By doing so, well-meaning parents, teachers, and other observers can inadvertently undermine the Victim's sense of meaning, community, and support, further contributing to her upset and despair. It is equally critical for adults not to take on roles that are overly active, directive, and instructive. Observers of social aggression can see the disruption, distress, and suffering that its interchanges engender and may understandably wish to bring such interchanges to a quick close and to smooth over differences. One can recognize an adult's wish to fix the problem and help a girl move away from her own discomfort in the process, but by doing so, the helper inadvertently returns to "making nice," a typical response but one that rarely addresses the real issues. What needs to be brought into sharp focus are "the meanings that the adult world does not like to hear" (Flashman, 2003, p. 73). Flashman (2003) suggests that when children who are humiliated or traumatized are helped to calm down, rather than to bravely explore the meaning of their experience, they may feel silenced and become confused. In order to avoid such pitfalls, it is essential that potential helping adults understand their own relational experiences. Only then can they be what children and adolescents need them to be: mentors and trailblazers, willing to take risks in relationships and speak their own truth (Underwood, 2003; Wiseman, 2002).

To help girls recover from the impact of social aggression, neither repairing relationships alone nor teaching girls how to talk with one another in more positive or supportive ways nor teaching social competency and conflict resolutions skills will suffice. The goal of any intervention or prevention activity related to social aggression must be to reconstruct the network of relationships that was damaged. The events must be examined, attending to the girl's loss of trust and security, shared and accepted meaning regarding the traumatic event, and connection to a sustaining peer group. Restoring security, trust, and a meaningful connection to others involves repetitive practice of those skills that are essential to a personal sense of well-being and to healthy interpersonal relationships. Attending to the primary experiences that are disrupted by social aggression, cultivating core strengths, and helping girls reconstruct their stories inoculates girls against the most troubling impact of such interpersonal trauma and can also establish preventive communities of support well in advance of those occasions when social aggression reoccurs.

STORYTELLING IN PLAY THERAPY

Storytelling is at the heart of all therapy. In play therapy, whether using puppets, art therapy, or miniatures in sand trays, children and adolescents reveal their daily lives and inner experience through their verbal and nonverbal stories. Therefore, whether in individual therapy, group therapy, or as part of a comprehensive intervention program in a school or other facility, the use of narrative techniques is highly recommended. Siegel (1999) writes, "The telling of stories has a central place in human cultures throughout the world. . . . What is so special about stories? Why are we as a species so consumed by the process of telling and listening to stories?" (pp. 60–61). Telling stories captures and relates the essence of personal experience. Whether reading a story, passing along anecdotes about one's family, or telling about experiences that reveal the unusual twists and turns of relationships, storytelling imparts the history and culture of families and groups, strengthening the memories and perspectives of parents or grandparents and initiating youngsters into the fold of their particular group. Telling a story lends structure to events that might otherwise seem random and meaningless and can be a profound medium for facilitating change through expressing and altering a girl's view of her personal history.

Whether directed or undirected, storytelling activities encourage, support, and strengthen a child's ability to reflect on how he or she is feeling and how others are experiencing shared events.

> One way that young children process their lived experience is through pretend play. By creating scenarios of imagined and lived experiences, they are able to practice new skills and assimilate the complex emotional understandings of the social world in which they live. Creating stories through play [helps the] mind to "make sense" of our experiences and consolidate this understanding into a picture of our selves in the world. (Siegel & Hartzell, 2003, p. 36).

Storytelling helps children acquire an ability to cope with challenges, stresses, and puzzling circumstances by encouraging them imaginatively to spin out their thoughts, daydreams, hopes, and fears. These images can be arranged and rearranged, and children can explore, review, fantasize about what fits, revise their stories, and gradually try out and integrate new perspectives and experiences.

Utilizing narrative storytelling techniques encourages the natural unfolding of the play therapy process with the aim of healing. The play therapist creates a safe environment within which girls can begin to identify painful experiences previously dismissed as not worthy of attention and to play with different scenarios that restructure interactions and suggest more positive outcomes. As a result of this process, girls who have experienced or participated in social aggression can come to understand their experience in its fullness and their reactions to the motivations of others who were involved. This ability to identify one's ideas and feelings and to recognize the different but equally meaningful experiences of others brings girls out of a fixed, angry, isolated, or shamed position and facilitates their return to emotional and interpersonal vitality—free to move around in their internal as well as their external world, no longer trapped in the web of known but unsatisfying relationships from which they were afraid to depart.

Storytelling not only helps children identify and resolve challenges they are currently facing; it also shapes the ways in which past experiences are remembered and recounted. Though it is widely known that a girl's self-narrative carries important implications for the way she will react and behave, it appears that the ways in which events are recalled and retold also influences establishing new schemas of understanding, feeling, and experiencing (Siegel, 1999). Storytelling influences interpersonal and internal experiences and perspectives and simultaneously changes the underlying neural pathways that transmit information to the brain, carving "enduring patterns of knowledge into the developing circuits of the mind" (Lewis, Amini, & Lannon, 2000, p. 99). Thus, the brain undergoes ongoing structural change based on experiences that are stored in memory. These memories become prototypes or schemas (i.e., neural templates) for understanding the landscape of who one is and the landscape of relationships. Essentially, girls memorize the lessons of relationships learned throughout childhood and seek out that model or "archetype" (Lewis et al., 2000, p. 150) in all relational encounters. As Lewis et al. (2000) and Siegel (1999; Siegel & Hartzell, 2003) observe, children are more likely to choose to remain in an unhappy or painful relationship that their "brain recognizes over the stagnant pleasure of a 'nice' relationship with someone" their neural networks do not recognize as an established relationship pattern (Lewis et al., 2000, p. 163).

Our neural networks establish a bias toward a certain type of experience, a certain type of response, and a certain interpretation of the meaning of events.

> Through repeated experiences [with others] . . . our mind creates models that affect our view of both others and ourselves. . . . The models create a filter that patterns the way we channel our perceptions and construct our responses. . . . [That is], through these filtering models we develop characteristic ways of seeing and being. (Siegel & Hartzell, 2003, p. 23)

These mental models reflect a girl's beliefs about herself and others and "create the themes the stories tell and organize the ways in which [girls] make life decisions" (Siegel & Hartzell, 2003, p. 51). For example, if a girl's social relationships have been undermined, her vigilance and reactivity to such events is heightened, and her experience will operate as a mental model or lens, the belief system that shapes what she will anticipate in future encounters with girls. Siegel and Hartzell (2003) suggest that "the shadows that . . . mental models cast upon our decisions and the stories we tell about our life can be made explicit through [such] focused self-reflections" as storytelling and journal writing (p. 52). "Such a conscious process can deepen self-understanding and may be a way to alter mental models" (p. 52) that facilitate ongoing change and development throughout life.

It is this bias that we are attempting to reshape through storytelling in play therapy, where participants can take on different roles, consider, practice, and encode the experience of different considerations, perspectives, actions, and outcomes, so as to open each child to new possibilities, emotional experiences, and relationship patterns. Clearly, this is one of the primary requirements of meaningful play therapy: to facilitate the acquisition of new images and possibilities that create new neural pathways over time that are used more and more frequently and gradually predominate in each individual's neural networks or schemas. If established patterns for understanding experiences and interpersonal relationships are not altered, previously well-established styles of responding to distress and relating to others remain fixed. Impervious to logic or alternate behaviors deemed more promising by adults, this type of emotional knowledge is doggedly implicit once it is encoded in the brain and comes to dominate each girl's worldview. What this tells us is that "describing good relatedness to someone, no matter how precisely or how often, does not *inscribe* it into the neural networks" that help to create a change in self-perception and relationship patterns (Lewis et al., 2000, p. 177). Instead, "as subtle changes accrue . . . experience methodically rewires the brain, and the nature of what it *has* seen dictates what it *can* see" (Lewis et al., 2000, p. 135).

Storytelling in play therapy presents opportunities to focus on a girl's narrative, providing the mindful, focused attention necessary for her to comprehend the meaning of experiences and creating the neurological opportunity to develop new patterns for seeking out and enjoying positive, meaningful relationships, developing new methods of understanding, and resolving relational distress. This approach fosters the reconstructive aspect of memory that enhances a child's narrative sense of self. That is, storytelling not only helps children to identify and resolve challenges they are currently facing, but it also facilitates the way in which past experiences are remembered and recounted (Siegel, 1999). Storytelling, role playing, journal writing, and interactive exercises all contribute to the ongoing experiences that "gradually transform a [girl's] neural configuration, changing [her] from who [she] was into who she is, one synapse at a time" (Lewis et al., 2000, p. 151). Lewis et al. (2000) observe, "The *sine qua non* of a neural network is its penchant for strengthening neural patterns in direct proportion to their use" (p. 143).

Further, storytelling between individuals who have experienced a rupture in their relationship is also potentially healing and facilitates conflict resolution. Siegel (1999) observes, "repair requires the recognition that a rupture has occurred in the attunement process, and the [subsequent] realignment of states between the two individuals" or the group of individuals involved (p. 291). The repair process is an interactive one, requiring the openness of all in attempts to reconnect after the rupture. Storytelling is thus an essential ingredient in rewriting one's personal perceptions and stories and in rewiring one's neural pathways to create change in one's schemas or internal working models that affect what one anticipates and how one is likely to behave, having an impact on change in the domain of "interpersonal neurobiology" (Siegel & Hartzell, 2003, p. 3). The opportunity to tell one's original story and try out new or revised stories creates a blueprint or template for new behavior. In editing our narratives, we change the organization and nature of our memories, and reorganize our brains as well as our minds. This is a central endeavor in many forms of psychotherapy (Cozolino, 2002), the process by which girls come to create new, healthier relational possibilities. These repeated opportunities to create new stories and a new self-narrative are essential to changing a girl's perceptions and behaviors.

Play therapy approaches that address the loss of security and trust, the disruption of connections to others, and one's personal understanding of the meaning of experiences can be readily adapted to various populations and settings, including individuals or groups of girls who are part of a social network, participating in therapy, or placed in residential centers, hospitals, park district programs, or after-school or school-based programs, and several approaches that work effectively with this population are described below.

PLAY THERAPY CONSIDERATIONS: WHO SHOULD PARTICIPATE?

It is often characteristic of school-based and other group programs to identify particular students with "problem behaviors" to participate in intervention programs. Although one can understand the temptation to select those students who are involved as Aggressors or Victims of social aggression and provide them with the skills needed to resolve conflicts and build strong interpersonal connections, decades of research and practice indicate that this is an inefficient and ineffective approach. School-based mental health initiatives, as described by Adelman and Taylor (1999), emphasize the importance of comprehensive, inclusive programs that embrace entire cohorts, addressing systemic issues within the systems in which they occur.

The early results of research conducted with The Games Girls Play©️ program clearly demonstrate the difficulties encountered if only problem girls are identified for inclusion in such a program as opposed to the powerful interactions encouraged and supported when an entire cohort participates. When only problem girls are selected for intervention, the group operates without the entire social network of participants, inevitably weakening optimal outcomes. Girls who view themselves as Aggressors tend to band together with little insight or motivation to explore their actions, while girls who view themselves as Victims are typically presented with suggestions for responding to bullies or ignoring what is said or done. In either case, there is no opportunity for girls in disagreement to explore their experiences and learn from one another. Rather, the identity with which they enter the group tends to remain fixed, with little room to participate in new experiences and create new perspectives. Particularly in cases of social aggression, it is the entire cohort that participates, even if most are only Bystanders. Since the roles that girls assume in the drama of social aggression are fluid, with the Queen Bee vulnerable to becoming a Victim, with Bystanders anticipating and dreading their turn as Victim, and Bystanders or Floaters moving back and forth between the Aggressor and her Allies and the girl or group currently under siege, it is suggested that group interventions include a cohort of girls (e.g., an entire classroom, an entire grade of girls) to incorporate all the players and shifting alliances. After all, girls know that they could easily be the next one targeted and that they occasionally treat others in ways that are hurtful, exclusionary, or humiliating.

PLAY THERAPY APPROACHES

Narrative techniques such as telling stories using interactive cards and journal writing as a means of identifying and expressing feelings and experiences are extremely helpful and important because they invite imagination as an intermediate step to action. By using these techniques, a girl can consider, revise, and reconstruct what will facilitate her desired outcome, consider what might impede that outcome, and reflect on her own emotions, beliefs, and ideas about the events that have occurred. It is in this potential space where the possibility for change exists and creativity occurs that can lead to effective problem solving, renewed hope, and, ultimately, resilience.

Three excellent techniques suited to narrative therapy that can be used in individual or group settings are the OH card sets, The Games Girls Play cards, and journal writing using pages designed with evocative images and messages that encourage a girl to tell her own story. Elements of these programs are incorporated below into two school-based programs created to use play therapy techniques in an intervention and prevention program specifically targeting social aggression among girls.

Using Visual Images to Enhance Storytelling in Play Therapy

The use of pictures to prompt storytelling is well established as a projective technique to understand better how an individual sees herself and the world in which she lives. Although storytelling can be facilitated in a variety of ways, the personal images and stories evoked by art invite girls into something deeply felt, resonate with timeless archetypes, and propel them toward new ways of seeing and being. Why use art to facilitate storytelling? Moore (1996) writes, "art facilitates gaining intimacy" with our inner sense of ourselves, "and if we live from such a deep place, alienation and anxiety diminish, replaced by a sense of connection to our humanity and that of others" (p. 202).

Using visual images to enhance the processing of emotional experiences can be extremely helpful. First, visual images engage the brain's left hemisphere, bypassing language centers and facilitating new emotional observations and connections. In the case of girls who are in the habit of saying things like "It really doesn't matter" or "I'm just making too big a deal out of this," when looking at a picture that evokes a memory of something that happened to them, creates an opportunity to experience an emotional response too powerful to deny. This helps girls understand the strength and truth of their perspective, even when its accuracy is denied or refuted by their socially aggressive peers. Second, most people (even children) rely on the left hemisphere of the brain, which processes language, much more than the right hemisphere, which processes visual-spatial stimuli. Between on-line chats, instant messaging, and phone conversations, children are bombarded with opportunities to exercise their left hemispheres, whereas the common visual-spatial experiences of the past, such as enjoying unstructured play for hours at a time, are in short supply. The combination of

> verbal and nonverbal expressions of emotion, activates and utilizes processing of both left and right hemispheres, as well as cortical and sub-cortical processing. This simultaneous activation may be what is required for wiring and rewiring through the simultaneous or alternating activation of feelings, thoughts, behaviors and sensations. (Cozolino, 2002, pp. 169–170)

Incorporating visual imagery into play therapy allows children to fully integrate the visual and verbal experiences encoded in the right and left hemispheres of the brain, which fosters a sense of wholeness and overall well-being.

The OH interactive card sets created by Moritz Egetmeyer and described by Kirschke (1997), are decks of standard-sized cards intended for creative and playful use. Each set is created by a different artist and is colorful, compelling, and evocative. Some feature human faces, some feature individuals interacting with each other or with the environment, some tap into magical and mythical themes, and some are abstract. All are highly sensitive to cultural and ethnic diversity. While these sets of cards were not intended to be therapeutic tools, therapists worldwide have found them helpful in their work with clients of all ages. Telling stories prompted by images such as those provided in the interactive card sets allows participants to experience art, with its accompanying archetypes, symbols, and iconic images, and then use these images to explore their own inner landscapes. Using the cards as prompts to tell stories creates a bond between players who work together and facilitates an integration of emotions, thoughts, and disparate feelings in the individual who works with the cards on her own or in a group. Below are some suggestions for using this tool when helping girls process the experience of social aggression.

Interactive storytelling cards are suitable for use with an individual, child, or adolescent and a therapist or for use in groups with or without a facilitator. Generally, in our work, card sets are used in the presence of a Shared Vision trained staff member who follows the storytelling process as it unfolds. Cards can be placed face up or face down in front of the participants. We initially thought the girls would prefer to select images from a face-up display but found they actually preferred selecting random, face-down cards for exercises whenever possible. Girls expressed liking the idea that they weren't "responsible" for the image with which they would begin a story, making initial storytelling efforts feel more impersonal and accidental and less revealing. Girls can also be instructed to tell stories that begin with "once upon a time" or "a long time ago," introductions that set the story safely in the past, inviting a more playful, make-believe atmosphere in which to explore their ideas, feelings, and relationships.

In exercises designed for groups of girls, each participant can tell part of a story and select other girls in the group with whom she will work out solutions to the challenge or dilemma she is describing. In these interactions, a girl can ask for assistance or suggestions about how to solve a particular problem, appointing other group members to assume the role of Bystander, Ally, or Aggressor and to pick a card or cards that help them to create their portion of the story. The conditions for group storytelling focus on exploring and establishing conditions of trust, security, and connection. This works equally well for girls involved in any aspect of social aggression since all the girls need and value security and support to maintain their place in the peer group.

As Jung noted regarding active imagination, it can be helpful in storytelling exercises to suggest that a girl or group of girls concentrate on a disturbing experience with social aggression and wait until a visual image appears with which to start a story. The girls "must make the emotional state the basis or starting point" of the story (Jung, 1917/1958, par. 167, as cited in Chodorow, 1997, p.7). Prior to asking a child to tell a story we might ask her to think about something currently stirring her thoughts or feelings or, more specifically, to select one or more images that feel related to something with which she is struggling. Then she could select card images to facilitate expressing the story she has in mind. As with active imagination, sometimes a card leaps out of the array, speaking to a storyteller before she knows what the story will be; on other occasions, the story is present, and the storyteller must seek out just the right cards to represent her ideas.

In our work with children experiencing social aggression as well as other challenges that prompt their referral to play therapy, they repeatedly tell us when presented with the opportunity to tell stories, "I didn't know I could do that!" or "I didn't know I was going to tell *that* story," surprising themselves with their creativity, accomplishment, and personal discovery and feeling pride and self-satisfaction at finding their own words. As Thomas Moore (1996) observes, "in psychotherapy, I have always believed that finding good words to describe a problem might be more important than coming up with explanations and solutions" (p. 243).

A general set of instructions guides the use of images and prompts that facilitate storytelling for an individual or group of girls (Lawrence & Jacobi, 2005). It is important in all group storytelling that participants accept each girl's story without alteration so that everyone can be listened to and experience others hearing their perspective. The facilitator and others present are encouraged to ask thoughtful questions that help clarify their understanding of the storyteller's perspective. Rather than inviting other participants to tell the storyteller what she ought to say or do, it is more helpful to suggest that she select another girl in the group to pick a card and tell a story about what might be helpful in the dilemma described. This serves to maintain support and create trust, respect, and connection. Although we are suggesting the use of particular card sets that facilitate storytelling, the girls might want to collect their own images from magazines, clip art, or their own representations to facilitate any of the exercises described. Images can be placed face down or face up, as the participants choose or as needed for a specific exercise. Girls can choose one or more images to complete their portion of the story. If a girl picks a card that is face down and she doesn't like the image or feel that she can tell a story in response, she is encouraged to pick other cards until she finds one that is suitable for her. The following describes various storytelling exercises suitable for individual or group use.

Ice Breaker

When groups of girls come together, their prior alliances or misalliances often dictate who will talk—or listen—to whom. In this playful exercise, any set of picture cards or images is placed face down in the center of the group. Each girl is asked to select a card or image that she will not look at until it is her turn to participate. One girl is asked to start a story in which the entire group will participate. The instructions are to look at the image on the card she selected and tell a story that uses associations with the image presented. One could suggest that the girls use such phrases as "once upon a time" or "long ago and far away" to emphasize the fantasy element of the story that is going to be told. Not only does this help girls feel that they do not have to talk about a specific problem right away, but it also helps them feel playful together. The girl to the right or left of the one who initiated the story is then asked to look at her card and continue the story. This process continues around the circle until each girl has an opportunity to participate in creating this group story. In this interactive, cooperative process that introduces the work of the group, each girl gets to hear some element of what she contributed to the story repeated by all the girls in the group.

Feeling and Coping

For this exercise, the OH interactive card sets suggested include the COPE, MYTHOS, and SAGA decks. Each participant is asked to select three cards: the first represents a problem that she has had with another girl or group of girls, the second represents her immediate emotional reaction to the problem, and the third represents how she could deal with her feelings and/or the problem. Each girl takes a turn showing the images she has chosen and explaining their meaning to her.

Finding Support

For this exercise, either the OH or PERSONA card set is recommended. Each participant is asked to select a portrait card that represents someone to whom she could turn for help and support if she was having a problem with a close friend or group of friends. Each girl in turn shows the portrait she picked and talks about her supportive helper. Girls can be encouraged to talk about the qualities they find in peers with whom they encounter difficulty, the qualities they look for in someone who can be helpful, and how they can seek out more supportive peers.

For this second exercise, the COPE, PERSONA, MYTHOS, or SAGA card set is recommended. A girl is asked to volunteer to relate a personal experience with socially aggressive behavior from the position of Aggressor, Ally, Bystander, Floater or Victim. Selecting cards that help her depict her experience, she is asked to choose four helpers, two who sit on either side of her to offer security and two who sit across from her to acknowledge the meaning of her experience. The volunteer assumes "responsibility for enlisting the help of others in creating her own safe environment" (Flashman, 2002, p. 79); she is encouraged to make use of her helpers, but they must check with her to see if the help they want to offer is what she needs. The helpers can either offer observations and responses on their own, or they can select one or more cards or images to explain how they see the situation, what they think would be helpful to its resolution, and what would be supportive to the girl telling about the experience. The other group members, observers of this process, are expected to contribute to this safe space within which new perspectives, new connections, and new outcomes can be established through attentive and respectful listening.

Friends and Enemies

The OH card sets PERSONA and HABITAT are recommended for this exercise, although girls may choose to use a combination of images from different sources.

Each girl is asked to select a card or two that represent people she would like to have as friends and another card or two that represent people she feels might be enemies. Each girl in turn shows her cards and explains why she chose them and how she views friendships.

Identities: The Masks We Wear

In this exercise, the PERSONA or HABITAT set or a combination of card sets and other images can be used. Each girl is asked to select three images: one that represents the me others see, one that represents the me no one sees, and one that represents the me the girl would like other people to know. Each girl in turn shows her cards and talks about her outer and inner identities. This exercise can be expanded to include the selection of an image of a girl or girls who they consider friends; participants talk about how they think this girl sees them and how this is similar to or different from how they believe others see them.

While we have found the OH card sets very useful to invite individual introspection and group discussion among girls about their experiences of social aggression, we were intrigued by the idea of creating a visually powerful game that focuses more specifically on these experiences. We wanted images of specific stressors associated with social aggression, such as exclusion, shunning, gossiping, and spreading rumors through e-mail and instant messaging, and to include the various roles girls can take on in these experiences—the Aggressor, the Ally or Sidekick, the Victim, the Bystander, the Floater, etc. After sharing our ideas with artist Kathie Schefer, who specializes in computer-assisted artwork with anime-like images that represent stressful situations associated with social aggression, we created The Games Girls Play card game.

This game contains two sets of cards: (1) a set of colorful and original visual images depicting girls (and occasionally boys) in different situations, suggesting various feelings that evoke the experiences of social aggression, and (2) a set of prompts. These prompts present a particular question or dilemma and ask the participant who has drawn the prompt on her turn to choose an image from the picture cards that will help her connect to the question or dilemma and respond to it. Girls can either draw a card from the prompts and select picture images that go along with that situation to tell a story, or they can select a picture image or series of images to tell a story about an event and what they believe the girls in that story, including the Aggressors, Allies, Victims, and Bystanders, are thinking, feeling, saying, or planning. Here, storytelling encourages girls to strengthen their sense of identity, respect and responsibility for self and others, effective communication, and positive relationships. Facilitators can encourage girls to consider what choices or actions would promote trust, security, and a sense of connection with others.

For example, a player might draw a prompt card that says, "The other girls begin talking badly about a friend of yours who was not invited to a sleepover. What do you say when they ask if you agree with them?" With a picture that represents girls with conspiratorial looks passing a note in class, a girl might tell a story to a prompt that says, "A girl who was recently ignored in the group sees two girls passing a note in class. How does she feel? What might she worry about?" Follow-up from a facilitator might include consideration of who could help in this situation, who or what might stand in the way, and what might help the girl feel reconnected to other girls. Suggestions about picture cards that might be appropriate or helpful are included on the prompt cards. Girls can also draw a card that describes the way in which a Bystander, Ally, Target, or

Aggressor might behave. They are then encouraged to tell a second version of their story from the perspective of a different role. These opportunities to play the roles of others help participants become aware of the perspectives of other girls and try out new behaviors and points of view as they explore the internal life of the characters in the events described. This moves storytelling beyond a linear exposition and fosters "collaborative or contingent communication [that allows] us to expand our own minds by taking in others' points of view and seeing our own point of view reflected in their responses" (Siegel & Hartzell, 2003, p. 80). Facilitating reflective dialogue and feelings of connection with others, these storytelling experiences support empathic communication, the foundation for an enhanced sense of security, insight, awareness, and the attunement to and compassion and respect for others that strengthen self-identity and the bonds among group members (Siegel & Hartzell, 2003).

The game includes many prompts, and their variety enables girls to explore all facets of their experiences. Negative and positive potential outcomes are included, and creating strategies for social problem solving is required. Some prompts are geared toward group play and interaction and are to be used specifically when the game is being played by a group of girls. For example, a player in a group might draw a prompt that says, "A girl has just been prevented from sitting at her regular lunch table. Choose a picture card to help you talk about how she feels, and then ask the player on your right to suggest what this girl could do about this." All players will have multiple turns to draw prompts and choose picture cards to help them perform the task set out by each prompt. It is important to keep in mind that the players are free to choose any picture card that strikes their imagination—the suggestions are merely aids to help players who might feel overwhelmed or have trouble choosing. It is also possible to play the game by drawing the picture cards at random from a face-down display, as they all evoke feelings related to the general topic of social aggression. Enhancing both self-awareness and empathy for the feelings of others is encouraged, as players are required both to express themselves verbally and to listen to others. The game offers girls multiple opportunities to play the roles of Aggressors, Allies, Bystanders, Floaters, or Victims and to look at events from multiple perspectives to develop an understanding of and empathy for the experiences of others. Storytelling interactions cultivate a network of relationships that support each girl's need for security and trust and create opportunities to look at events from multiple perspectives in order to develop understanding of and empathy for the experiences of others, fostering problem solving at individual and interpersonal levels.

The authors suggest that a group's initial experience with The Games Girls Play card game take place in the presence of an appropriate adult facilitator—a therapist, teacher, or counselor. Even a caring parent who wants to help his or her daughter process a challenging social experience might be the right facilitator for a particular girl. The game can be played in a group or one-on-one. Once girls get an idea about how the cards can be used to explore and address their personal experiences and develop some expressive and listening skills, they can play the game among themselves without a facilitator. Certainly, the use of images that directly relate to social aggression facilitates storytelling about this particular type of problem, whatever their source. It is our hope that these innovative therapy tools, which combine visual stimulation and verbal expression, will be useful both to girls experiencing the challenges of social aggression and to those helping them to develop effective coping skills.

Journal Writing to Enhance Storytelling in Play Therapy

An additional means of effective intervention for girls entangled in social aggression is the use of therapeutic journal writing. Journal writing, the use of reflective writing, is a highly effective way to explore and bring clarity to concerns and to assist personal development. Journal writing affords girls opportunities to recall challenging social experiences, express complicated emotions, and explore the meanings they create for relational losses. Through this introspective exercise, girls put their internal experiences into words and pictures and are prompted to create their own narrative version of emotionally charged events and interactions. Using journals, girls are able to form and view various perspectives, establish meaning and personal authenticity, and continue the healing process following the hurtful impact of social aggression. Research has demonstrated that "the writing down of material about emotionally traumatic experiences can lead to profound psychological and physiological changes associated with resolution" (Siegel & Hartzell, 2003, p. 27). Girls state that they like writing in journals because they can say whatever they think or feel without fear of being judged (Brown, 2003). Journal writing, however, serves more than the purpose of getting out what a girl is holding in without threat of reprisal. It is an extremely effective means by which a girl can develop her own narrative version of events and consider how to enter and maintain future relationships, and it contributes to change at the levels of interpersonal neurobiology and interpersonal relationships.

Therapeutic journaling can be either a structured or an unstructured activity. Several journals on the market (*Me and My Friends* [Klutz, 2004], or *The Games Girls Play Journal* [Lawrence, Condon, & Nicholson, 2004]) present girls with a combination of directive prompts and suggested exercises aimed at generating innovative ways to understand both successful friendships and episodes of social aggression. For instance, a girl may be asked to write about the ups and downs of female friendships. Other exercises may prompt her to recall a particularly memorable episode of social aggression, inviting her to describe the players involved in the event, her understanding of how the event unfolded, and both her actual and desired reactions to the event. In this way, girls are provided opportunities not only to retell experiences of, for instance, social exclusion or rumor mongering, but also to include what they wish they could have said or done and the outcomes they hope to create in the future. Additional journaling activities involve less structured prompts that simply provide the writer with an image depicting girls engaged in social aggression. The writer is given ample space to respond to the image in any way she chooses. Through these exercises, girls are actively engaged in activities that help them decipher the components of healthy relationships and the dynamics of social aggression and facilitate their engagement in social problem solving. These activities serve to reestablish the lost meaning, security, and trust that contribute to the traumatic impact of social aggression and strengthen girls' abilities to forge positive friendships in the future.

The use of journal writing can supplement both individual and group treatment, as it provides girls a safe space outside of the treatment hour to revisit or continue the therapeutic work. This may be particularly valuable for girls who are less apt to give voice to their feelings in a group setting, but benefit from a more private place to begin processing challenging or overwhelming emotions. Over time, this exercise in self-reflection and mindfulness about relationships facilitates growth in both individual and group treatment settings by:

- Offering new opportunities to reflect upon social aggression occurring within a girl's circle of friends
- Confirming a girl's trust in her version and experience of social events
- Facilitating healing of traumatic losses associated with social aggression
- Constructing novel ways of interpreting, understanding, and responding to socially aggressive acts in the future
- Cultivating a self-awareness that strengthens trust in one's own perspective and personal narrative

- Encouraging resilience to navigate social challenges successfully and move away from socially toxic relationships with confidence
- Awakening a girl's motivation to engage in healthy, supportive relationships

School-Based Intervention and Prevention Programs: Two Models

The Games Girls Play and Project P.E.E.R are both 10-week school-based intervention and prevention programs designed to be implemented with girls in middle school and high school. With a focus on helping girls recognize what social aggression is, what it feels like, how to deal with it, and how to move on to new friendships with optimism, the programs foster a sense of connection between girls and a sense of meaning about their experiences within a secure environment where trust can be established. While no one is suggesting that all girls must come to be good friends as a result of their participation, the programs facilitate acceptance of different points of view, respect for others, and respect for oneself.

The Games Girls Play

The Games Girls Play is part of a series of programs designed to address social aggression. This school-based or after-school 10- to 12-week program incorporates storytelling, journal writing, didactic training, professional coaching of peer groups, role playing with peers, and rehearsal and practice of new social skills. These elements in combination have been soundly demonstrated to be essential to effective intervention and prevention program training in a variety of school settings. Whereas storytelling activities contribute to developing a supportive, secure group environment, journal writing encourages program participants to be aware of their own emotions and reflect on relationships with peers when they are away from the group, thereby increasing a girl's sense of confidence and increasing her understanding of self and others.

We have learned through our experience working with children in a variety of school and clinical settings using play therapy that there are specific core strengths that facilitate positive peer relationships and creative problem solving strategies. We have identified six Core Strengths that help girls participate in healthy social relationships: (1) strong identity: know who you are and what you stand for; (2) respect: care for yourself and care for others; (3) resilience: bounce back from stress and change; (4) responsibility: at home, at school, with friends, in the community; (5) effective communication: solve problems and create solutions; and (6) positive relationships: work well, play well (Shared Vision, Inc., 2005). Our extensive experience shows that these qualities can be cultivated through play therapy in order to effectively address the profound impact of social aggression on girls' relationships. Developing these competencies helps girls restore their sense of trust, security, and connection and reconstruct the stories of their experiences in order to establish their meaning and significance. Such exercises conducted within a group support the interactional processes that are typically dismantled in the wake of social aggression.

- Week 1 begins with the girls enacting a skit from a prepared series of interchanges that represent typical social aggression interactions. This introduces girls to the issues involved in these destructive, hurtful behaviors and helps them recognize varied ways in which the messages of social aggression are communicated. Girls begin to identify qualities they look for in a good friend and characteristics they bring to their relationships. All remaining weekly activities incorporate such interactive experiences as storytelling and journal writing exercises that support the development of the six Core Strengths.
- Weeks 2 and 3 focus on the development of a strong identity, effective communication, and respect for self and others.
- Week 4 activities facilitate skill acquisition and experiences that emphasize listening and developing empathy.
- Week 5 activities focus on responsibility, building supportive groups, emphasizing team building, and considering how to become part of new groups.
- Weeks 6 and 7 directly address bullying, teasing, and social aggression, helping girls focus on identity, effective communication, respect, listening, and responsibility as these strengths affect how one might experience and respond to such behaviors.
- Week 8 emphasizes resilience, helping girls explore how they might bounce back from hurtful encounters.
- Week 9 consolidates the ongoing program focus on positive relationships within small groups and within the larger classroom.
- Week 10 concludes the group program with a focus on positive problem solving that invites girls to incorporate all of the six Core Strengths in their efforts to resolve difficulties in old relationships when possible and to recognize their abilities to face new challenges, engage in

new relationships, and revise their understanding of how relationships work best for them.

In the 12-week model, the first week is devoted to conducting pretest measures that identify the strengths and limitations each girl experiences relative to the six Core Strengths and explore each girl's awareness of the behaviors that characterize social aggression and its effect on her and her relationships. Week 12 is devoted to posttest measures to evaluate changes that occur over the course of this intervention and prevention program. Storytelling and journal writing activities are incorporated each week. These weekly exercises are designed to address the specific issues, social skills, and core strengths that are the focus for that week's discussion.

Project P.E.E.R.

The acronym P.E.E.R. stands for *Promoting Empathic Empowering Relationships*. Girls take part in a variety of activities, including a skit using a script that describes various interactions characteristic of social aggression, interactive exercises, role playing, and journal writing to allow each girl to explore her own experiences, ideas and reactions in a more private manner. All exercises are designed

- To help the participants learn about the behaviors in which they are engaging that are described as social aggression
- To practice techniques designed to assist development of effective coping skills to deal with peers with whom they do not get along
- To channel aggressive energies into rewarding, effective interactions

In order to understand fully the intensity and ramifications of social aggression, it is important to recognize and validate the importance of female friendships. To facilitate this, participants discuss the various roles, responsibilities, thoughts, and feelings friends maintain in everyday interactions. The girls also engage in open dialogues about their emotionally significant peer relationships. A particular focus of the weekly sessions is to raise awareness about the undermining behaviors in which some girls participate. This focus is intended to help girls identify what they value in a friend, how to evaluate the type of friend they are to others, how to recognize any behaviors they might engage in that are hurtful or destructive to others, and what they might do to resolve differences or more effectively choose girls who have the qualities necessary to be their good friends. The groups are always provided a variety of vignettes describing social aggression to foster discussion. Our experience suggests, however, that although girls enjoy these generic prompts, they quickly set aside the general vignettes provided and talk about their specific experiences, interactions, and concerns.

Once the participants establish a sense of meaning about their experiences and the program exercises support a growing sense of trust and connection, the girls are ready to learn the skills that will help them know and respect themselves and others. Interactive exercises facilitate listening, empathizing, recognizing and expressing their emotions, and integrating effective conflict resolution strategies. When the girls believe that their peers are listening to and empathizing with them, they begin to feel more comfortable recognizing and expressing their genuine feelings, even such feelings as anger and jealousy that society does not encourage girls to express. The more the girls feel understood and at ease expressing their feelings, the better able they are to resolve their conflicts. Rather than shy away from confrontation out of fear that their peers will not listen or will fail to understand their perspective, participants learn how to resolve their conflicts in a respectful, effective, and genuine manner. The girls begin to learn how to express their points of view and their similarities and differences in a spirit of discovery and support rather than trying to gain power and control over one another.

CONCLUSION

The behaviors that characterize overt and covert social aggression are often overlooked and their impact dismissed or minimized. Spreading rumors, shunning, isolating and excluding a girl from her former group of friends, gossiping, and sending anonymous e-mail or instant messages all serve to separate girls from their peer group. Yet, girls are often told that they are taking an incident too seriously, that they are making more of not being included than was intended by their friends. When their perceptions are not validated or affirmed, girls may feel that they cannot trust their own judgment or appraisal of social situations, and their sense of the meaning of events is confused. However, social aggression *is* intended to disrupt the network of relationships and friendships on which girls rely to establish their sense of connection through meaningful relationships with others and to secure their core identity. Play therapy that introduces such interactive exercises as storytelling including card sets, role playing, skits, and journal writing facilitates restoration of trust, security, and girls' connections to each other that are disrupted by social aggression.

REFERENCES

Adelman, H., & Taylor, L. (1999). *A sampling of outcome findings from interventions relevant to addressing barriers to learning*. Los Angeles: School Mental Health Project, Department of Psychology, UCLA.

Brown, L. M. (2003). *Girlfighting*. New York: New York University Press.

Chodorow, J. (Ed.). (1997). *Encountering Jung: Jung on active imagination*. Princeton, NJ: Princeton University Press.

Cozolino, L. (2002). *The neuroscience of psychotherapy: Building and rebuilding the human brain*. New York: Norton.

Flashman, A. (2003). Israeli and Palestinian teachers learn about children and trauma: Security, connection and meaning. In O. Ayalon, M. Lahad, & A. Cohen (Eds.), *Community stress prevention* (Vol. 5, pp. 69–81). Israel: Community Stress Prevention Center.

Galen, B. R., & Underwood, M. K. (1997). A developmental investigation of social aggression among children. *Developmental Psychology, 33*, 589–600.

Herman, J. (1992). *Trauma and recovery*. New York: Basic Books.

Kirschke, W. (1997). *Strawberries beyond my window*. Victoria, British Columbia: OH Publishing—Eos Interactive Cards.

Klutz Press. (Ed.). (2004). *Me and my friends: The book of us*. Palo Alto, CA: Author.

Lawrence, M. M., Condon, K., & Nicholson, E. (2004). *The games girls play journal*. Oak Brook, IL: Shared Vision, Inc.

Lawrence, M. M., & Jacobi, K. S. (2005). *The playfulness of storytelling: A manual of interactive techniques*. Oak Brook, IL: Shared Vision, Inc.

Lewis, T., Amini, F., & Lannon, R. (2000). *A general theory of love*. New York: Vintage Books.

Moore, T. (1996). *The re-enchantment of everyday life*. New York: HarperCollins.

Shared Vision, Inc. (2005). *The games girls play program manual*. Unpublished document.

Siegel, D. (1999). *The developing mind: How relationships and the brain interact to shape who we are*. New York: Guilford Press.

Siegel, D., & Hartzell, M. (2003). *Parenting from the inside out*. New York: Jeremy P. Tarcher/Putnam.

Simmons, R. (2002). *Odd girl out*. New York: Harcourt.

Thompson, M., & Grace, C. (2001). *Best friends, worst enemies*. New York: Ballantine Books.

Underwood, M. K. (2003). *Social aggression among girls*. New York: Guilford Press.

Wiseman, R. (2002). *Queen Bees and wannabes*. New York: Three Rivers Press.

CHAPTER 10

Culturally Competent Play Therapy with the Mexican American Child and Family

ROBERTO ROBLES

According to the President's New Freedom Commission on Mental Health (2003) people of color will comprise at least 40% of the U.S. population by 2025. In certain metropolitan areas, this is already the case. The commission has further noted that the

> mental health system has not kept pace with the diverse needs of racial and ethnic minorities, often underserving or inappropriately serving them. Specifically, the system has neglected to incorporate respect, or understanding of the histories, traditions, beliefs, languages, and value systems of culturally diverse groups. (2003, p. 49)

The American Psychological Association (APA, 2005), the Association for Play Therapy (APT, 2000), and the National Association of Social Workers (NASW, 1996) have all adopted guidelines that address ethnic and cultural diversity. One principle identified by the APA (2005) concerns development of interventions that complement the client's background. The APT (2000) indicates that a play therapist should use interventions geared to the client's culture. The NASW (1996) outlines several principles in its code of ethics with regard to responsibilities social workers have to their clients, such as providing culturally sensitive services.

Demographically, Hispanics/Latinos account for a sizable percentage of the nation's population growth:

> The nation's Hispanic population reached 41.3 million as of July 1, 2004, according to national estimates by race, Hispanic origin and age released

today by the U.S. Census Bureau. Hispanics, who may be of any race, accounted for about one-half of the national population growth of 2.9 million between July 1, 2003, and July 1, 2004. The Hispanic growth rate of 3.6 percent over the 12-month period was more than three times that of the total population (1.0 percent). (Bernstein, 2005, p. 1)

According to Ramirez and De La Cruz (2002) more than one in eight people in the United States is currently of Hispanic origin (p. 1). In the West[1], 44% are Hispanic and 19.2% are non-Hispanic white (Ramirez & De La Cruz, 2002, p. 2). In the South[2], 34.8% are Hispanic and 33.3% are non-Hispanic white (Ramirez & De La Cruz, 2002, p. 2). Of this subgroup, the majority (nearly two-thirds) is of Mexican origin.

These numbers speak for the need for the mental health profession to address the unique needs of Mexican Americans, specifically the Mexican American child. Canino, Earley, and Rogler (1980), Rogler, Malgady, Costantino, and Blumenthal (1987), Martinez and Valdez (1992), and Hinman (2003) have all identified the need to develop and provide appropriate approaches for culturally diverse child and family populations.

The focus of this chapter is the Mexican American child and family; however, the literature cited includes information about Hispanics and Latinos in general. The primary aim of this chapter is to identify and describe specific tools and techniques that can be used with the Mexican American child and family. These ideas might be transferable to children and families of other Hispanic descent. This chapter by no means covers all aspects of working with the Mexican American child and family. A brief review of the literature is presented that covers assessment issues and play therapy with the Hispanic/Mexican American child. Following this, a discussion about how to engage the family is provided and some tools and techniques a therapist can use to conduct a culturally congruent assessment and treatment are identified. Case examples are provided to illustrate the use of these tools and followed by a discussion about treatment retention issues and measures that may help maintain necessary ongoing involvement of Mexican American children and families in the treatment process. Finally, future research needs are laid out.

LITERATURE REVIEW OF ASSESSMENT ISSUES

A few studies are reviewed below regarding the Mexican American child and family, including a detailed review by Mejia (1983). The Mexican

American family is not static, but dynamic, and there are multiple types of Mexican American families as there are multiple types of all American families (Arroyo, 1997; Ramirez, 1998).

Ramirez (1998) has written in depth about what seems to characterize the Mexican American family. He cites several features and offers suggestions with regard to facilitating engagement of families in the treatment process. He notes, for instance, that Mexican American families have strong extended families. Godparents may play important roles as part of the extended family—a child may have a different set of godparents for nearly every major religious event (baptism, first communion, confirmation, marriage)—if the family is Catholic (Arroyo, 1997).

With regard to parent–child relationships, Ramirez (1998) states that the household is centered on the preschool-age child. He goes on to describe how the relationship between the child and his or her parents may be perceived as more important than the relationship between mother and father. He also notes that children are treated differently based on their sex; parents place more restrictions on their female adolescents than on males of the same age (Ramirez, 1998). This system is often a source of conflict for female adolescents, who clearly verbalize the inequity of this situation.

Arroyo (1997) also discusses the Mexican American child and family as well. Some of issues he identifies and discusses are language, racial and ethnic identity, and family structure. He reports that the Spanish-speaking child tends to identify with traditional Mexican culture at a higher level than the non–Spanish-speaking child. Bernal, Knight, Garza, Ocampo, and Cota (1990) also document this finding. Arroyo notes that there has not been much research on the acquisition of racial and ethnic identity in Mexican American children, even though by age six or seven these children can identify to which group they belong (Bernal et al., 1990). In terms of family structure, Arroyo (1997) identifies how Mexican American family members assist in the raising of children.

A few authors have identified characteristics found in the Mexican American family. Some Hispanic males espouse *machismo*, which is characterized by the adult male exhibiting and exerting dominant authority over his family and females (Falicov, 1998; Ramirez & Arce, 1981). Mejia (1983) also discusses this phenomenon. Regarding family values, many Hispanic families value interdependence rather than independence. Sue and Sue (1999) and Phinney (1996) have also documented how many Mexican American/Hispanic families value interdependence and place family needs above individual needs. Mexican American families have and exhibit preferences for particular children. For example, it is not uncommon for Mexican American parents to place a higher value on lighter skinned children (Hopkins, Huici, & Bermudez, 2004) and male children. This may stem from early Mexican history when the darker skin tone was associated with indigenous peoples who were thought to be inferior. Another equally important phenomenon is acculturation. Within families and among different families, there are often different levels of acculturation; this can lead to a problematic relationship between parents and their children (Sluzski, 1979). Arroyo (1997) provides several scales that can help define acculturation levels in children and adults.

The manner in which someone seeks help in times of need often sheds light on how much he or she espouses traditional beliefs. It is common for the Mexican American family to seek help through the church or within the family. When this fails, parents seek other providers, such as *curanderos* (folk healers).

MENTAL HEALTH SERVICES IN MEXICO

In order to comprehend the health-seeking behaviors observed in Mexican American families, it is crucial to understand who provides services in Mexico and how. In Mexico, there are at least four systems that provide mental health–related services to children and families. In the larger urban areas, el Sistema Nacional para el Desarrollo Integral de la Familia (DIF) (the National System for the Integral Development of the Family) provides a number of mental health and social services to individuals and families who do not have other means (DIF, 2005). The DIF is equivalent to the department of social services, alcohol and drug department, services for the disabled, and county mental health combined. The second system is known as el Seguro Social (Social Security) and provides a full range of services to state and federal employees, similar to a Health Maintenance Organization (HMO). For example, if a child has a mental health condition, the primary care doctor can refer the child to specialty mental health services. The third system is the private sector: psychiatrists and psychologists. Social workers do not provide psychotherapeutic services in Mexico, as they do in the United States. Services generally can be easily accessed in well-populated urban areas if the families are open to seeking them and have the means to cover the transportation costs; however, those families who live in rural areas have fewer options. In rural areas, families often rely on obtaining help from one another, the church, or *curanderos*, which, together, constitute the fourth type of system.

SEEKING HELP IN THE UNITED STATES

Once in the United States, some Mexican American parents seek traditional providers before seeking services from a mental health professional. When the family seeks a *curandero*, the treatment might consist of practicing an elaborate ritual. For instance, the *curandero* might pass an uncooked egg or herbs over the child's body for a cleansing, while reciting a prayer. Tharp and Meadow's (1973) article discusses their study with 250 Mexican American families. They examined traditional ailments and folk remedies provided by *curanderos* and found that the majority of the participants believed the supposed origins of several Mexican folk diseases, including those of emotional nature, such as *susto*, which occurs when the self and the body separate; *bilis*, which occurs when the body's four positions become unbalanced; *mal ojo* (the evil eye) and *mal puesto*, which occur when an individual is victimized by witchcraft. Through the process of acculturation, those traditional beliefs change.

Researchers have indicated that there is both a high and low rate of belief in *curanderismo*, *Espiritismo*, and *Santería* for Latinos. Baez and Hernandez (2001) provide a concise overview of the literature about these three practices. *Espiritismo* is a spiritual belief system in which a person can become subject to good or bad spirits. Practitioners use various methods to treat an individual. *Santería*'s origins are from *Ifa*, a religion practiced in Nigeria; it is more common in the Caribbean than in Mexico.

It is important to explore these belief systems tactfully, but in depth. Simply asking about this area is not sufficient. Mental health professionals often determine if the client has beliefs in *curanderismo*, *Espiritismo*, or *Santería* but nothing else. These providers might very well quickly assess by Western standards what is going on and begin to treat the condition rather promptly. This might carry a negative consequence for the individual, particularly if he or she has a life-threatening condition that requires a thorough workup.

Not all Mexican American families seek traditional providers before consulting Western providers. Some parents may seek professional mental health services first, then decide on a traditional provider after. When Mexican American families seek treatment, some do so cautiously.

LITERATURE REVIEW OF PLAY THERAPY

This section includes some basic information about play therapy principles and reviews the play therapy literature as it relates to the Mexican American, Latino, and Hispanic child. According to Axline (1947) and

Landreth (1982) the child expresses him- or herself and his or her problems through play.

Child therapy literature dealing with Hispanic children is minimal. There are basically two groups of literature: empirically based and nonempirically based. Costantino, Malgady, and Rogler (1986) and Trostle (1988) conducted empirical studies. Costantino et al. (1986) studied 210 Puerto Rican families, dividing them into three groups. One group was treated with *cuento* therapy, another group with traditional therapy, and the third group received no treatment. The *cuento* therapy treatment approach is based upon the use of Puerto Rican traditional stories to help bicultural children value and cope with being in two worlds. Using this model, they found that aggression and anxiety were considerably reduced with the *cuento* therapy group and that the children improved in the area of academic comprehension. Trostle (1988) studied 48 Puerto Rican children newly arrived in New York. He looked at how group play sessions affected free play, self-control, and social ratings and found that children who had group play sessions fared better than the control group children.

The second set of literature, which is nonempirically based, describes techniques and strategies or provides models to be used with the Hispanic child. Martinez and Valdez (1992) developed a structured play therapy model to be used with Hispanic children. In this model, children are expected to discover themselves by using different structured situations that involve cultural elements to help the children strengthen their ethnic identity. One way Martinez and Valdez propose to engage the children is to talk to them in Spanish, even though they might speak English functionally. They also provide a list of materials to be used with the Hispanic child.

Hopkins et al. (2004) discuss their work with sexually abused Hispanic children. They report that there is a need to incorporate several modalities (individual, family, and group) when treating this population. They emphasize the importance of becoming familiar with Hispanic culture and how it manifests in the individual family. They also identify several factors that the therapist should be aware of when working with the Hispanic family, such as respecting the family's values.

ENGAGEMENT

When the Spanish-speaking Mexican American family seeks treatment in public clinics, they may encounter posters and magazines in Spanish and, if they are lucky, pre-intake forms in Spanish. In the private sector, the family might find similar media, but what happens once the family enters the office? What messages are conveyed to the family by the therapist? Does the therapist have symbols that reflect the Mexican American family's experiences? Martinez and Valdez (1992) believe it is important to have items that the Mexican American family can identify. Hinman (2003) indicates that the physical setting where treatment is provided is often overlooked. She goes on to state that when the therapist only provides toys that speak to the dominant culture, it might

> serve as an inhibitor of communication for ethnic minority children. The use of toys that reflect Caucasian values may serve as an indication to the child that he or she is in a majority culture setting and his or her behavior needs to conform to what is considered appropriate in such a setting. (p. 117)

When the therapist shows sensitivity to the Mexican American family by displaying pictures and games that the parent recognizes, the parent feels welcomed in a nonverbal manner.

There are several ways to engage the Mexican American child and family in therapy; the first and most important involves making a connection with the family. With the Mexican American family, some argue that it is important to practice what is known as *personalismo*. Ramirez (1998) defines this as projecting personal contact and warmth to the family. *Personalismo* could be shown by greeting the father with a handshake followed by one for the mother and a gentle touch on the child's shoulder. In this manner, the therapist also conveys respect for the family hierarchy (Ramirez, 1998).

Beginning the session with light conversation prior to discussing sensitive topics (Hopkins et al., 2004) conveys to the parents that the therapist is *bien educado* (well-educated) in the social graces of the culture. With the underprivileged family, one might ask about any barriers that the family encountered on the way to the appointment. For instance, did they have any transportation problems or trouble finding the office? McCabe (2002) recommends that the therapist address the possible barrier issues at the beginning of the session. When a therapist asks about these issues, he or she conveys a genuine interest to the family.

To conduct a thorough assessment, ask about language, indigenous background, immigration status, religion, and treatment approaches. When evaluating the Mexican American family and child, it is vital to put aside preconceived notions and stereotypes. For instance, one should not assume that the parents speak Spanish or that the child speaks English.

For those therapists who speak Spanish fluently, it is important initially to use the formal rather than the informal verb tense when working with the family. Later, once rapport is established, the therapist may ask the parents about switching to the informal verb tense. The child may or may not address the therapist in the formal manner. Mexican American children are strongly encouraged to respect their elders, however. One way the child may demonstrate this is by using the formal verb tense.

With regard to language, some Mexican American parents may be bilingual (in Spanish and an indigenous language) or trilingual (indigenous language, Spanish, and English). It is estimated that 13% of the Mexican population belongs to an indigenous group, and there are 62 recognized indigenous languages that are spoken in Mexico (Mexican Government, 2005). Please note that, generally speaking, in Mexico acknowledgment of indigenous roots is often frowned upon. It is important to recognize that Mexican American children of Mexican-born and -raised parents may disagree about the need to acknowledge the indigenous connection. Exercise caution when exploring these issues.

When asking about immigration and indigenous background, take note that both can elicit strong internal reactions from parents, so tread lightly. The family that has documentation may feel stereotyped; the undocumented family might worry about being reported to Immigration and Naturalization Services (INS). Do discuss confidentiality and its limits under the law. McCabe (2002) recommends addressing this issue at intake. An appropriate way to do this might be to inquire about the child's contact with the grandparents, allowing parents to disclose whether they reside in the United States or in Mexico. If the parents are from Mexico, ask about which state they come from and whether it is a rural or urban area. This could provide the therapist with valuable information, as those from rural areas have less access to therapists. Assessing for religious beliefs and practices is also important. Not all families are Roman Catholic. However, many Mexican American families are aware that the *Virgin de Guadalupe* (the Virgin Mary) is Mexico's patron saint. She is honored on December 12 throughout Mexico and the United States.

Traditional treatment approaches need to be explored as well. One way to initiate this discussion is by asking how the family would attempt to remedy their child's problems in Mexico or how the child's grandparents would go about seeking assistance for the child. Ask if the parent or the child was ever treated by a *curandero*. Ramirez (1972) notes that *curanderos* can treat individuals who have guilt, fear, or somatic complaints. Other families seek religious intervention by talking with a priest or pastor. Some may even consider paying homage to a revered saint in exchange for granting their child or themselves a cure for a condition. It is interesting to note that, according to Edgerton and Karno (1971), the vast majority of Mexican Americans interviewed in their study pray to relieve mental problems. It is uncertain what a current study would reveal.

According to Martinez and Valdez (1992), Ramirez (1998), and Hopkins et al. (2004), it is also important to examine acculturation levels for each family member, as they may all be different. Such dynamics might reveal some interesting juxtapositions when taken into consideration. Take, for example, the following Mexican American family: a Mexican-born national who has worked for several years as an agricultural worker on the same U.S. farm and frequently returns to Mexico in the winter months. He obtains legal residency for his wife and children, who live in a rural area of Mexico. The wife and children immigrate to the United States. During the winter months, the father obtains unemployment insurance, but this does not meet the family's needs. The wife seeks and obtains employment. With time she takes in the culture of her coworkers and slowly becomes more acculturated than her husband, who has not needed to acquire new behaviors because he has had little contact with the host culture. The wife might become conflicted over her role, and the husband might experience his wife's normal adjustment to the host culture as an incursion into his comfort zone. Conflict might ensue if the couple does not engage in ongoing dialogue about the changes. Meanwhile, the couple's children continue to become educated consciously and unconsciously by the host culture. This family, with great hesitation, might seek mental health services for a child and not understand how the different acculturation levels affect its members. Acculturation levels can be very different. It behooves the therapist to investigate the acculturation matter carefully.

When the assessment is complete, the therapist needs to consider what modality will best address the child's problems. Some authors (Ramirez, 1972; LeVine & Padilla, 1980; Martinez & Valdez, 1992; Hopkins et al., 2004) propose that to maintain the family's cultural equilibrium, providing family therapy rather than individual therapy to the child is important.

The majority of parents expect that the therapist will share with them concrete treatment recommendations before the end of the session. Sometimes therapists do not do this and non-Mexican American parents will pursue this information. Because the Mexican American family may defer to the therapist as an authority, they may not question the treatment decision (Ramirez, 1998), for example, not sharing much after the first meeting. Encourage the parents to ask questions freely about the process

(Hinman, 2003) since they might not feel it is their place to do so, like other parents do.

Although parents might expect some form of family therapy, play therapy may also be indicated. It is important to outline the ideas behind play therapy strategies in a manner that the parent can understand. For instance, the therapist might explain that the use of play activities helps the child uncover internal conflicts by projecting onto the play his or her internal experience. Schaefer and O'Connor (1983) state that the use of toys helps the therapist unravel the child's personality and family dynamics.

TOOLS FOR PROVIDING CULTURALLY APPROPRIATE SERVICES

Play therapy approaches are plentiful; some have greater utility with the Mexican American child than others. Dollhouse, sand tray, and art are just a few of the tools therapists employ. Play therapy games are also available to engage, assess, and treat children who have any number of problems; however, most were developed with little or no attention to cultural diversity. Little is available for the Spanish-speaking child and family. Those games that are available do not take into account the Mexican American culture. Further, they presume that the parent and child have some Spanish literacy skills, which may or may not be the case.

CULTURALLY APPROPRIATE SERVICES

Critics of mental health services have voiced the need for Hispanics to have therapeutic services that take into account their culture (Padilla, Ruiz, & Alvarez, 1975; Rogler, Blumenthal, Malgady, & Costantino, 1985). To date, the mental health field has made some strides in meeting this objective. Rogler et al., (1985) outlined three approaches to providing culturally sensitive services. The first involves incorporating bilingual/bicultural staff into the pool of mental health providers. The second recommends that therapy be congruent or modified to include individual cultural values (Cohen, 1972; Padilla et al., 1975), and the third involves making adaptations to therapy that match the individual's culture. The authors' first recommendation has been met; there are bilingual Hispanic mental health providers in several agencies, but it is unclear to what extent. With regard to recommendations two and three, anecdotally it appears as if several of my mental health professional colleagues of color have implemented them.

Two tools have been developed to meet the specific needs of the Hispanic child. Malgady, Costantino, and Rogler (1984) developed Tell Me a Story (TEMAS), similar to the Thematic Apperception Test (TAT). This is a projective test that consists of 23 colorful cards that show African American or Latino characters in a metropolitan setting. The participants are expected to resolve the conflict depicted in the cards. Malgady et al. found that the children were more verbal on the TEMAS than the TAT. The other tool is a form of therapy known as *cuento* therapy discussed earlier.

PLAY MATERIALS AND TECHNIQUES TO BE USED WITH THE MEXICAN AMERICAN CHILD

Drewes (2004), Hinman (2003), and Martinez and Valdez (1992) strongly recommend that the therapist have culturally diverse toys in the office. When treating the Mexican American child and family, it would be helpful to have traditional Mexican children's games available. Castillo (2005) reflects on her memories from her childhood when she and her playmates played with traditional Mexican games that reinforced Mexican American culture. A few Mexican board games can be used for assessment and treatment purposes. *Juego de la Oca, Serpientes y Escaleras*, and *La Lotería* have been played by Mexican families for more than 200 years (Monsiváis, 1991). They can be purchased in any Mexican American minimarket. The first two board games have images such as Mayan pyramids on them. *La Lotería*, a Bingo-style game that uses images instead of numbers and letters, is a family game as well as a learning tool in Mexico. A brief history of each game is provided in the following section. The first bilingual/bicultural child therapy game, called *Historia de la Lotería*/Lotto Story©, which I developed, is also discussed.

There is debate with regard to when *Juego de la Oca* (Game of the Goose) originated. Some say that it originated in the 11th century in Germany, while others say it originated in Italy (Sirauras, 2005). In the 16th century, a copy was sent to King Phillip II of Spain (Sirauras, 2005). When it arrived in Mexico, the game was modified to reflect the culture (e.g., Mayan temple images were added). This game can be used to establish rapport with the child and family. The parent might recognize it and consequently be put at ease.

Serpientes y Escaleras (Snakes and Ladders) originated in India and was developed to teach children about religion (Masters, 2005). Like the

American version, it rewards good deeds and punishes misdeeds; however, the images in this game are quite graphic. For instance, it shows a child who ends up in the hospital bandaged with some blood on his head because he ate too much candy. The Mexican version has images specific to the Mexican culture, such as a skull and a Mexican cowboy.

La Loteria started off as a colonial Spanish card game. It arrived in Mexico during the last half of the 18th century and was originally played as a parlor game by the socially elite (Sánchez, 1997). Since then it has been incorporated in all sectors of the Mexican population and is as popular as Monopoly is in the United States. This game is also used in gambling at carnivals. In the state of Oaxaca, poetic verses are shouted out at a family gathering or in a gaming room. If one verse is "I'm the _____ and I've arrived although you can't see me; I haven't come to borrow, not even to eat," the one described would be "*el Diablito,*" the little devil. Yet another way to play the game would be using riddles and rhymes. For example, one would be expected to identify the image for the riddle "one that dies by the mouth" as the fish. Castillo (2005) documents that playing *La Loteria* is not only about fun but a way for the family to be together. Martinez and Valdez (1992) describe using the game in the traditional manner with a family and how it helped children increase their Spanish-speaking comfort level.

Historia de la Loteria/Lotto Story is a projective storytelling assessment tool and game that is similar to *La Loteria* (see Figure 10.1). I developed it after trying and failing to locate a bilingual and bicultural game that could be used with children who do not read Spanish and parents who have limited literacy skills. This game contains several images that are found in the traditional game, such as *el nopal* (the cactus) and *la muerte* (death). It also contains other images, such as gun, drugs, broken heart, and knife. The game instructions for the game are provided below in the Case Examples section.

THERAPEUTIC USES OF *JUEGO DE LA OCA,*
SERPIENTES Y ESCALERAS, AND *LA LOTERIA*

Once the therapist has engaged the child and family in traditional play with the abovementioned games, he or she can utilize the games to conduct an assessment or treatment.

With *Juego de la Oca,* during the course of the play the child will land on several spaces; wherever the child lands he or she is asked to identify a thought, memory, or feeling that is evoked by the image on that space. For example, if the child lands on the image of the jail, the therapist might

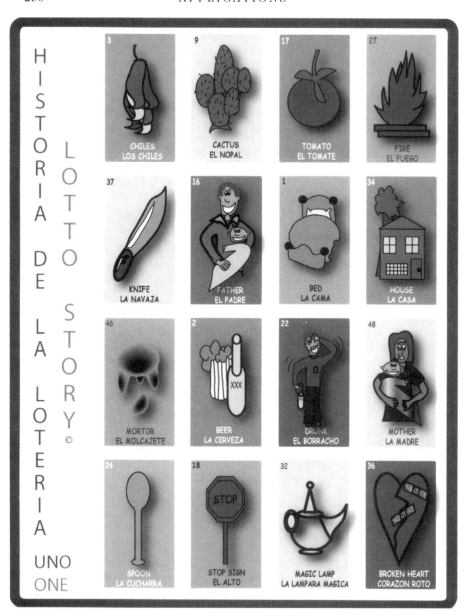

FIGURE 10.1. *Historia de la Loteria*/Lotto Story: 1 of 10 cards. Game includes 52 individual cards and emotion pegs.

explore what feeling or memory is evoked when the child thinks of a jail and perhaps ask the child if he or she has ever met anyone who went to jail. If the child lands on a typical Hispanic iconic image, such as the bull or a Mayan temple, the therapist can explore ethnic identity information by asking if the child can identify it. For instance, a 10-year-old Mexican American girl identified the Mayan temple as an Egyptian pyramid. When asked why she thought it was Egyptian, she said that at school she and her classmates were studying Egypt. For a child who might be struggling with self-acceptance issues related to his or her ethnic background, the therapist could share a little about Mayan history in Mexico.

With the *Serpientes y Escaleras* board game, when the child lands on an image that conveys a misdeed, the therapist can explore if he or she has ever engaged in the behavior displayed. If the child acknowledges the misdeed, the therapist can ask the child to describe what consequence he or she experienced as a result of the misdeed after he or she traveled down to the snake's head. If a child who frequently misbehaves lands on a positive behavior space, the therapist can encourage him or her to make better behavior choices and highlight the forthcoming reward to be had when the child climbs up the ladder. With repeated opportunities, the child might associate engaging in positive behaviors with rewards.

The *La Loteria* board game can be used as a projective tool. It is an excellent alternative to the Thematic Apperception Test (TAT). It can also be used the way toys are used in a sand tray, the sand tray being the table or floor area where the cards would be displayed. Unlike with the TAT, the child is instructed to develop a story based on several images that he or she chooses. Through the storytelling activity, the child reveals his or her dynamics as well as information about his or her family. This game can be used in a structured or nonstructured manner.

In an individual session, the therapist places all of the 52 picture cards face up on the desk or the floor. Depending on the child's ability and age, the therapist asks the child to select a specific number of cards of his or her choice from which he or she will develop a story in a semistructured format. The therapist can also instruct the child to develop the story about his or her family or any individual family member depending upon the need.

Case Examples

The following case examples are a mix of descriptions and discussion to emphasize how the abovementioned games can be used in various manners. The identities of the children and families have been concealed.

Miguel

Miguel is an 8-year-old boy who was born to his Mexican American father and Caucasian mother in a California city. His parents divorced a year prior to the referral after his mother discovered her husband was abusing drugs. After the divorce, child protective services (CPS) became involved and Miguel and his siblings were placed in protective custody for a short period of time. Miguel's mother brought him to treatment at the urging of the CPS social worker and identified him as withdrawn and aggressive with his brother.

In an assessment meeting, Miguel was asked to select eight cards from the 52 on the table and develop a story using them. He ended up developing two stories with the same cards. He selected the *alacrán* (the scorpion), the *indigena* (the indigenous man), the *diablo* (the devil), the *muerte* (death), the *soldado* (the soldier), the *calavera* (the skull), the *araña* (the spider), and the *bailador* (the dancer). See Figure 10.2.

> This a story about a scorpion that killed an Indian. One day when the Indian was walking down a field, he saw a scorpion. He tried to put it in a jar, but he was too late, and the scorpion stung him with a poisonous sting, and then he died and never came back to his family, and then soon they found out he was dead, and then after 3 years he turned into a killing skeleton, and then he became a devil because someone killed his son. The devil will kill; this is a different story.

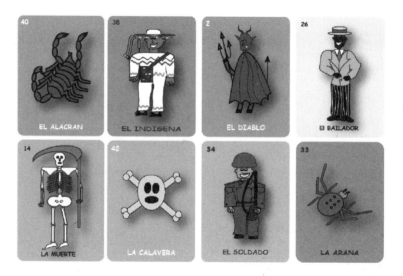

FIGURE 10.2. Renditions of the Loteria cards Miguel selected during the assessment meeting.

Story number two follows.

> This is about two men: a dancing man and a soldier. One time these two men—a black man who can dance very well and a soldier who never died in war—and one time they saw this black widow and they went out to find a bug to eat, but when they got back there was three more webs, so they caught the insect and put it in the web, and the other three spiders bit them with poison with really deadly venom, and then they died and they were soon sons of the devil because they did not get any insects for the other three.

Themes Presented in Miguel's Story. Various themes emerge in Miguel's story, including death, separation, aggression, and danger. Perhaps Miguel continues to struggle with being separated from his mother; it is likely that he still worries about this happening again.

Miguel was seen a few weeks later. In his next session, Miguel presented as anxious, as he moved about considerably in the playroom. Prior to this visit, Miguel had observed his family members fight while he and his siblings were visiting their father. Miguel attempted to intervene and was hurt. He called 911, and the police, the fire department, and an ambulance were summoned. What follows below is clinical material from that session.

Once in the playroom, he saw that I had the *Loteria* cards, and he asked if we could play the game again. I asked him to pick out eight cards, and he asked me, "Do you speak Spanish? Really good?" Before he selected the cards, he commented on the *muerte* (the death) card and stated, "I know this guy. He is the grim reaper." He then proceeded to select eight cards and divide them into two groups for two different stories. See Figure 10.3 for cards he used in the first story.

> The drunk man was really drunk. He had torn shoes and a torn vest, and then the next day he got drunk at night and he saw a spider that glowed

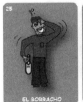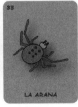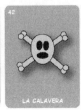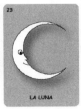

FIGURE 10.3. Renditions of the Loteria cards Miguel chose for his first story in his second session.

in the dark, and then he tried to look at it. The spider got really close and he tried to feed it but the spider bit him—it was poisonous—it was a black widow. And then he died in 5 minutes because he did not make it to a hospital, and he died at night after the moon was up with a little star.

He then began to assemble the cards for the next story (see Figure 10.4). He stated:

> This is going to be really short. The music man was playing music when he saw a scorpion in the middle of this song, and then the scorpion stung him and he died and became the grim reaper.

I decided to add to the story from the remaining cards on the table. Miguel walked away and went to the dollhouse; he returned with some funny glasses and a sword. I then proceeded to add to the story (see Figure 10.5), stating:

> The nurse (*la dama*) came in. Then the nurse went to go and check on the soldier (*el soldado*) to check if he was dying from the bullets to his heart. She saw her coworker's hand (*la mano*), and the nurse (*la dama*) told her she would check on the soldier. Why don't you check on the drunken man because he looks like he needs your help?

Miguel brought with him a toy highway patrol car that he incorporated into the game, and he drove it on top of the table as he searched for another card to add to the story. He grabbed *la calavera* (the skull) again and stated, "The coworker's hand was on the floor because it was bleeding because he cut it off" (see Figure 10.6). Miguel returned to the theme

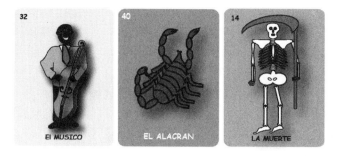

FIGURE 10.4. Renditions of the Loteria cards Miguel chose for his second story in his second session.

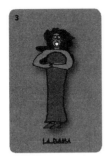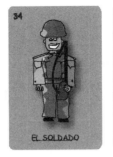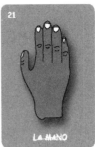

FIGURE 10.5. Renditions of the Loteria cards I chose to add to Miguel's story.

of danger. After Miguel asked that the toy highway patrol vehicle be used and stated, "The nurse saw a container," I added *el cazo* (the dipper) (Figure 10.7). Miguel added, "With blood in it?" and I responded by continuing, "and took the hand to the coworker's body and put it back together and she felt good about that." Miguel then shifted his story theme. He got *la corona* (the crown) from the remaining cards on the table and stated, "Then the lady felt like a queen" (see Figure 10.8). I added *el violoncello* (the violin) from the remaining cards on the table and stated, "And someone started to play the violin" (see Figure 10.9). Miguel added, "that was big," and I added, "because the lady was better and the drunken man was still alive." Miguel selected *la luna* (the moon) from the remaining cards on the table and added, "but because someone was playing the violin it was already night" (see Figure 10.10). I stated that it was the end of the story, but Miguel protested and I decided to add more to the ending. Perhaps Miguel felt as if the story had not been finished or began to experience some discomfort with a happy ending. I added, "The next morning

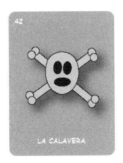

FIGURE 10.6. Rendition of the Loteria card Miguel added next.

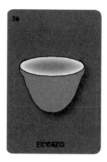

FIGURE 10.7. Rendition of the Loteria card, the dipper.

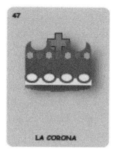

FIGURE 10.8. Rendition of the Loteria card, the crown.

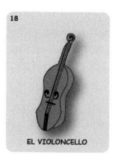

FIGURE 10.9. Rendition of the Loteria card, the violin.

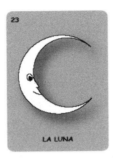

FIGURE 10.10. Rendition of the Loteria card, the moon.

the drunken man, the lady who played the big violin, and the two nurses heard the bird sing outside the window, and they were all very happy because no one died—the end." Miguel seemed comfortable with this ending. Perhaps he expected that things would take a turn for the worse or considered adding to the story but decided against doing so.

Diego

Diego is a 9-year-old Spanish-speaking Mexican boy. He and his mother and sibling emigrated from a rural area in Mexico to a California city to be with his father. His mother brought him to see me at the urging of a teacher, who thought he appeared anxious. He was instructed to Draw-a-Person (DAP) of his choice. He sketched a 9-year-old named Tom. Diego was then instructed to develop a story about something that happened to Tom using nine cards, as determined by Tom's age. He selected the nine from the 52 placed on the table (see Figure 10.11). He stated in Spanish:

> Tom was seated and he was hot because the sun was very hot, and the clouds became dark and it began to rain, and he got an umbrella and it stopped raining, and he sat down under a tree and he saw a skull, and he got scared because a spider had crawled on him, and he got scared until his heart wanted to come out, and then it became green like a pear. He went out eating and he saw some bushes, and he saw a heron also a frog, and he went to his house.

The Draw-a-Person activity is meant to represent the child's projections of himself. Diego's story describes how things can change rather quickly. Diego's life changed rather quickly when he moved to the United

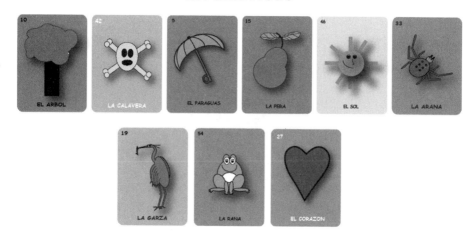

FIGURE 10.11. Renditions of the Loteria cards Diego selected.

States. Tom was able to secure shelter from the rain—an umbrella—soon after it stopped raining. Diego's story reveals that he is able to seek assistance when things get dark. Soon after, Tom became so scared that "his heart wanted to come out," but able to go to his house, where I imagine he sought protection. Diego comes from an intact family, and his story demonstrates that he is able to take care of himself. He is much healthier than the other children presented.

David

David is a 10-year-old Mexican American boy who lives with his parents and sister in a California city. Although bilingual, he preferred to speak English in his sessions with me. He was asked to develop a story without any prompts using 10 cards from the 52 placed on the table (see Figure 10.12 for the cards he chose and Figure 10.13 for the order he put them in). He stated:

> This is a tree, and a bird flew down to the tree. Then a deer came and started eating. Then another bird flew down and got into a fight with another bird. Then they were fighting because they wanted to get the watermelon. A man came and got the watermelon and he started eating it. Then a spider came. Then it bit him in his hand. Then a star fell from the sky. Then the moon became the king because he got the crown.

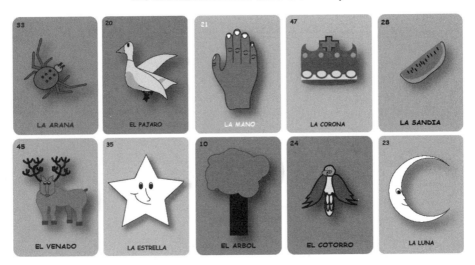

FIGURE 10.12. Renditions of the 10 Loteria cards David chose first.

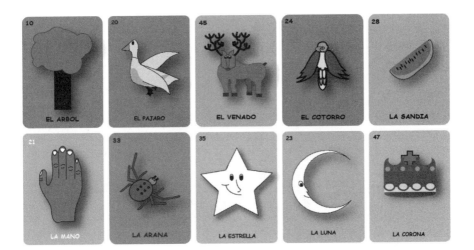

FIGURE 10.13. The order in which David put his cards (renditions of the Loteria cards).

David was asked to put the cards back on the floor and to develop a story about his father. He grabbed 10 cards (see Figure 10.14) and appeared confused. He kept them in his hand for a while before beginning to tell his story. He tentatively stated, "My dad got 10 cards then he gave one each to each person. He asked everyone to put the cards down and whoever had the last card would win." He failed to develop the story using the cards as instructed. Perhaps he was becoming defensive—it was too close to home and/or to his issues (as explained below). I provided him with the same instructions, and he responded by stating, "Like last time?" He then stated:

> There was a boat. Then he wanted to try it on but his bones were falling apart. Then he ate a pear, but it fell because he did not have skin—it fell. Then a scorpion came and started to sting him, but then he kicked it, but when he kicked it his bones fell. Then he needed to cross the river. The shrimp came and he grabbed the shrimp and his arm fell. Then he heard a parade and people played a drum. Then he saw the frog and he wanted to eat it. Then he ran toward it but his other leg fell. Then he found a crown, put it on. Then his head fell down. Then the bird came along and it thought that his ribs were a house. Then birds laid there and then other birds came along.

David asked me, "Can I change a card?" He was allowed to switch *la garza* (the heron) for *la chalupa* (the canoe) from the remaining cards on the table (see Figure 10.15). He then stated:

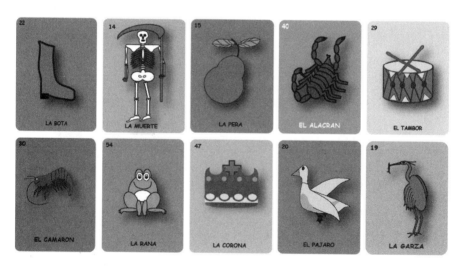

FIGURE 10.14. Renditions of the next 10 Loteria cards David chose.

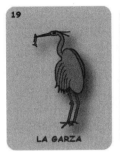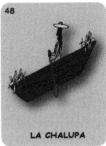

FIGURE 10.15. David switched the heron for the canoe (renditions of the Loteria cards).

> Then the lady saw the bones. Then she started yelling, and people came, and they thought somebody killed someone, and they tried to find out who did it for a whole bunch of years.

I asked David, "Did they ever find out?" He stated:

> No, because it came back from the dead. Then it wanted to go to the village to scare them but his bones were falling—that should have been in the beginning of the story. He tried to grab a shrimp but his head fell in the water.

I asked, "Do you worry about your dad?" He shared, "A little bit—that something might happen to him, like get into a car accident." He was asked about what other worries he has and he shared, "I might not pass a test or . . . that's it." He became noticeably uncomfortable, and I stated, "It is too fast to let me know about all your worries today. We can go slowly."

Family work was conducted with David's mother. These sessions primarily consisted of providing psychoeducational information to her to increase her understanding of her child's problems.

THERAPEUTIC USES OF THE *HISTORIA DE LA LOTERIA*/LOTTO STORY

As mentioned earlier I developed *Historia de la Loteria*/Lotto Story to meet the needs of the Mexican American child and family. This assessment and therapy game is played in the same manner as *La Loteria* and has images such as *día de los muertos* (Halloween), *el oficial* (the police officer), *la droga* (drugs), *corazón roto* (the broken heart), and *los chiles* (the chiles) (see Figure 10.16). Another way to use *La Loteria* and *Historia de la Loteria*/Lotto Story involves placing all the cards face up on the floor or desk and having the child place "emotion pegs" on top of the cards based on the feeling that is evoked by viewing the image on each card. Emotion pegs include six different faces (see Figure 10.17).

Case Examples

Lisa

Lisa, an 8-year-old Caucasian girl, was also removed by CPS and reunited with her parents. I turned the *Historia de la Loteria*/Lotto Story cards face up on the table and asked Lisa to place at least one emotion peg on top of the a card that corresponded with the feeling evoked for her when viewing the image. She placed a sad emotion peg on top of the judge card (see Figure 10.18). When asked how she decided to place that particular peg on the judge, she shared, "I don't like that job because they separate moms and dads from their children." She also placed a sad emotion peg on top of the knife card and described how sad she was when she could not take her bunny with her because it died (see Figure 10.19).

Cassandra

Cassandra is a 7-year-old Mexican American child, who was also removed by CPS and placed with her paternal grandmother after her parents refused to participate in the CPS treatment plan. She was instructed to develop a story using seven cards (the number of cards was based on her age). She selected the cards in Figure 10.20 and stated:

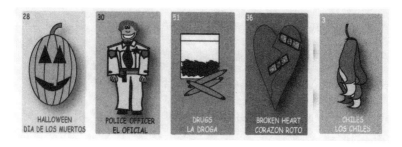

FIGURE 10.16. Some cards from *Historia de la Loteria*/Lotto Story.

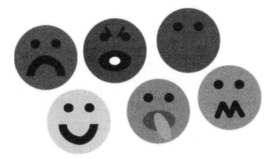

FIGURE 10.17. Emotion pegs.

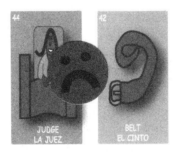

FIGURE 10.18. Sad emotion peg on judge card, placed by Lisa.

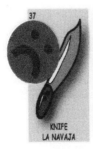

FIGURE 10.19. Sad emotion peg on knife card, placed by Lisa.

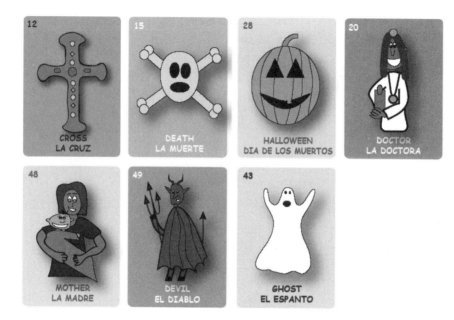

FIGURE 10.20. The cards Cassandra selected.

Once upon a time the there was a mother and a baby. The mother asked her baby "Would you like something to eat?" The baby said "Yes." The mom told her baby about Halloween, which would be the next day. The baby moved her head. The mother's baby was sick and she called her doctor. The doctor told the mother to put her baby to sleep because she has a fever. The mom went to bed and the doctor left. But before the doctor left, the mom asked the doctor what to give her baby to eat. Food and milk, and then she took the blanket off the baby and she went to sleep. Mom got lost and Dad looked around for her. A ghost took her away. Dad, the devil, went to jail and the baby's mom died because she went into hot pool of rock.

Cassandra's mother was mentally ill in addition to actively abusing methamphetamine and alcohol. The child described her experience with her mother through the story. She described her mother as "lost" and dying in a "hot pool of rock." This tool helped identify some of internal issues.

CONCLUDING REMARKS

Latino (Hispanic and Mexican American) youth are highly underrepresented in the public mental health system (McCabe et al., 1999). This might be related to providers not making services available, or, possibly, when these youth do seek assistance they do not believe the services are helpful. When Latinos do seek help, most drop out after one session (Huey, 1998). McCabe (2002) looked at premature termination issues with Mexican American children in the San Diego County community mental health service agency. In her discussion, she recommended that therapists explore and address with families what barriers they encountered before arriving at the appointment, hoping that this might decrease the dropout rate within this group. I hope that the ideas presented here will help keep the Mexican American child and family in treatment until it is time for termination by helping the family feel welcomed.

I have provided background information to help therapists increase their understanding of the Mexican American family so that there is an increased sensitivity to it. Clearly, Mexican American families are not homogeneous. Therapists who work with children and families who are unlike themselves should strongly consider modifying the manner in which they provide services. For instance, with the Mexican American family it is important to take into account that family therapy might be more acceptable than individual therapy, and it is important to acknowledge the family hierarchy. When the therapist does not speak the parents' language, it is important to provide the family with an interpreter. Having background about the Mexican American family helps the therapist provide culturally sensitive engagement.

This chapter has also identified four psychotherapeutic tools to use with the Mexican American child and family. Therapists who use these tools can provide more culturally responsive and appropriate therapy to the Mexican American child and family if they are used as suggested. When the therapist acknowledges the client's culture, the Mexican American family feels welcomed, honored, and understood.

The clinical material presented in this chapter was selected to highlight the use of native games and the game I developed to conduct assessments and treatment. For instance, Miguel's vignette highlighted how *La Loteria* can be used to aid in the assessment process as well as providing treatment similar to a sand tray. The children depicted in the clinical examples represent a diverse sample: Miguel is the child of a divorced Mexican American father and a Caucasian mother. David is a child of

Mexican-born and -raised parents. Cassandra is the child of a divorced Mexican-born and -raised father and a Mexican American mother. Diego is a Mexican-born child with Mexican-born parents, and Lisa is a Caucasian child. The tools identified clearly can be used with children of diverse backgrounds.

Different theoretical orientations are helpful to understand the work to be done with the Mexican American family. Awareness of narrative therapy principles, family therapy ideas, and psychodynamically informed therapies are three orientations that have been helpful for me when working with children and families. For instance, family therapy helps the family maintain its unity. Narrative therapy ideas help the therapist identify the child's story and how to help the child develop a healthier story. Psychodynamic theories help the therapist understand why the child projects his or her story onto the story activity.

Juego de la Oca, Serpientes y Escaleras, and *La Loteria* are not Mexican games per se, for the origins of these games are found outside of Mexico, but they were adapted to suit the Mexican people when the Spanish introduced them to Mexico. *Historia de la Loteria*/Lotto Story, developed from American and Mexican cultures, now joins those three games.

There is a saying in Spanish: *la cultura cura no locura* (culture cures; it does not make one crazy). We should always look at the richness of culture as we continue to develop innovative ways to help children and families in an optimal manner. Empirical research is needed to determine in what ways the tools outlined in this chapter are effective with regard to treatment outcomes. When a therapist takes into account a family's culture, he or she can become more culturally competent, as part of a *lifelong process.*[3]

NOTES

1. Alaska, Arizona, California, Colorado, Hawaii, Idaho, Montana, Nevada, New Mexico, Oregon, Utah, Washington, and Wyoming.
2. Alabama, Arkansas, Delaware, District of Columbia, Florida, Georgia, Kentucky, Louisiana, Maryland, Mississippi, North Carolina, Oklahoma, South Carolina, Tennessee, Texas, Virginia, and West Virginia.
3. Ideally, before working crossculturally, it is important to have some information about the client's culture. Many therapists strive to become culturally competent. To achieve this goal it is important first to understand one's own cultural background. Please see Gil (2004) for more information about the process by which a therapist becomes more culturally competent.

REFERENCES

American Psychological Association. (2005). *APA guidelines for providers of psychological services to ethnic, linguistic, and culturally diverse populations.* Retrieved August 17, 2005, from www.apa.org/pi/oema/guide

Arroyo, W. (1997). Children and families of Mexican descent. In G. Johnson-Powell (Ed.), *Transcultural child development: Psychological assessment and treatment* (pp. 290–304). New York: Wiley.

Association for Play Therapy. (2000). *Voluntary play therapy practice guidelines.* Retrieved August 17, 2005, from www.a4pt.org/forms/Voluntary_Play_Therapy_Practice_Guidelines.pdf

Axline, V. (1947). *Play therapy.* Cambridge, MA: Riverside.

Baez, A., & Hernandez, D. (2001). Complementary spiritual beliefs in the Latino community: The interface with psychotherapy. *American Journal of Orthopsychiatry, 71*(4), 408–415.

Bernal, B. E., Knight, G. P., Garza, C. A., Ocampo, K. A., & Cota, M. K. (1990). The development of ethnic identity in Mexican American children. *Hispanic Journal of Behavioral Sciences, 12*(1), 3–24.

Bernstein, R. (2005). Hispanic population passes 40 million. U.S. Census Bureau News (DB05-77). Retrieved August 17, 2005, from www.census.gov/Press-Release/www/releases/archives/population/005164.html

Canino, I. A., Earley, B. F., & Rogler, L. H. (1980). *The Puerto Rican child in New York City: Stress and mental health* [Monograph, no. 4]. New York: Hispanic Research Center, Fordham University.

Castillo, G. G. (2005). *Traditional Hispanic children's games disappear.* Retrieved August 17, 2005, from epcc.edu/ftp/homes/monicaw/borderlines/11_traditional_hispanic.htm

Cohen, R. E. (1972). Principles of preventive mental health programs for ethnic minority populations: The acculturation of Puerto Ricans to the United States. *American Journal of Psychiatry, 128*, 1529–1533.

Costantino, G., Malgady, R. G., & Rogler, L. H. (1986). *Cuento* therapy: A culturally sensitive modality for Puerto Rican children. *Journal of Consulting and Clinical Psychology, 54*(5), 639–645.

Drewes, A. A. (2004). Multicultural play therapy resources. In E. Gil & A. A. Drewes (Eds.), *Cultural issues in play therapy* (pp. 195–205). New York: Guilford Press.

Edgerton, R., & Karno, M. (1971). Mexican-American bilingualism and the perception of mental illness. *Archives of General Psychiatry, 24*, 286–290.

Falicov, C. J. (1998). *Latino families in therapy: A guide to multicultural practice.* New York: Guilford Press.

Gil, E. (2004). From sensitivity to competence in working across cultures. In E. Gil & A. A. Drewes (Eds.), *Cultural issues in play therapy* (pp. 3–25). New York: Guilford Press.

Hinman, C. (2003). Multicultural considerations in the delivery of play therapy services. *International Journal of Play Therapy, 12*(2), 107–122.

Hopkins, S., Huici, V., & Bermudez, D. (2004). Therapeutic play with Hispanic clients. In E. Gil & A. A. Drewes (Eds.), *Cultural issues in play therapy* (pp. 148–167). New York: Guilford Press.

Huey, S. J. (1998). *Therapy termination among black, Caucasian, and Latino children referred to community mental health clinics.* Unpublished doctoral dissertation, University of California, Los Angeles.

Landreth, G. L. (1982). *Play therapy: Dynamics of the process of counseling with children.* Springfield, IL: Thomas.

LeVine, E. S., & Padilla, A. (1980). *Crossing cultures in therapy: Pluralistic counseling for the Hispanic.* Monterey, CA: Brooks/Cole.

Malgady, R. C., Costantino, G., & Rogler, L. H. (1984). Development of a Thematic Apperception Test (TEMAS) for urban Hispanic children. *Journal of Consulting and Clinical Psychology, 52*(6), 989–996.

Martinez, K. J., & Valdez, D. M. (1992). Cultural considerations in play therapy with Hispanic children. In L. A. Vargas & J. D. Koss-Chioino (Eds.), *Working with culture: Psychotherapeutic interventions with ethnic minority children and adolescents* (pp. 85–102). San Francisco: Jossey-Bass.

Masters, J. (2005). *The online guide to traditional games moksha-patamu (snakes and ladders).* Retrieved August 17, 2005, from www.tradgames.org.uk/games/Moksha-Patamu.htm

McCabe, K., Yeh, M., Hough, R., Landsverk, J., Hurlburt, M., Culver, S., et al. (1999). Racial/ethnic representation across five public sectors of care for youth. *Journal of Emotional and Behavioral Disorders, 7,* 72–82.

McCabe, M. M. (2002). Factors that predict premature termination among Mexican-American children in outpatient psychotherapy. *Journal of Child and Family Studies, 11*(3), 347–359.

Mejia, D. (1983). The development of Mexican-American children. In G. J. Powell (Ed.), *The psychosocial development of minority group children* (pp. 77–114). New York: Brunner/Mazel.

Mexican Government. (2005). *Diversidad etnolingüística* [Ethnolinguistic diversity]. Retrieved August 17, 2005, from www.indigenas.presidencia.gob.mx/print.php?id_seccion=90

Monsiváis, C., (1991). Ecclesiastic loteria [Ecclesiatic lottery]. *Artes de Mexico, El Arte de la Suerte, 13,* 53–55

National Association of Social Workers. (1996). *Code of ethics of the National Association of Social Workers.* Washington, DC: Author.

New Freedom Commission on Mental Health. (2003). *Achieving the promise: Transforming mental health care in America. Final Report* (DHHS Pub. No. SMA-03-3832). Rockville, MD: Author.

Padilla, A. M., Ruiz, R. A., & Alvarez, R. (1975). Community mental health services for the Spanish-speaking/surnamed population. *American Psychologist, 30,* 892–905.

Phinney, J. S. (1996). When we talk about American ethnic groups, what do we mean? *American Psychologist, 51*(9), 918–927.

Ramirez, M. (1972). Towards cultural democracy in mental health: The case of the Mexican-American. *Interamerican Journal of Psychology, 6,* 1–2.

Ramirez, O. (1998). Mexican American children and adolescents. In J. T. Gibbs & L. N. Huang (Eds.), *Children of color: Psychological interventions with culturally diverse youth* (pp. 215–239). San Francisco: Jossey-Bass.

Ramirez, O., & Arce, C. H. (1981). The contemporary Chicano family: An empirically based review. In A. Baron (Ed.), *Explorations in Chicano psychology* (pp. 3–28). New York: Praeger.

Ramirez, R. R., & De La Cruz, P. (2002). *The Hispanic population in the United States: March 2002, current population reports.* Retrieved August 17, 2005, from www.census.gov/prod/2003/p20-545/pdf

Rogler, L. H., Blumenthal, R., Malgady, R. G., & Costantino, G. (1985). Hispanics and culturally sensitive mental health services. *Research Bulletin, 8,* 1–11. Hispanic Research Center, Fordham University.

Rogler, L. H., Malgady, R. G., Costantino, G., & Blumenthal, R. (1987). What do culturally sensitive mental health services mean?: The case of Hispanics. *American Psychologist, 42*(6), 565–570.

Sánchez, A. R. (1997). Estetica de la suerte [The esthetics of fortune]. *Artes de Mexico, El Arte De La Suerte, 13,* 22. Mexico, DF: Artes de Mexico y del Mundo, S.A. de C.V.

Schaefer, C. E., & O'Connor, K. J. (1983). *Handbook of play therapy.* New York: Wiley.

Sirauras. (2005). *El juego De La Oca.* Retrieved August 17, 2005, from www.sirauras.iespana.es/sirauras/temas/juegosmesa.htm

Sistema Nacional para el Desarrollo Integral de la Familia (DIF). (2005). Menores, adolescentes, adultos mayores, personas con discapacidad [Children, adolescents, older adults, disabled persons]. Retrieved August 17, 2005, from www.dif.gob.mx/grupos.html

Sluzski, C. (1979). Migration and family conflict. *Family Process, 18*(4), 379–390.

Sue, D. W., & Sue, D. (1999). *Counseling the culturally different: Theory and practice* (3rd ed.). New York: Wiley.

Tharp, R. G., & Meadow, A. (1973). Differential change in folk disease concepts. *Interamerican Journal of Psychology, 7,* 55–63.

Trostle, S. L. (1988). The effects of child-centered group play sessions on the social-emotional growth of three- to six-year-old Puerto Rican children. *Journal of Research in Childhood Education, 3*(2), 93–106.

CLAYtherapy

The Clinical Application of Clay with Children

PAUL R. WHITE

Many counselors want to work with children. Most think it would be easier and more fun than working with adults. Child counselors will agree that children are more fun than adults, but troubled children are more therapeutically difficult by far than any adult.

The primary modality of therapy with children is one of the several forms of play therapy. Play therapy sounds fun but is extremely difficult. It brings children to treatment who have not yet completed their psychological, educational, or even neurological development. These children bring near impossible-to-solve life issues combined with severe, sometimes multiple, diagnoses. They often are resistant, usually without a grasp of the clinical procedure and fearful of this mysterious and unprecedented process they are forced to endure. They come to an unknown adult, not of their choosing, and are asked to talk and play with him or her behind closed doors.

The counselor enters this process from the other direction, equipped with complex psychological abstraction and theoretical constructs that are difficult to apply at best, expecting to meet the child's needs by developing a problem-solving and personal relationship that resolves the child's life stressors and/or diagnostic symptoms. In short, the counselor is asked to take this underdeveloped and inexperienced child of just a few years old from a state of emotional or mental disorganization to one of organization through the use of puppets, sand, paint, figurines, and clay. Play therapy is indeed difficult (Reid, 1986).

Since the inception of play therapy, clay has always been an element noted and suggested as a necessary instrument of therapists. Clay is one of those tools used by the counselor to bring about the aforementioned adult–child relationship followed by the child's transformation from disorganization to normalization. Clay or play-dough is listed again and again in nearly every play therapy text, journal article, or teaching seminar, from the inception of play therapy, as a primary device to bring about this transformation and to assist with this psychological encounter (Freud, 1971; Moustakas, 1953).

Every recognized author on the subject of play therapy, from Axline (1947) to Landreth (2004), recommends that the play therapist secure play-dough as a tool of the trade, but there are only minimal guidelines, directions, suggestions, or applications for its clinical use. When there is direction, it is brief and nonspecific, usually supporting nondirective expressive play intended to reveal inner struggles or unspoken themes. Another frequently stated application is its use as a safe outlet for aggression, allowing the child to pound, squeeze, and knead out his or her hostility, much like a primal scream (Hart, 1992).

There are volumes of books, papers, dissertations, studies, and seminars on the clinical use and application of sand, drawing, puppets, storytelling, and dollhouses, but there is practically no equivalent for the clinical application and effectiveness of clay beyond initial expression and aggression reliever.

This lack of data, the absence of clinical scrutiny and empirical analysis, is a glaring void, but this leaves opportunity and an invitation to discovery and innovation. CLAYtherapy is a response to that void. It is a child-friendly, clinically supportive application of an old friend to all children: clay.

BEFORE CLAYtherapy

Before I discovered CLAYtherapy, I had used clay or play-dough in my practice with children. It was effective regardless of the clinical setting in which I found myself or my agency's objectives. Having been trained in the nondirective school of play therapy, I had always encouraged children's self-expression and nondirective free play with clay. Expressive play is a window into the child's internal processes and secret thoughts; children will reveal many emotional conflicts, experiences, and unresolved anxieties through nondirected free play. If the therapist is patient and uses clinical observation skills, he or she can observe not only major clinical themes but many subtleties and nuances through the expressive play process, especially with clay.

However helpful the nondirective clay process, I can remember always wanting to put this free play, reflective, tracking process aside and make something from play-dough that resembled something real and then to make that structured process just as therapeutic as nonstructured play. I wanted to respond to a child's direct request to make a bear, a bird, or a boat instead of saying, "You're saying you want to make a boat." I wanted to teach the child to build a specific creature like an African elephant, a farm animal, a jet plane, or a wheeled vehicle. I wanted to use this powerful medium to enhance my relationship with children, to make counseling not so boring, and through play-dough identify emerging clinical conflicts and concepts. I wanted to make the process of working with clay more directive, more therapeutic, and more fun.

No matter how hard I tried, I couldn't respond to these desires because I had no formal training in three-dimensional freeform arts, no innate art skills, and definitely no clay-to-clinical skills. Clinical clay skills were nonexistent at that point. I had no idea of how to make a dog, how to make that dog clinical, or how to make the making of that dog clinical. When I attempted to ignore and disregard these three "how to's" and build anyway, I always failed. Transforming play-dough into objects and then giving that process clinical value was an enigma.

ANCIENT CLAY

Clay is primal. From the beginnings of civilization, clay has been a substance associated with people. We mark our time with its archaeological shards. We fill our museums with its surviving remnants. We adorn our homes with its shapes, its utility and beauty. Clay finds its way into our literature, our religion, and our language:

> Imperial Caesar dead and turned to clay may stop a hole to keep the wind away.
>
> —SHAKESPEARE, *Macbeth*, Act I, Scene 1

> And man is made from the clay of the earth. . . .
>
> —GENESIS, 1:24

Mud pies, mud tires, mud packs, mud slides, mud slinging, and mud wrestling.
—Fifth Annual Mud-Wrestling Convention

From the earliest of times, we have used its versatile properties to meet our many needs. Clay hardened in early wood-fired ovens formed primitive domestic vessels. The same oven eventually made roof tiles, then storage jars, fine china, and finally porcelain. Ground into powder and mixed with tallow, clay formed paint used to create mysterious symbols and enchanting animals on cave walls across primeval Europe. These evolved into the elegant frescoes of the Sistine Chapel during the Renaissance.

We use clay today in many of the same ways our ancestors did. From its flexible properties, we make cements, paints and adhesives. We use it for plumbing, roofing, and floor tiles. We have rediscovered clay and employ it in medicines, chemicals, computers, bonding agents, and surfaces of artificial joints. We use clay in the space shuttle, from its electrical insulators and filtering components to its protective skin. Clay is with mankind more now than ever.

MODERN CLAY AND CLINICAL TREATMENT

Clay has a place in the world of counseling. Play therapists have traditionally used natural clays and, more recently, synthetic modeling clays because it's a substance children know well. Children like clay, and if they don't have it, they will play with pudding, pie dough, or mashed potatoes. Place a lump of clay in front of any child from any period in time or any place in the world and watch the inevitable interaction between child and material.

Today modeling clay comes in many forms, both natural and manmade. They are either water or oil based. The manmade commercial forms of clay are usually given a name to identify them as some form of dough—Fun-Dough, Kid-Dough, and of course Play-Doh®. Play therapists use both the factory-produced and homemade forms of dough, depending upon their clinical mission and personal taste. Clay or playdough is found in practically every school, counseling office, and home in our world.

I find Play-Doh brand play-dough to be the most useful and beneficial to the counseling environment.[1]

Every therapist in every child-centered clinical treatment environment on the planet uses some form of clay to engage children and
enhance the therapeutic process. This time-honored medium of expression and universal toy responds to the most primal and basic need of the
child: to play. Most children entering the counseling process are delighted
to see their old friend play-dough as part of the counselor's accessories,
sitting quietly on the shelf waiting for the next boy or girl.

Clay has always been a toy of children and more recently a tool of
play therapy. Counselors use clay as a means to enhance the therapeutic
relationship and support the clinical process. Clay provides children with
a natural method of connection and expression.

FROM TOYS TO CLINICAL TOOLS

A universal direction of child care researchers and therapists over the last
several decades has been the discovery and acquisition of techniques and
strategies with which to engage children in treatment. This has resulted
in a stampede to rediscover the rudiments and role of *play* in the child's
developmental process and then to link that connection to a child's natural
attraction to traditional *toys*. The final step in this process is to bring those
three components together in the development of clinical tools.

This three-way connection is the basis of all clinical tools used in play
therapy today. We have made the toy-to-clinical tool transition with many
counseling rediscoveries like hand puppets, dollhouses, miniature people, sandboxes, stuffed animals, board games, and storybooks. We have
then transformed these into a myriad of clinical tools, filling mail-order
catalogs and play therapy rooms with effective props and aids to enhance
and support our clinical work with children.

There has long been a need to rediscover similar methods in the
transformation of clay into a more effective clinical tool. This basic toy
and friend of children has been patiently waiting in the wings for its turn
to go beyond its passive ice-breaker, aggression-reliever role to center
stage as a primary tool of treatment. The problem is that, to date, there
has been no rediscovery process to make this transformation possible.
The existing professional community and its research institutions have
not made this toy-to-clinical tool connection, thereby bringing clay to the
attention of the established play therapy community or the next generation of child therapists.

The best example of this process is sand tray therapy. Once upon a
time, we did not apply sand trays and little creatures as we do today. At

some point, a counselor brought a sandbox and a handful of figurines into the playroom, and over time another old friend of children, sand, became an irreplaceable clinical tool.

SNAKES AND BALLS

Most counselors, either just beginning or with years of experience, are not artists. Most would define themselves as "artistically challenged" and have received no art background or training in their educational experience. Most cannot effectively draw, paint, or sculpt or teach children to do the same. More important, they cannot interface clay with treatment.

They cannot teach problem solving, trauma resolution, consequences for actions, or anger control through clay. They cannot provide metaphors with clay that enhance a child's self-esteem, promise a resolution to grief, or build the clinical relationship through their clay work with children. This isn't because they wouldn't like to, but because until now no one knew how.

In the early years of my career, I was not unlike all other therapists when it came to the clinical application of toys of any kind, especially clay. I was child-centered. I used clay purely as an expressive non-directive tool. I had no idea of clay's therapeutic usefulness beyond its expressive role or how to construct clay creatures. Like all other therapists, I made snakes and balls and snakes and balls and snakes and balls. It wasn't because I or the child didn't want to make elephants, dinosaurs, or roses, but because we didn't know how. I had no idea how to get past my lack of art skills, so we made snakes and balls.

With great effort, we made some things, but even our best attempts resulted in difficult to distinguish frogs and dogs. Our creatures' bodies were disproportionate, or their legs fell off, or they were smashed by our well-meaning fingers in the very process of construction. Most of our creatures were best described by one of my young patients, when she said, "All our dinosaurs look like funny cows with no horns."

I knew that play-dough was primal. I knew that all children liked it and I knew that it had promise of great therapeutic value beyond its expressive role. What I didn't know was how to tap it. I became discouraged, but I didn't give up.

Play-dough has always been a clinically useful and pleasant experience for the children I served. For me, it had been an unequalled ice-breaker in my first session with them. When playing with clay, they have always had some form of nondirect clinical experience, usually positive. Occasionally, major insightful experiences spontaneously and totally unexpectedly emerged from them in the presence of clay. All the children demonstrated a universal attachment to its feel, its smell, its place in their childhood. *Was I to let this child-friendly, naturally engaging, untapped gem of therapy languish as a mere accessory to play therapy?* Not if I could help it. I had to find a way for me, the nonartistic therapist, to develop a user-friendly relationship with this stuff. So began a 15-year quest that eventually elevated humble clay to a revolutionary new level of clinical application in the play therapy community. At the beginning, I could see clay therapy, but I had not yet conceived CLAYtherapy.

When sharing the idea of clay therapy and this clay-to-clinical transition with my colleagues, I received a consistent response: "Good idea, Paul, but, how would you do that?" I soon realized that if play-dough were ever to become more useful as a clinical tool, to me and the children I served, it would need to grow up. Play-dough had to move from its traditional role of "pound out your aggression" and enter the 21st century. Clay would have to experience that magical conversion, that transformation from toy to clinical tool in a similar manner to puppets, storybooks, and sand. Clay therapy would have to meet both the scrutiny of the therapeutic community and daily clinical engagement with children and come out a winner.

For this transformation to happen I sorted out *two* major obstacles and *seven* basic questions. Over the years, I found those obstacles and questions difficult enough by themselves, but each time I resolved or answered any I was led to yet more questions. I determined that if all these obstacles could be hurdled and the questions answered then I would be well on my way to making play-dough more clinically useful for me and the children I served.

The two obstacles were:
1. The actual construction process of creatures
2. Their clinical application

The seven original questions were:
1. How to control the volume of clay in a creatures various parts
2. How physically to hook the pieces together to stay together
3. How to make our projects look like the creatures we had intended
4. How to make clay construction simple for children
5. How to make the clay-play process interactive

6. How to link therapeutic value to the specific clay creatures and the clay-play process
7. How to get children past the barrier of artistic impairment

THE DISCOVERY AND DEVELOPMENT
OF CLAYtherapy

One November day, an 11-year-old boy and I were playing with play-dough while we talked about some rather serious problems, their solutions, and his choices in the matter. As we talked and played, he asked me, "Mr. White, can you make a dinosaur?" I replied, "I can't make a dinosaur. I don't know how," and he said, "Can you try?" I tried, and, as always, I could not convert the vision in my brain to a three-dimensional clay dinosaur. He said, "Thanks for trying," and we continued. After more weeks of talking and making snakes and balls and snakes and balls, it came to me, just as the flux capacitor had come to Dr. Emmett Smith in the movie *Back to the Future*, making time travel possible. If I made a ball of play-dough, smashed it flat as a pancake, and cut it into wedges like a pie, then I could control the volume of a creature's parts by controlling the size of the wedges.

I did just that, and it didn't work. I adjusted the wedge size, and it didn't work, but I kept adjusting the wedge sizes, and finally it worked! *I made a dinosaur with proportioned body parts!* By this method, I eventually was able to determine the exact volume of dough for any dinosaur's parts with trial and error.

I had discovered the answer to my first question, how to control the volume of the various parts. My young client and I made another dinosaur and another and another. They were a bit rough, but they were the proper proportions and could be called dinosaurs because they resembled dinosaurs. I called the wedged division process "pie-portions."

Next came a way to overcome one of the two obstacles, how to achieve clinical application, or value. After a few weeks of dinosaur making we divided our jointly made dinosaurs in half and each took four or five. As the boy was leaving that day, he said, "I can take these home, Mr. White, and they will remind me of what we have been talking about." Eureka! Clinical value! Since that day, I have been making dinosaurs, hooking them to the clinical process, and sending them home with the boys and girls I serve. I was now well on my way to answering the rest of my questions.

Over the next several years, I overcame the other obstacle and learned not only the answers to those original seven critical questions, but to hundreds of other questions I never would have imagined. Answering those led me to a whole array of even more questions and another major obstacle: I had made the process work for me, but I had to discover a way to make it work for children, how to make all this fit the therapeutic definition of play therapy, and how to teach clay therapy to my peers.

Some of the new questions dealt with construction issues, like how long to make an elephant's legs, how to connect those legs securely to its body, how to make a rose have realistic petals, how to make an airplane's wings look like an airfoil, and how to make treads on a car's tires. Other questions dealt with clinical issues, such as how to teach a child problem resolution, self-esteem enhancement, anger control, and patience through the use of play-dough. Over the past 15 years, all these construction questions and clinical applications were addressed, answered, and developed as play-dough emerged from simple toy to revolutionary clinical tool and clay therapy evolved into CLAYtherapy.

CLAYtherapy exists today as a single play therapist's body of knowledge. It encompasses the discoveries and developments of the clay play process over those first 15 years. It is housed in a single book[2] with hundreds of drawings and pictures to assist in making the 12 projects and contains more than 50 clinical direct and indirect applications. The construction and clinical application skills can be mastered by anyone in a relatively short period. CLAYtherapy has been embraced internationally by thousands of child-treatment professionals. It is used in numerous educational and clinical environments with children of various ages experiencing a wide variety of diagnostic, emotional, and situational needs.

The entirety of the book cannot be presented within this brief chapter, but a few of its discoveries and applications should provide you with an idea of its scope.

NINE OF THE DISCOVERIES AND APPLICATIONS OF CLAYtherapy

Artistic Impairment

Artistic impairment is a concept most adults, especially counselors, identify with. Most say, "I'm all thumbs." Most child counselors are not trained with art materials as art therapists are, yet soon after graduation or employment, we are immersed in an environment of crayons, paint, puppets, and clay. Our first reactions to this challenge are verbal. Counselors make statements claiming artistic impairment and digital atrophy. They get into denial, self-debasement, or other forms of evasion and avoidance behavior. Sometimes counselors use the self-convincing child-hood phrase "I can't," or they say, "My sister got all the art genes in our family."

However convincing we are about our lack of art skills, we all can learn to do art things. We all have brought our brain and hands together to make or do something constructive or creative at some point. We all have made something as a child, learned a new skill in college, or taken on hobbies as an adult. We all do something; macramé, cook, paint, play an instrument, quilt, carve wood, garden, fly fish, sing, compute, dance, mess with gadgets, sew, or craft. The most important point is, there was a time when we could not do those things and said to ourselves, "I can't."

We all respond to our children when they say "I can't" with encour-agements like "Make an effort," "Practice," "Yes, you can," "How do you know you can't?" and "You don't know until you try." I encourage all my artistically impaired would-be play-dough counselors to give those same encouragements to themselves.

Snakes and Balls

When considering play-dough, many counselors proudly say,"I can make snakes and balls," indicating their elementary mastery of at least two clay objects. This is actually a wonderful statement of clay ability because CLAYtherapy teaches that if you can make snakes and balls, all you need to do is add one more shape, and then anything can be made. If a thera-pist or a child can make one more shape, a cone, they can make almost anything, plant or animal, natural or manmade. Think about it. A pig's body is an oval, egglike ball with four squatty cylindrical legs (short snakes), triangle ears (smashed cones), and a curly tail (skinny snake)—snakes and balls and cones! A dinosaur starts with a ball. One end of the ball is formed into a cone for a tail. The other end of the ball is formed into a snake for a neck with a lump on the end (small ball) that becomes the head. Its legs are like the pig's, only longer. A few details with a crayon and a seashell, and the kid has a dinosaur. A jet is not as complex as it may seem at first. Jets are made with 12 cones; if you can make a cone, you can make a jet. A snail is a snake rolled up with two balls for eyes. Everything—cars, elephants, roses, and frogs—is little more than snakes and balls and cones.

Tablespoons and Tools

In CLAYtherapy, most projects are made from a heaping tablespoon (HTS) of play-dough. An HTS is about all most little hands can comfortably handle. A pie-portion with an HTS of clay makes animal legs that fit perfectly into holes made by a Crayola crayon. An HTS is just enough play-dough to make projects like planes and cars that can be measured with a Bicycle-brand playing card and takes about a week to dry with minimal or no cracks. Every standard can of play-dough (Play-Doh) has approximately eight HTSes. An HTS makes success more possible for children and self-esteem a more frequent occurrence during the counseling process.

Through CLAYtherapy, children are introduced to the concept of tools. Play-dough itself is a tool, as are crayons, fingers, water, playing cards, seashells, bottlecaps, cassette tape boxes, screws, pen caps, plastic spoons, pencils, coffee stirrers, and dozens of other everyday items. They all go in a toolbox to which we can add tools. We teach children to make tools, we give tools, we share tools, we learn to use tools, and we develop tools of our own design. Play-dough tools are a metaphor and subtle precursor to the problem-solving and life tools that soon will be taught and transferred from counselor to child.

Cracks, Color, Connections, Construction, and Clinical Application

CLAYtherapy teaches the would-be clay counselor everything he or she needs to know to be successful with play-dough and to teach children the same. Construction is taught by teaching the child: "Piece by piece, first things first, and there is nothing we can't fix." The child and counselor learn to prepare the various clay parts, connect them in sequence, and be patient if something goes wrong. Children learn new skills like how to avoid cracks, how to patch them up, and how to not let cracks or crack disasters affect the outcome. They learn how to use water and the mechanical connection of twirling to ensure parts stick together. They learn to judge size, estimate volume, and move from abstract to practical thought. They learn to make any color of clay in the rainbow, to keep their clay supple and their projects safe, and how to get play-dough out of the carpet.

Naturally a Tool

For countless generations, if you gave a child a lump of clay, he or she naturally and immediately began to roll, fold, and mash it. This natural physical connection can be seen any day in any preschool, elementary school, or middle school. It is a natural and primal friendship between children and a basic element of their earth: clay.

The natural clinical applications became obvious from that first child when he said, "I can take these home, Mr. White, and they will remind me of what we have been talking about." When the counselor sits with a child in the play process, the counselor is invited into and becomes part of that natural, primal child–clay connection.

Natural clinical applications are usually subtle and nondirective. Sometimes they start nondirect and are converted by the counselor into direct clinical value. For instance, I have converted this natural nondirect process to a direct one by saying to nearly three generations of children things like, "You can take that frog home and put her on your shelf, and she will remind you of our discussion about controlling your depression," or "What a nice car we made. You can take it home, and it will remind you of the three things you learned today about controlling your anger," or "A boy has to be patient when solving his problems, just like he is when making a play-dough elephant. It's hard at first, but it gets easier as time goes by."

A Tool of Discovery

All therapists discover what works and what doesn't with children. They experience the theory-to-application process that can only come from years of engaging hundreds of children in eyeball-to-eyeball problem solving and discovery. They learn to mix and match nondirect and direct play therapy. Through years of application, observation, and trial and error, I have experienced that discovery process. The difference between me and other therapists is that I have performed this discovery process with one extra element: Play-Doh.

I have taken numerous therapeutic theories learned or read in my formal training and converted and reformed them into techniques using play-dough. Over the years, I have engaged my young clients directly and nondirectly in my play-dough research. I have discovered and applied CLAYtherapy techniques to a wide variety of diagnosis encountered over a 35-year period. I have watched, listened, applied, modified, and reapplied the use of play-dough to thousands of children from all quarters of the client and diagnostic spectrum, both public and private, inpatient and out-, office and home, willing and unwilling, young and old. Through this process, I have developed, discovered, conceived, and invented dozens of techniques and strategies that bring play-dough to bear as a clinical tool. This conversion of play-dough from a universal toy and first-session icebreaker to a dynamic and unequaled partner in the clinical treatment of children has been the single most valuable asset to my work.

Following my initial discovery, after I became confident with this new approach, I eventually began to engage my clients. At first I only engaged older elementary-school-age children with this new tool. I purposefully avoided younger children due to my belief that they responded exclusively to nondirective play therapy. I avoided latency-age and older children because of their emerging abilities of speech and reason and their usual avoidance of traditional play. As the years passed and I became more proficient with this new therapy, however, I found it increasingly useful for both younger and older children. I discovered that my methods could be utilized both in directive and nondirective environments and that I and my small following of "clay heads" were able to use my discoveries with a wide variety of ages, clinical environments, personal styles, and diagnostic needs. This discovery/conversion process continues, and I am constantly testing, discovering, probing, teaching, and reprocessing the elements of CLAYtherapy.

How Can CLAYtherapy Enhance Clinical Relationships?

Most of what happens between a child and therapist is relationship. Unlike adults, children have to like their therapist. Without connection between them, therapy with a child is difficult. Too often, I have seen counselors watch a child randomly play with clay while repeatedly attempting parallel conversation and failing. It fails because the child is more comfortable with parallel play than the therapist. It fails because there are two dynamic and parallel processes happening at the same time, and they need to complement, not compete with, each other. It fails because the therapist doesn't know how to combine the powerful clay attraction with his or her clinical expectations and therapeutic direction. With CLAYtherapy, there is a built-in mutual connective process between the child's play needs and the counselor's treatment direction. In CLAYtherapy, the counselor engages the child with something the child wants to be engaged with (clay). Children have never seen creatures and vehicles like those they see in the clay therapist's office. It doesn't matter their diagnosis, the extent of their trauma, or how resistant they have been to therapy in the past; they can't wait to make or have me make and teach them to make these marvelous creatures.

Counselors can teach a child wonderful things about life and living by using clay as a tool. When counselors use clay, they speak to the genetic code within the child that says, "Children need adults. Adults teach children. This is an OK process." Children don't know why this clay/talk process is so meaningful; it just is. It is not unlike a prehistoric adult squatting at the clan's firepit with a child, teaching some bit of knowledge to promote mastery or ensure survival. This primal, adult–child, student–teacher, clay/talk process is about as natural as it gets, and the child has to respond because he or she is a child.

Through mutual clay play, a conversation between child and counselor automatically emerges. Dialogue doesn't have to be forced or fabricated, but happens naturally when the counselor is revealing, demonstrating, and teaching this dynamic and engaging clay process and the child is asking, learning, and experiencing his or her own trial and error. This manner of interaction links the adult with the child through a hands-on, verbal, nonintrusive, problem-solving counseling process. It sets the stage for additional therapy, establishes teacher and student roles, and supports transference. It is nature at its best.

Metaphor Galore

In play therapy, metaphor is a commonly used tool. Sometimes we remain in a metaphorical process for much of the therapeutic experience. Other times, we slowly coax the child or follow the child's invitation into his or her avoided or uncovered reality and then back into metaphor. Sometimes we never come out of metaphor. It's one of those balance things we learn to do in counseling.

With clay, there is both nondirect and direct metaphor galore. We allow children to choose what to make or choose if they want to play with play-dough at all. They select their favorite color and/or favorite animal. Together, we seek solutions to the problems of making a frog, monkey, or dog. We discover the secrets of making a dinosaur's teeth realistic or a rose petal thin. We use the tools we have at hand—crayons, bottlecaps, shells—to solve the problems of play-dough. If we don't have a tool, we make one. We transfer the skills of one project to resolve the issues of the next. We learn that life is better understood if we go from simple to complex.

We cooperate, mirror, reflect, and clarify. We communicate critique and compliment children on a job well done. We experience frustration, anger, and failure. Children learn new skills. Through sitting close and rolling and mashing clay together, children can experience good touch from the counselor. They do their part to make a project, and we do our part. We can talk eyeball-to-eyeball. We talk of trusting your eyes and hands to get correct sizes of and balance among parts. Trust of adults, feelings, and friends are a short distance from there. Being the boss of the clay is easily converted into being the boss of your behavior, your feelings, and your thoughts. Clay teaches responsibility. For the abused child, being the boss of his or her body and feelings is a wonderful, empowering lesson to learn. And all this comes from simple play-dough.

Making the creature look just right too much has meaning for the obsessive child. Doing first things first has usefulness for attention-deficit/hyperactivity disorder and Asperger syndrome children who are having difficulty with impulse control or sequencing. The attachment disordered child receives lessons in trust, deference, and cooperation. The angry child, when making a play-dough project, has to deal with all the same precursor anger elements with play-dough that he would in school or life: frustration, lack of skills, no tools, bad habits, bad problem-solving information, wanting to give up, lack of success, and not listening to adults. With play-dough, the child gets to turn every one of those around. He gets to fail and start again. He gets to be successful and enhance his self-esteem. He gets to control his emotions and build a problem-solving relationship with a significant adult. Mastery over the clay becomes mastery over life issues. The child thinks, "If I can master this play-dough thing, then maybe I can master my bad dreams, my anxiety, my behavior, my fears, and my depression." It is a very small step from play skills to life skills. Children learn to visualize, create, fail, and try again without the penalties of real-life situations. Clay has all this and much, much more.

Problem Solving

After establishing a therapeutic relationship with their clients, most of what counselors do is solve problems for children or teach them to solve their own. The most important word in that last statement is *"teach."* We forget sometimes that our role in therapy is largely that of teacher—teaching children to identify, understand, and change their feelings, to make decisions and control impulses, to accept new ways of thinking, to individuate, to believe in themselves, to get along with others, and, of course, to problem-solve.

The nice thing about clay is that making stuff from it involves teaching. Making things from clay isn't always easy; life is hard, but if you know how to solve problems, it becomes easier. If children allow us to teach them to make things out of play-dough, then they usually allow us to teach them about life. Children often seek solutions to life problems from their teachers at school because they have a history of solving other kinds of problems with their teachers. They trust their teachers, which is why they often go to those same teachers before parents or even school counselors with their fears, anxieties, or thoughts of self-harm. This is also why some school counselors are less than successful with children—because they haven't gone through the basic process of problem solving with simple things before attempting to tackle difficult ones.

All children need a basic problem-solving process that they can employ automatically when dealing with life issues big and small. I use a four-step process: step-by-step, secrets, tools, and practice. With the help of play-dough, this process can be taught over and over in a pleasant and easily remembered format.

1. *Step-by-step*. Every problem children will ever have, every problem anyone has ever had is solved by a series of steps, first things first and second things second. This fundamental concept is easily taught through play-dough. First you make a ball. Then you squish it into a pancake. Next, you cut the pancake into sections. Then you make a ball from one of the pancake sections and form it into a cone, then a cylinder, etc. You make body, head, legs, and details step by step.

2. *Secrets*. All problems have secrets. Knowing the secrets makes problems easier to solve. Adults in every culture for countless generations have known the secrets to life and living, and it's their job to teach these secrets to the children or that culture dies; it's simple anthropology. There are secrets to finding water in the desert, fish on the flats, or eatable roots. There is a secret to reading the weather. There is a secret to a jump shot, to driving a stick-shift car, to making friends, and to mending a broken heart.

With CLAYtherapy, we first teach the simple secrets of making things out of play-dough. We hope that if children will allow us to teach them those play secrets, then they will allow us to teach them some of the weightier secrets of life and living (e.g., secrets to understanding divorce, controlling depression, recovering from abuse, and feeling better about oneself).

3. *Tools*. Tools make the secrets happen. For a child, talking to adults differently than to his or her friends is a tool. Identifying and controlling anger, depression, and inferiority is a tool. Learning and reducing the three parts of obsessive–compulsive behavior is a tool. Making good friends is a tool. We teach children to use tools to solve the problems of play-dough with seashells, crayons, pen caps, and playing cards. It's a short step to solving real-life problems with the tools taught through counseling.

4. *Practice*. Every parent knows the necessity of teaching children practice, and every child knows the need for practice, whether it be at video games, sports, or lyrics to songs. There is no better medium than

play-dough to learn this. Making things with play-dough is difficult at first, as is problem solving. Many a child's first projects have gone flying across my office. When children say things like "I can't, Mr. White. It's too hard," it is an invitation to learning because we as adults know they can, and we know that with practice they'll get better.

CASE EXAMPLES

Introduction of CLAYtherapy

CLAYtherapy can be introduced at any phase of treatment. It is especially useful in the first meeting with the child because it introduces the concepts of "talk some, play some" and that counseling can be a learning experience and still be fun. The play process parallels the therapeutic process when the counselor talks about the beginning, middle, and end of clay projects like the dinosaur, pig, or airplane. This three-stage process parallels the three phases of treatment. Clay play begins the process of the adult helping the child problem-solve, make decisions, and express feelings. It begins the relationship between helper and child, between student of life and teacher of life. It gives something for today and a promise for tomorrow, like a clay creature today and the promise of another next time, as well as the promise of additional adult–child hook-ups, problem resolution, relief of stress, and growth of self esteem. Therapy gives intangibles to take home, while clay provides take-home tangibles.

Dinosaurs and Divorce

Susan is a bright, engaging, usually articulate 9-year-old girl of divorcing parents. The divorce is imminent. It is more than she can bear to have her parents apart, her family dismantled, and her world torn asunder. She avoids talking about her emotions and pretends that her parents will be getting back together any day. She is having major eating, interpersonal, sleeping, and academic disturbances. She welcomes therapy and is quickly engaged. When she does begin to talk, she is overwhelmed by the flow of emotions. The thought of her parents divorcing is too painful, the consequences too scary, the future totally unknown, and the perceived process dismal. Susan is full of fear, anger, loyalty, betrayal, avoidance, worry, unrealistic hope, resentment, and blame, all at the same time. She vacillates from accepting reality to retreating into her fantasies. When she does talk of her reality, she becomes anxious, tearful, depressed, and hopeless. Her expressions are full of statements like "I just can't fix all these feelings . . . they are just too much . . . make them go away . . . this will never end . . . it's too big . . . I don't know how . . . I want to leave now . . . etc." Then she usually will withdraw into memories of better times or her fantasies or totally shut down.

I ask, "What is your favorite animal?"

She replies, "Penguins," and smiles.

I say, "Can you make a penguin from play-dough like mine on the shelf?"

She replies, "No, that would be hard."

"OK," I say. "Can you make a ball from this black piece of play-dough?"

"Yes, I can make a ball," she says. "That's easy."

"Can you make a penguin?" I ask.

"No, I can't make a penguin," she replies, with a somewhat anxious, questioning look.

"Oh," I say. "Can you roll that black ball in the palms of your hands into an egglike shape that is bigger at one end and smaller at the other?"

"Yes, I can do that," she says. "That's easy too."

"Can you make a penguin?" I ask.

She thinks, "Is this guy deaf?" Then she says, firmly, "No, I can't make a penguin!"

"Oh," I say. I proceed to ask her to make two small yellow balls (feet). Then I ask her to make two small black balls with blunt cones at each end, each smushed a bit (wings). I help her attach them with water and a crayon. Then I ask her to make a white ball, roll it into a cone, smash it, and attach it to the black egg (a tummy apron). Then she makes the tiny white eyes and the yellow beak. She splits the beak with a playing card and voilà, a penguin.

"I can make a penguin. I can!!!" she says, smiling.

I wait for the right moment and ask, "Can you fix the pain, the fear, the worry, and all the other feelings you told me about that come with your parents' divorce?"

"No, I can't, Mr. White." Sadness and hopelessness returns, with a pretearful face.

"Can we take all those terrible and confusing feelings and fix them one at a time, part by part, fear by fear, worry by worry, piece by piece, just like we made the penguin, and I'll help just like I helped with the penguin?"

Susan is quiet; I can almost see the wheels turning in her head. She looks up . . .

"Yes, I could do that," she says. "I want to do that." She smiles. "Good," I say. "Let's get to work."

Anger and Airplanes

Anger is one of the common denominators of working with children. We hope to teach children about anger: where it comes from, how to cope with its powers, and how to control its coming and going. In devising analogies and metaphors to respond to anger in children, play-dough is a helpful partner to the counselor. Play-dough provides not only the obvious elements of *expression* of anger through rolling, folding, and pounding, but also the less obvious elements of *recognition, modulation,* and *control* of anger and its two cousins, frustration and aggression.

Recognition of Anger

When opening a new can of play-dough, a child learns that clay directly off the shelf is not ready to form into stars and cars. Clay has a crystalline structure when taken directly from the can. The moisture content of play-dough is inconsistent from factory to store shelf or store to store. When making any creature or vehicle from play-dough, we learn to take the clay from the can and make several balls with no cracks to ensure that the clay is soft and has enough water content. If the clay is dry, we knead in some water. I ask, "Is the clay soft enough yet?" or "How's the moisture?" or "How do you/we know when the clay is ready to make something?" Clay has to be soft enough to form into balls, snakes, and cones. It has to be free of small cracks so they don't develop into big cracks as it dries.

I teach the children that the choice isn't just wet or dry, but that there are many variations of water content between the two extremes. And they learn how to remove the cracks by rolling the clay between their hands so they can feel it softening. They develop sensitivity to the substance and cultivate an awareness of its physical moods. They learn to recognize its various states, to know its variations in structure, moisture content, and readiness to use. They become the boss of the clay.

It's a small jump to convert clay knowledge into anger-awareness knowledge. A child has to be aware of his or her anger, to recognize its various states, to know whether it's present or absent, soft or hard, big or small. A child has to know and recognize the difference among anger, aggression, and frustration. He or she needs to develop sensitivity to his or her anger, an awareness of its presence, and a responsibility for its growth or control. He or she has to feel it coming and going, recognize its triggers, and sense frustration building and when lack of control gives way to aggression. A child has to become the boss of his or her anger.

Modulation of Anger

In time, children learn the difference between hard and soft clay, when a little is better than a lot, and that there are infinite points of hardness, amounts, details, and colors when creating clay projects. They learn the different number of cranks (revolutions) between their palms needed to make a certain amount of clay soft. They learn to take a little bit of clay or a lot, depending on the project. They learn to modulate the time in session needed to make a dinosaur or cow, how to pace themselves, follow the sequence of construction, and apply the secrets of simple to complex clay construction. As therapy continues, the counselor converts all this and more into clinical value.

Children learn the difference among states of anger, how anger evolves from frustration, and how aggression results from lack of anger control. They learn that anger isn't either off or on, hard or soft, but an infinite number of places on a continuum, just like clay. They learn that they can take out a little bit of anger or a lot depending on need or not take it out at all. They learn the process of solving life's problems, whether simple or complex. They learn to become the bosses of their anger.

Control of Anger

A child has to learn frustration control when dealing with clay. Clay will want to go its own way, just like children, just like anger. Sometimes clay goes flying across the room due to a child's lack of control. Through CLAYtherapy, we teach control, sometimes directly, sometimes quietly and nondirectly. We start with control of moisture, volume, color, and time, and we teach the amount of pressure necessary to connect parts without deforming the animal being made.

While we are teaching control of clay, we teach control of self— control of what we make, who does what, how much the adult does versus how much the child does, who is in control of the session, and who controls what and when things happen. CLAYtherapy teaches frustration control. When things don't come out the way we wanted them to, when they fall apart or crack, we have to control our anger and our sadness. We learn how to control ourselves when our pet dog eats our best play-dough car or our little sister breaks our best pig. Through play-dough, children learn they are the boss of their own behavior!

Airplanes and Anger

My favorite anger control CLAYtherapy approach is airplanes. Airplanes have a lot of power, in their construction, engines, avionics, and even bombs, if it's a military aircraft. An airplane can fly fast, high, and far. But it has to obey the laws of physics and the rules of flying; there are rules to follow and consequences for breaking the laws of nature or society. It has a ceiling above which it can't safely go. It can't fly once it runs out of gasoline. The pilot has to obey the instructions from the tower, the base, and his or her boss. An airplane has wonderful powers, but it also needs control or responsibility.

How is a boy or girl like an airplane? A child or teen has to obey the rules of nature and society as he or she goes about the business of growing. Boys or girls have to control and be responsible with their powers. Children have power in four places:

1. In their muscles (behavior)
2. In their brains (thoughts)
3. In their mouths (words)
4. In their hearts (feelings)

I say, "Think of the times you've gotten into trouble. Most of the time, it's because you didn't control your powers." And, "Take that airplane we made home and put it on your dresser. Every time you look at it, think of what we talked about today: controlling your powers." Once the child learns the lesson of the airplane and anger, the counselor can expand that concept to other feelings that need control like sadness, worry, fear, and anxiety.

CONCLUSION

Professionals in every child-centered discipline seek to improve their clinical skills and techniques with children. Experienced counselors are constantly seeking innovative methods to enhance their therapeutic intervention and treatment proficiency. New counselors seek techniques to compensate for limited experience and assistance in their development of clinical methodology. Most counselors in office, school, or clinic, whether experienced or recent graduate, use some form of play therapy with children. Most of them use clay, but few have learned how to use it effectively. *CLAYtherapy pulls together the play needs of the child with the treatment needs of the therapist.*

CLAYtherapy is an unequaled tool in helping children with problem-solving skills, self-esteem enhancement, decision-making processes, and control of impulse and anger. Any clinician providing short- or long-term therapy, intervention, or supportive services to children will welcome CLAYtherapy to his or her skill-building toolbox. CLAYtherapy reduces children's fears of counseling, grabs and holds their interest, provides a wide array of clinical connections, establishes an immediate problem-solving environment, complements the ongoing treatment plan, strengthens the clinical relationship, and is fun. CLAYtherapy is used with children from kindergarten through middle school.

CLAYtherapy is in its infancy. To date, its utilization has been limited to a few thousand counselors working within the crucible of day-to-day clinical engagement. I continue to discover additional applications, advance its parameters, and teach its application. Its eventual effectiveness and contribution to the broader play therapy community is yet to be known. I have issued an open invitation calling for suggestions, questions, recommendations, and challenges, and I welcome empirical scrutiny and academic review to determine the range of CLAYtherapy's therapeutic effectiveness, its acceptance by treatment professions, and its placement in the toolbox of play therapy.

NOTES

1. I use the universal word "clay" or "play-dough" in teaching CLAYtherapy. Both terms refer to the many natural or manmade clays, putties, and doughs or play-dough products on the market. They all have their pros and cons, and the user should select his or her favorite substance based on treatment needs. I have used every substance and find my CLAYtherapy techniques adaptable to them all. I have used dozens of homemade play-dough recipes with CLAYtherapy over the years. I no longer use homebrewed play-doughs. I use Play-Doh brand for three reasons:

   - Children seem to do best when they have the same consistency, smell, and feel from project to project, session to session. Homemade dough just can't be made to such consistent standards.
   - Children are already familiar with and have had positive experiences with Play-Doh at home, school, church, shelter, aftercare, and day camp.
   - In these days of malpractice litigation, I have to be careful in concocting something in my kitchen that might cause a child to have an allergic reaction in my office. Therefore, I use the standard in the industry: Play-Doh.

2. *CLAYtherapy*®: *The Clinical Application of Clay with Children*—This 150-page manual—with color pictures, line drawings, and text, teaches counselors to employ CLAYtherapy and to become proficient in its use. It is accompanied by a disk that shows step-by-step construction of the first four projects in the 12-creature inventory. *CLAYtherapy*® was published in 1989 by The Weebstar Press. Copies are available through my office (phone: 815-636-9742) or at my website (www.PlaytherapyCLAY.com).

REFERENCES

Axline, V. (1947). *Play therapy*. Cambridge, MA: Riverside Press.

Freud, A. (1971). *The writings of Anna Freud, 1966–1970, Vol. 7*. New York: International Universities Press.

Hart, R. (1992). *Therapeutic play activities*. St. Louis, MO: Mosby Year Book.

Landreth, G. (2004). *Play therapy interventions with children's problems*. Northvale, NJ: Aronson.

Moustakas, C. (1953). *Children in play therapy*. New York: McGraw-Hill.

Reid, S. E. (1986). Therapeutic use of card games. In C. E. Schaefer & S. E. Reid (Eds.), *Game play* (pp. 257–276). New York: Wiley.

Time-Limited Play Therapy to Enhance Resiliency in Children

DEBRA MAY

This chapter explores to what extent a 12-week time-limited play therapy intervention might help a child to enhance or develop the resilience factors of self-esteem, self-efficacy, and problem-solving skills, with a particular focus on the presentation of two cases, a 7-year old boy and a 10-year old girl.

There is little doubt that children have to cope with a variety of obstacles and difficulties as they enter each new developmental stage, but what about the difficulties that are born out of life's unpredictability and adversities? Whichever kind of difficulty it is, the child will have to negotiate with her inner self and others as she draws on what resilience she already has. But what of the child who has little resilience or sense of herself?

It has long been understood that in order for children to thrive and reach their potential they need to grow and be nurtured in a predictable and loving environment (Ainsworth, Blehar, Waters, & Wall, 1978; Crittenden, 1995, 1996). While most children are in this situation, there are also those who merely survive the relationships they have with their carers and environment. For some children, it is a daily struggle to cope with the volatility of their parental problems, such as homelessness, lack of money, family violence, mental health difficulties, and substance abuse. These problems are often further compounded by the added pressures of new relationships imposed by their families or circumstances (Harington, 1994; Rutter & Sandberg, 1992) as well as by trying to learn and develop new skills socially, educationally, culturally, or linguistically (O'Hara & Anderson, 1991).

HOW DO CHILDREN SURVIVE?

Winnicott believed that children were predisposed to "seek an external stability without which they may go mad" (1964, p. 228). If they do not receive the care and security they need at home, they look for it from members of their extended family, neighbors, friends, or at school. But what if it is not there in the measure they need? If children have an unpredictable relationship with their parents or carers leaving them with attachment difficulties (Carr, 1999), they may subsequently struggle to find any emotional and psychological meaning or safety in a relationship with another person.

A resilient child is able to integrate his or her experiences on a cognitive and emotional level and cope with the stresses of life's adversities without his or her normal development being impaired (Fonagy, Steele, Steele, Higgitt, & Target, 1994). Longitudinal studies of children's resilience have found that although not all children are vulnerable to the same adversities, one-third grow up to be psychologically and socially well adjusted (Garmezy & Rutter, 1983; Hetherington & Blechman, 1996; Rutter, 1981, 1990; Wang & Gordon, 1994; Werner, 1989, 1992).

WHAT IS RESILIENCE?

The three main models for understanding resilience are:

1. The "challenge" model, which views increased stress factors as potential enhancers of resilience that serve to stimulate the child to master skills, with the view that most people have a "self-righting mechanism" (Lifton, 1994).
2. The "compensatory" model, which focuses on the deficits in a child's environment and his or her individual protective factors to predict risk versus vulnerability outcomes (Gilligan, 1999a, 1999b; Rutter, 1985). Rutter focused on the individual protective factors that could be developed within a child, rather than the familial and environmental issues affecting him or her.

3. The "conditional" model, which looks at the personal characteristics of individuals, including whether they have the personality to cope with the stresses caused by adversities (Garmezy, Masten, & Tellegen, 1984).

The compensatory model is often criticized for its focus on what is wrong in a child's life rather than what is going right, which makes it hard for the child to change his or her coping strategies on his or her own (Selekman, 1997). On the other hand, Rutter's model (1985) focuses on the individual protective (rather than familial and environmental) factors that can be developed in a child. He claims that the protective factors moderate the negative effects of life's adversities and stresses and make a child more resilient.

Rutter's work in this field has been used and adapted by many professionals seeking to help children. The UK government has used it in its assessment framework to assess children's sources of vulnerability and resilience (Department of Health, 2000). Gilligan has used it as a basis for his work on how to build up children's resilience in the public care system (Gilligan, 1999a, 1999b). Seymour and Edman (1996) have also used Rutter's model successfully to develop family play therapy.

Rutter (1985) furthermore advised that children should be seen in a developmental context, as some will naturally develop the following resilience factors as they age and gain understanding of adversities and how to deal with them. Those who do not may need to be helped by others. According to Rutter (1985), the resilience factors are:

- The cognitive ability to appraise and attach meaning to an experience
- A coping strategy of being proactive or reactive
- A child's self-esteem and feelings of self-efficacy as well as a range of problem-solving skills
- A child's cognitive set, influenced by secure relationships and positive experiences as well as temperamental attributes
- A child's ability to adapt to and influence interactions
- The accumulation of positive experiences of encountering stress competently and appropriately

Play therapy is well placed to help children develop their sense of self as well as the factors listed above in Rutter's model. However, this is too broad a scope to focus on in a time-limited play therapy intervention. Instead, the focus for the intervention is on the development of self-esteem, self-efficacy, and problem-solving skills, which can serve to enhance each other. The possible linking of these resilience factors can be seen when a child has the ability to think up creative or constructive ways to solve problems; if this is then acknowledged by others, the child's sense of self-efficacy is improved, which in turn helps develop his or her self-esteem (Howe, Brandon, Hinings, & Schofield, 1999).

The focus of this chapter does not allow me to explain the importance of how a child's sense of self is first arrived at, other than to assert a belief that the care the child receives from birth, both physically and emotionally, within a caregiving relationship, is a key factor (Howe et al., 1999; Coppersmith, 1967). It is within this relationship that the child is given the opportunity to learn about him- or herself as likable, capable, and able to solve his or her own problems effectively. From this healthy position and view of self, a child feels free to explore his or her environment and develop relationships with others.

Winnicott (1971) claimed that it is only in play that a child's sense of self emerges and is allowed to develop as well as a sense of the other, which Cattanach (1997) defines as "the rest of the world, both people and objects" (p. 51). Both are equally necessary for the child's understanding to develop (Dunn, 1998). This discovery is facilitated through the process of play therapy, as the child has the freedom to explore his or her struggles and frustrations of the various roles and situations he or she has encountered and might be fearful of and gain some form of mastery or healing.

Research in the area of play therapy is increasing and has shown that as children are allowed to explore and develop their sense of self, their symptomatic behavioral difficulties are considerably reduced compared with control groups who do not have play therapy or any other intervention (Kot, 1995, as quoted in Ray & Bratton, 1999; Post, 1998, as quoted in Ray & Bratton, 1999, and Tyndall-Lind, 1999). It is often argued that the children's behavior improved due to the adult attention they received as opposed to the process of therapy, but Trostle (1988) and Schmidtchen, Hennies, and Acke (1993) found that the children who participated in play therapy showed a marked increase in person-centered competencies compared to the control group, who participated in a social education program.

In play therapy, a child's sense of self can be identified as it is projected from the child's internal working models onto the toys or the therapist through the child's use of narrative and play. From this, the play therapist gathers a baseline of the child's self-esteem, self-efficacy, and problem-solving skills and monitors what happens to these through the 12-week intervention. This requires a clear view and definition of these three resilience factors.

Self-Esteem

There are different ideas about how self-esteem is developed, for example, through a looking glass self, which, like a mirror, reflects a person's sense of worth through the opinions of significant others (Cooley, 1902). While it is argued that children gain their understanding of self through their relationships with significant others (Dunn, 1988), it would seem that this is only part of the answer, as there are children and adults who have had positive relationships with their significant others, yet lack a positive self-esteem. There remains the issue of whether the developing child's individual goals and aspirations are achieved or not. James said that the match between these two resulted in a "self-love," producing a positive self-esteem (Block & Robins, 1993; James, 1890).

Neither of the above explanations allows for the fluctuations of emotion and experience in relation to social interactions generally and specifically in conjunction with the child's sense of achievement. Govier's (1993) definition of self-esteem is more useful—he terms self-esteem as self-trust, in that if you didn't accept and trust yourself it was unlikely you would like yourself. This seems to me a healthier concept than one that does not self-evaluate and change, and could be seen, for example, with a child who is confident about social situations and enjoys learning at school but is also realistic about his or her strengths and shortcomings. With this in mind, the following criterion is applied to describe a positive self-esteem: "The self as lovable and self as likable as viewed by the child" (May, 2002).

Self-Efficacy

Some might argue that it is difficult to separate self-esteem and self-efficacy because they are inextricably linked (Howe et al., 1999). While it is agreed that they influence each other, they are separate factors, with neither more important than or possibly able to achieve before the other.

There are different views on how a person achieves self-efficacy. Gura (1996) maintained that children achieve self-efficacy when they are capable of solving social, physical, and practical problems that they face in social relationships or schoolwork and have control over these matters. Bandura (1977) used a social learning approach, making a case that people are constrained by how they perceive their behavior affects others as well as themselves. Kelly's (1955) personal construct theory contended that people are not victims of their past or present circumstances; rather, self-efficacy depends on how they have constructed meanings in their world. These are not set and can be reconstructed, such as through the different narratives and stories the child co-creates with the therapist in their play. This enables the child to internalize them and create potentially healthier methods of coping as he or she begins to experiment with new ways of seeing and achieving success. From this, the following criterion is used for self-efficacy: "The self as capable and able to affect and influence what happens to her socially, physically, and practically" (May, 2002).

Problem-Solving Skills

The important question is not whether children have a repertoire of social problem-solving approaches, as it could be argued that otherwise they wouldn't have survived. Rather, the question it is whether these skills are helpful to the children's sense of well-being, both individually and socially, or whether they are simply an adaptation, an inadequate response to a problem that may well "induce negative reactions in other people" (Rutter, 1985, p. 607). Therefore, this resilient factor is described as: "The self seeking solutions to problems or risks and successfully or unsuccessfully completing the task" (May, 2002).

TIME-LIMITED PLAY THERAPY

There are several names and models used for play therapy with a fixed number of sessions (Cattanach, 1994; Johnson, 2001; Ryan & Needham 2001; Sloves & Peterlin, 1994). They share some commonalities, such as a given number of sessions with the end date irrevocably fixed, as well as a general consensus that a time-conscious approach can be therapeutically beneficial to the child (Johnson, 2001; Wilson, Kendrick, & Ryan, 1992).

Sloves and Peterlin's model (1994) uses a focused directive approach for 12 sessions. It is "a highly structured, aggressively managed, interactive treatment modality" with the therapist as a "co-equal with the child" with an emphasis throughout the intervention on strengths, not weaknesses (p. 31). This is only possible if the child has experienced good enough parenting and is able to "conceptualize time" as the ending is built into the therapy from the beginning (p. 32). This is assessed at the referral and in the first two therapy sessions with the child. It also discourages regression and a negative transfer onto the therapist.

Critics of this model would argue that it can be problematic for some children who may need a longer intervention in which they can negatively transfer onto the therapist and explore earlier developmental stages in their play. Sloves and Peterlin's model (1994) may not be suitable for children who prevent themselves from engaging in the play therapy due to their consciousness of its end and the feelings of separation and loss or rejection this may evoke. The other issue children's willingness to let a therapist usurp their cues. To this end, Guerney (1983) advocates that the child work at his or her own pace in the therapeutic process (p. 30) and Gardner (1993) suggests that time-limited play therapy cannot bring about any permanent change for the child (p. 25).

In the end, a combination of Sloves and Peterlin's model (1994) and Ryan and Needham's model (2001) was used, as shown below.

- Meeting with referrer
- Introduction letter to parents
- Semi-structured interview with the child's parent(s)
- Introduction letter to child
- Meeting with family and child
- Meeting with the child's teacher
- Play therapy agreement between the child and therapist
- 12 time-limited play therapy sessions of 50 minutes each
- A review after six sessions

This is a child-centered model and can use either a focused or a nondirective approach, depending on whether the child is able to engage with the therapist quickly within the first two sessions when the core themes are identified. If the child is able to do this, then the focused approach could be used; if not, then the therapist would need to use a more nondirective approach. Such a model also encompasses the child's different systems, including school, parents or the child's main carers, and any other people involved with the child.

In order for children to receive the time-limited play therapy intervention, they had to be displaying moderate behavioral difficulties either at home or at school. At the same time, they had to be receiving emotional and physical support from their parents. This was assessed by speaking to the referrer about his or her knowledge of the child's family. An initial visit was also made to the parents to gather background on the child and family. The suitability of the intervention for the child was assessed within the first two therapeutic sessions by determining whether each child could quickly engage in the therapeutic process as well as his or her ability to sequence events in play, narratives, and stories.

In order to gather a baseline of the child's resilient factors mentioned above, the themes from each play therapy session were analyzed in the children's play in the sessions. Kohut (1984) suggests these are indicators that the child "has not given up hope of having these needs met" (p. 95). The construction of a theme has been based on Landreth's (2001) definition: "a recurrence of certain events or topics in the child's play, either within a play experience, such as during a play therapy session, or across several play experiences or sessions" (p. 11).

CASE EXAMPLES

Gemma

Gemma was 10 years old at the time of the referral. She was mixed race. Her father was black British and her mother white British and her skin was light brown. She had dark brown eyes. Gemma was her mother's first child. She witnessed domestic violence between her mother and father when she was 2 years old; her father hit her mother, and her mother stabbed him with a knife. This episode ended the relationship between her parents. Gemma saw her father occasionally when her mother arranged it. He had three other children by two other women. Gemma was due to meet one of these children for the first time at the time of the referral. Gemma's stepfather was also black British.

Gemma had not attended nursery school, as her mother felt she did not like it. Since the reception class, Gemma had attended five schools, and her attendance was reported as good. At the time of the referral, her school was concerned that she was increasingly picking fights with other girls on the playground and appeared to have difficulty maintaining relationships. Her teacher described her as a bright girl who had been in the top sets for all her subjects up until the previous year but had become increasingly uninterested in her learning.

• *Had Gemma's self-esteem been enhanced or developed by the end of the 12 sessions?* Gemma showed through her play in the first session that she knew how to make friends and go off and explore with them. This is a very good indicator of healthy self-esteem. Her play showed that this ability was adversely affected as she focused more on others' opinions of her with negative projections. Through play, Gemma explored her identity as a child in a family, as part of a group of friends, and as a black girl in a predominantly white culture. At the final session, she was able openly to talk about the effect of the racism she felt in her everyday life at school and at home. It is thought that Gemma's self-esteem had developed prior to the intervention to where she saw herself as likable. This had been upset, probably due to the unpredictability of her friends and how from Gemma's perspective one minute they liked her and the next they hated her and hit her. Another possible reason for the disruption in her self-esteem was developmental. Gemma was approaching adolescence and could need more independence from her mother. By the end of the 12 sessions, Gemma's self-esteem had been enhanced again.

- *Had Gemma's self-efficacy been enhanced or developed by the end of the 12 sessions?* The repetitive themes in this category showed Gemma had a sense of self-efficacy and knew she was capable of going away and returning. She also was able to seek out the affirmation she needed. Her play showed that this resilience factor was only affected in a more negative and needy way when connected in the play with her family or in a joint play therapy session with her mother. Was this due to Gemma's developmental stage and need for independence and a feeling of being overpowered by her mother's needs? Again, it was thought that Gemma had previously developed a positive sense of self-efficacy, where she saw herself as capable of effecting change, and that this probably had been disrupted, which had also adversely affected her self-esteem. On the other hand, it could have been a result of difficulties in her relationship with her mother, who had experienced complications in her pregnancy and was making increasing demands on Gemma.

- *Had Gemma's problem-solving skills been enhanced or developed by the end of the 12 sessions?* Problem-solving skills were the least developed resilience factor for Gemma at the start of the intervention. She mainly used magical solutions to solve problems at first, but gradually, through the 12 weeks, Gemma explored using different problem-solving skills in her play. From this, she was able to develop the ability to negotiate with others in her play.

Jack

Jack was 7 years old at the time of his referral. He was average height with a slightly built frame. He had blue eyes and fair hair. Jack's early history was largely unknown and anecdotal. He was raised by his mother, who separated from his father when Jack was a baby. She apparently moved several times during Jack's young life and had several partners during this time. There were also concerns about his mother having a drinking problem and possibly an issue with drugs.

Eventually, Jack moved to Ireland with his mother and stepfather. During this period, he did not have contact with his father. Prior to this, Jack had seen his father every weekend. It was this that precipitated

Jack's father seeking a residence order, after which Jack was brought back by his mother's partner to live with his father. At the time of the play therapy, Jack had had no contact with his mother for more than 2 years.

Jack had attended two previous schools, where he was reported to have had problems. At one, he had been permanently excluded for apparently carrying some of his faces into the classroom. It was not possible to verify these reports due to his reports being sent to his school in Ireland and lost in transit.

His father worked shifts locally. Jack's stepmother looked after him together with two other young children, ages 3 years and 10 months, the latter being Jack's half-brother.

Jack's paternal grandmother had regular contact with the family, and Jack spent one night a week with her. Jack showed difficulty trusting his stepmother, and their relationship was often difficult, which caused a strain on her relationship with Jack's father. They did accept support from the education welfare officer who referred Jack for play therapy.

- *Had Jack's self-esteem been enhanced or developed by the end of 12 sessions?* By the end of the twelve sessions there was little evidence of an increased positive self-esteem for Jack. There was only evidence of him trying to develop his sense of self as he explored conflicting aspects of physical and emotional needs that went back to a much earlier developmental stage of infancy, "trust versus mistrust" (Erikson, 1963). This could also have been compounded and confused for Jack by the added theme of his separation from and loss of his mother, which Jack only allowed himself to explore at the end of the 12 sessions.
- *Had Jack's self-efficacy been enhanced or developed by the end of 12 sessions?* Jack had been able to make a clear distinction between goodies and baddies and had shown in his play that the confusion he showed in who to trust in this area had been resolved. By session 4, Jack continued to explore his feelings particularly in relation to an aggressor. This was seen with the goodies fighting the baddies and killing him or them, depending on the narrative. Was this in relation to his mother's partner, who had physically abused him, or was he exploring being able to rescue his mother from the aggressor? The effect of physical abuse left him with little energy to explore his emotions; he would have used his survival skills instead and possibly as a result felt frequently overwhelmed by feelings of helplessness.

Jack did not develop self-efficacy during the 12 sessions, although he had begun to lay a foundation for self-efficacy as he explored his self in relation to others and events.

- *Had Jack's problem-solving skills been enhanced or developed by the end of the 12 sessions?* Jack had started play therapy with confusion about how to problem-solve, and he spent the 12 sessions exploring his feelings about events and who and what he could trust. By the end of the 12 sessions, Jack had shown slight shifts in his play, not burying everything (e.g., good and bad) and being prepared to explore some painful parts of his self.

CONCLUSION

Rutter (1985) described the three identified resilience factors as "cognitive sets" and not a "fixed personality trait"; as such, they "may change with altered circumstances" (p. 603). This explains Gemma's results, as she had previously developed the cognitive set, but, as a result of difficult circumstances at home and at school, it had been altered.

In addition, the results from the above case studies agree with the Sloves and Peterlin model of time-limited play therapy (1994), in that it is only possible if the child is able to engage with the therapist quickly and participate in a focused intervention directed by the therapist, as Gemma did. Otherwise the kind of focused, aggressively structured play their model suggests is appropriate, as was the case with Jack. Also, this model is firmly against the child regressing, and it could be argued that Jack would always have needed long-term play therapy. Both children represented different needs, and both required preventative work.

Another important factor is that both Gemma and Jack had supportive parents to help them and support them through any therapeutic process. Both Gemma's and Jack's parents received individual support with their personal issues from another professional and at the same time their child attended play therapy. This is a well-known way of producing optimum results for the child in therapy (Killough-McGuire & McGuire, 2000, p. 185). Due to parents having different needs, this support was offered in different ways in my research. In Gemma's case, her mother was heavily pregnant, so an outreach worker visited her weekly at home and worked with her on an adaptation of a parenting program that was cognitive in approach and focused on the parent being positive about his or her child. Jack's parents had support from an educational welfare officer whom they trusted and were able to work in a client-centered way (Rogers, 1991) on some delicate issues in their relationship. An unexpected outcome by the end of the 12 sessions was that both children had improved relationships with their parents.

Finally, as established in the case studies of Gemma and Jack, it is almost certain that Gemma had previously developed aspects of the identified resilience factors (Rutter, 1985) and the 12-week intervention served to enhance these, whereas Jack had an underdeveloped sense of self and had not been able to develop any of the identified resilience factors before the intervention and so would need a much longer intervention. It is important that children are screened appropriately for such an intervention and that their parents are willing and able to engage with the play therapist with ongoing support from a separate professional at the same time.

REFERENCES

Ainsworth, M. D. S., Blehar, M., Waters, E., & Wall, S. (1978). *Patterns of attachment and psychological study of the strange situation.* Hillsdale, NJ: Erlbaum.

Bandura, G. (1977). Self-efficacy: Toward a unifying theory of behavioural change. *Psychological Review, 84,* 191–215.

Block, J., & Robins, R. W. (1993). A longitudinal study of consistency and change in self-esteem from early adolescence to early adulthood. *Child Development, 64,* 909–923.

Carr, A. (1999). *The handbook of child and adolescent clinical psychology: A contextual approach.* London: Routledge.

Cattanach, A. (1994). *Play therapy: Where the sky meets the underworld.* London: Jessica Kingsley.

Cattanach, A. (1997). *Children's stories in play therapy.* London: Jessica Kingsley.

Cooley, C. H. (1902). *Human nature and the social order.* New York: Scribner.

Coppersmith, S. (1967). *The antecedents of self-esteem.* San Francisco: Freeman.

Crittenden, P. (1995). Attachment and psychopathology. In S. Goldberg, R. Muir, & J. Kerr (Eds.), *Attachment theory: Social, developmental and clinical perspectives* (pp. 367–406). Hillsdale, NJ: Analytic Press.

Crittenden, P. (1996). Research on maltreating families: Implications for intervention. In J. Brier, L. Berliner, & J. Buckley (Ed.), *The APSAC handbook of child maltreatment* (pp. 158–174). Thousand Oaks, CA: Sage.

Department of Health, Department for Education and Employment and Home Office. (2000). *Framework for the assessment of children in need and their families.* London: The Stationery Office.

Dunn, J. (1988). *The beginnings of social understanding.* Oxford, UK: Blackwell.

Erikson, E. (1963). *Childhood and society.* New York: Norton.

Fonagy, P., Steele, M., Steele, H., Higgitt, A., & Target, M. (1994). The Emmanuel Miller Memorial Lecture 1992: The theory and practice of resilience. *Journal of Child Psychology and Psychiatry, 35,* 231–257.

Gardner, R. A. (1993). *Story telling in psychotherapy with children*. Northvale, NJ: Aronson.

Garmezy, N., Masten, A. S., & Tellegen, A. (1984). The study of stress and competence in children: A building block for developmental psychopathology, *Child Development, 5*, 97–111.

Garmezy, N., & Rutter, M. (Eds.). (1983). *Stress, coping and development in children*. New York: McGraw-Hill.

Gilligan, R. (1999a). Children's own social network and network memers: Key resources in helping children at risk. In H. Mill (Ed.), *Effective ways of helping children* (pp. 70–88). London: Jessica Kingsley.

Gilligan, R. (1999b). Enhancing the resilience of children and young people in public care by encouraging their talents and interests. *Child and Family Social Work 4*(3), 187–196.

Govier, T. (1993). Self-trust, autonomy and self-esteem. *Hypatia, 8*(1), 99–120.

Guerney, L. F. (1983). Client-centered (non-directive) play therapy. In C. E. Shaefer & K. J. O'Connor (Eds.), *The handbook of play therapy*. New York, Wiley.

Gura, P. (1996, Summer). What I want for Cinderella: Self-esteem and self-assessment. *Baece Early Education*. Unpublished research paper, Roehampton Institute, London.

Harington, R. (1994). Affective disorders. In M. Rutter, E. Taylor, & L. Herson (Eds.), *Child and adolescent psychology*. Oxford, UK: Blackwell.

Hetherington, E. M., & Blechman, E. A. (Eds.). (1996). *Stress, coping, and resiliency in children and families*. Mahwah, NJ: Erlbaum.

Howe, D., Brandon, M., Hinings, D., & Schofield, G. (1999). *Attachment theory, child maltreatment and family support*. Basingstoke, UK: Palgrave.

James, W. (1890). *Principles of psychology* (Vol. 1). New York: Holt.

Johnson, S. P. (2001). Short-term play therapy. In G. Landreth (Ed.), *Innovations of play therapy* (pp. 217–234). Philadelphia: Brunner-Routledge.

Kelly, G. A. (1955). *A theory of personality: The psychology of personal constructs*. New York: Norton.

Killough-McGuire, D., & McGuire, D. (2000). *Linking parents to play therapy*. Philadelphia: Brunner-Routledge.

Kohut, H. (1984). *How does analysis cure?* Chicago: University of Chicago Press.

Landreth, G. L. (2001). *Innovations of play therapy*. Philadelphia: Brunner-Routledge.

Lifton, B. (1994). *The journey of the adopted self: A quest for wholeness*. New York: Basic Books.

May, D. (2002). *To what extent might a social construction approach within time-limited play therapy develop or enhance resilience in a child?* Unpublished master's dissertation, Roehampton, University of Surrey.

O'Hara, M., & Anderson, A. (1991). Welcome to the postmodern world. *Networker, 15*, 19–25.

Ray, D., & Bratton, S. (Eds.). (1999). *Update: What the research shows about play therapy*. Denton: University of North Texas.

Rogers, C. (1991). *Client-centred therapy*. London: Constable.

Rutter, M. (1981). *Maternal deprivation reassessed* (2nd ed.). Harmondsworth, UK: Penguin.

Rutter, M. (1985). Resilience in the face of adversity: Protective factors and resistance to psychiatric disorder. *British Journal of Psychiatry, 147*, 598–611.

Rutter, M. (1990). Psychosocial resilience and protective mechanisms. In J. Rolf, A. Masten, D. Cicchetti, K. Nuechterlein, & S. Weintraub (Eds.), *Risk and protective factors in the development of psychopathology* (pp. 181–214). New York: Cambridge University Press.

Rutter, M., & Sandberg, S. (1992). Psychosocial stressors, concepts, causes and effects. *European Child and Adolescent Psychiatry, 1*, 3–13.

Ryan, V., & Needham, C. (2001). Non-directive play therapy with children experiencing psychic trauma. *Clinical Child Psychology and Psychiatry 1359–1045*, 437–452.

Schmidtchen, S., Hennies, S., & Acke, H. (1993). To kill two birds with one stone? Evaluating the hypothesis of a twofold effectiveness of client-centered play therapy. *Psychologie in Erziehung und Unterricht, 40*, 34–42.

Selekman, M. D. (1997). *Solution-focused therapy with children*. New York: Guilford Press.

Seymour, J. W., & Edman, P. (1996). Family play therapy using resiliency model. *International Journal of Play Therapy, 5*, 9–30.

Sloves, R. E., & Peterlin, K. B. (1994). Time-limited play therapy. In K. O'Connor & C. E. Schaefer (Eds.), *Handbook of play therapy, Vol. 2: Advances and innovations* (pp. 29–57). New York: Wiley.

Trostle, S. (1988). The effects of child-centered group play sessions on social emotional growth of three- to six-year-old bilingual Puerto Rican children. *Journal of Research in Childhood Education, 3*, 93–106.

Tyndall-Lind, A. (1999). *A comparative analysis of intensive individual play therapy and intensive sibling group play therapy with child witnesses of domestic violence*. Doctoral dissertation, University of North Texas, Denton.

Wang, M. C., & Gordon, E. W. (1994). *Educational resilience in inner-city America: Challenges and prospects*. Hillsdale, NJ: Erlbaum.

Werner, E. E. (1989). High-risk children in adulthood: A longitudinal study from birth to 32 years. *American Journal of Orthopsychiatry, 59*, 72–81.

Werner, E. E. (1992). *Overcoming the odds: High risk children from birth to adulthood*. Ithaca, NY: Cornell University Press.

Wilson, K., Kendrick, P., & Ryan, V. (1992). *Play therapy a nondirective approach for children and adolescents*. London: Bailliere Tindall.

Winnicott, D. W. (1964). *The child, the family and the outside world*. Harmondsworth, UK: Penguin.

Winnicott, D. W. (1971). *Playing and reality*. London: Tavistock.

CHAPTER 13

Coping with Disaster

Psychosocial Interventions for Children in International Disaster Relief

ERIKA FELIX
DAVID BOND
JANINE SHELBY

Before the tsunami, nature was a gift for us. We were proud to have such a beautiful gift. But today the situation is different. I feel like crying. I am helpless because our happy home was washed away by the sea and now we have to ask someone else for shelter. My mother used to prepare tasty meals, but now we have to keep in hunger for several meals. I have very sad memories, which I can never forget. My friends and my relatives lost their lives. The sound of weeping, crying, and shouting are still in my ears. We can't bring those lives back. We never thought an incident like this would ever happen, even in dreams, but I don't hate or blame the sea. I will not weep by thinking of what I lost. I wish to live with what I gain.

—TEENAGE SRI LANKAN TSUNAMI SURVIVOR

Following devastating disasters, such as the tsunami that struck southeast Asia on December 26, 2004, many mental health professionals feel an urgent desire to help. In fact, mental health professionals are increasingly being called to serve in disaster relief operations and are doing so admirably. Mental health workers can be a vital component of the overall recovery process (Jacobs, 1995) as illustrated by the young tsunami survivor whose prose describes her experience of disaster and postdisaster integration. Some, however, are volunteering without adequate preparation, realistic expectations, or a systematic approach for intervening in the often chaotic and overwhelming postdisaster environment (Weine et al., 2002). When adequately trained, international volunteer mental health professionals can provide needed psychological assistance, but without adequate training and preparation, well-intentioned mental health professionals may harm or hinder the recovery process (Weine et al., 2002). The aim of this chapter is to provide concrete, practical information about the realities of disaster mental health relief work with children, including guidelines for and examples of empirically supported psychosocial interventions, discussion of the transportability of these interventions to diverse international settings, and pragmatic tips to assist interventionists develop reasonable expectations and cultural sensitivities pertaining to their work.

HISTORY AND EVOLUTION
OF DISASTER MENTAL HEALTH

The evolution of disaster mental health relief is relatively recent compared to the traditional humanitarian aid response to the physical needs of disaster survivors. Jacobs (1995) reviewed the historical developments that contributed to the creation of a national disaster mental health plan, including the collaboration between the American Red Cross (ARC) and the American Psychological Association (APA). In brief, Jacobs (1995) reported that modern disaster mental health response started in 1942, following the Coconut Grove fire that led to Lindemann's (1944) crisis theory, which influenced subsequent crisis response efforts for decades. The traditional 6-week period in which many crisis intervention programs offer services is directly based on Lindemann's observation of the duration of the crisis period. By 1982, Congress mandated the ARC to respond to every national disaster; however, it was not until 1988 that the ARC began developing a protocol for the provision of disaster mental health services. Eventually, the ARC developed a mental health protocol for both survivors and response personnel and corresponding training for mental health services workers. Although this was a step toward developing a more systematic means of delivering crisis intervention, the main focus of this protocol was responding to other ARC workers' job-related stress. This focus limited the training and preparation that mental health workers received regarding postdisaster response to survivors. Also, the ARC model to date does not provide a specific protocol for intervention with young survivors, although it offers some suggested tools for interventions, such as the use of therapeutic coloring books.

Historically, nongovernmental organizations (NGOs) providing disaster relief services have offered a variety of health services and supplies, but very few have offered crisis or acute intervention programs to survivors. During the last 15 years, play-based activities for children have become popular in mass care settings where large numbers of children are sheltered. Many NGOs offer art and other activities, such as puppet shows or other forms of entertainment, but the objectives of such activities are often unclear (e.g., Is the objective psychological intervention, diversion, or amusement?). Outcome evaluation of these activities is rare, and the quality of training that interventionists receive ranges widely. Manualized treatments and those with demonstrated efficacy remain relatively scant (for a review, see Vernberg, 2002). In summary, although there is burgeoning interest in providing psychological intervention to young survivors of disaster, there are few evidence-informed protocols for delivering such services, there is a lack of awareness of those that exist, and most literature on the subject involves general guidance (e.g., "encourage children to talk about their feelings") rather than specific intervention strategies. As a result, international efforts to provide psychological intervention often vary widely in terms of their objectives, quality, standardization, and level of reliance on available research evidence.

CONSIDERATIONS FOR PSYCHOSOCIAL RELIEF EFFORTS POSTDISASTER

In preparing to volunteer for a disaster mental health mission, interventionists should begin by consulting established guidelines on the provision of mental health services postdisaster. A brief summary of several of these protocols is offered below. Interventionists should also become familiar with factors that are believed to promote adaptive recovery and those that increase the risk for posttraumatic stress. This knowledge can affect the assessment process and the selection of interventions. Finally, interventionists should consider myriad cultural issues when interacting with the host culture and in the selection of intervention activities. A summary is detailed below.

Guidelines

The Disaster Mental Health Institute at the University of South Dakota (Jacobs, 1995; Reyes & Elhai, 2004), International Society for Traumatic

Stress Studies (ISTSS; Weine et al., 2002), National Center for Posttraumatic Stress Disorder (PTSD), National Center for Child Traumatic Stress (NCCTS), and World Health Organization all offer guidelines for the provision of mental health services postdisaster. These organizations offer general suggestions for intervention in the immediate, short-, and long-term aftermath as well as guidelines for training local counselors. These organizations caution against the belief that doing anything is better than doing nothing, as there is potential for the intervention to produce iatrogenic, or harmful, effects. For example, a well-meaning interventionist may inappropriately engage a survivor in an intervention that requires mental reexperiencing of the trauma before the interventionist has established that the survivor possesses adequate coping skills or social support systems to tolerate the potential stress of such an activity. Due to this and other risks, the interventionist is obliged to understand the common issues that occur during postdisaster adjustment and the integration process, assess the survivor's coping and resources, and use empirically supported, established interventions.

For the provision of training to local counselors or helpers, the ISTSS guidelines (Weine et al., 2002) advocate setting up a structure of ongoing supervision to promote sustainability and avoid harm. In Sri Lanka, local psychologists reported that paraprofessionals previously received 2 days of training by an organization that promoted the use of an advanced psychotherapeutic technique. Attempts by Sri Lankan paraprofessionals to apply the technique produced disastrous results. Without provisions for ongoing supervision to ensure the technique was implemented properly, survivors were inadequately assessed and treated, paraprofessionals were disheartened, Western mental health technology lost credibility in the eyes of a foreign system, and, on a broader level, new problems were created as traumatized survivors needed assistance to recover from their postdisaster intervention. Consequently, the few local psychologists and psychiatrists available had to reinstruct the poorly prepared paraprofessionals to refrain from using the technique without additional supervision and training.

Aspects of Recovery

Survivors, like the young person described in the opening paragraph, often show resilience and strength postdisaster as they cope with expected posttraumatic and grief symptoms (Norris, Byrne, Diaz, & Kaniasty, 2001; Watson & Shalev, 2005). Others show increased risk for developing clinical levels of maladjustment (Norris et al., 2001; Watson &

Shalev, 2005). Several factors interact to influence whether a child will develop clinical levels of posttraumatic stress or show postdisaster resiliency. Silverman and La Greca (2002) organize these factors into the following four groups: (1) aspects of the traumatic exposure, (2) preexisting characteristics of the child, (3) characteristics of the postdisaster recovery environment, and (4) the child's psychological resources. Traumatic exposure includes the extent of destruction, threatened or actual loss of life, and disruption of activities of daily living (e.g., displacement from home or school). The scope of devastation directly relates to the length of recovery for communities and individuals. The level of exposure children experienced to loss of life or threatened loss of life—as well as community destruction—affects the likelihood of developing PTSD. Likewise, disruption of daily activities, such as school closure, affects child functioning. Therefore, reestablishing educational programs, resuming normal roles and routines to the extent possible, and engaging in structured activities on a scheduled basis in mass care settings can help children return to a feeling of normalcy. The second factor, preexisting characteristics of the child, includes demographic characteristics and predisaster functioning. The third factor, characteristics of the postdisaster recovery environment, includes protective factors, such as the availability of social support, and risk factors, such as the occurrence of major life events or stressors (e.g., parental job loss, moving homes). Finally, the child's own psychological resources, such as adaptive coping skills and self-efficacy, influence psychological outcomes. Predisaster coping and global level of functioning are related to young survivors' capacity to cope postdisaster.

These interacting characteristics should be considered when planning the scope, duration, and type of interventions used in psychosocial disaster relief efforts (Silverman & La Greca, 2002). For example, universal interventions to promote adaptive coping and normalize common reactions may be helpful initially to most survivors, but those who had preexisting mental health problems and children who are showing marked signs of traumatic stress will need more targeted services (Vernberg, 2002). In addition, since having good communication skills, strong self-efficacy, and positive coping skills are all protective factors (Silverman & La Greca, 2002), mental health interventions that promote these skills and traits can provide lasting benefits and are considered to have less potential to do harm.

A broad program of psychological services including family and community interventions can increase the effectiveness and lasting impact of mental health relief services (Vernberg, 2002). For example, helping caregivers and community members provide effective social support to each other and children can create lasting benefits, as perceived social support has been related to better outcomes postdisaster (Silverman & La Greca, 2002). Likewise, helping parents cope with their own PTSD symptoms can help prevent them from transmitting their anxiety and avoidance reactions onto their children, thereby decreasing the intensity or duration of the children's symptoms.

Cultural Issues

Prior to delivering interventions, it is imperative to gather as much information as possible about the culture, religion, politics, social structure, and ethnic composition of the devastated region in order to best understand the context within which relief efforts are to be provided. If the interventionist is unfamiliar with the culture, it is particularly important that he or she engage in universal principles of sensitivity, such as approaching everyone with humility and respect. Also, it is helpful to assess the situation, observe the behavior of others, and inquire about typical strategies used to promote mental health before implementing interventions. Interventionists should also obtain feedback from persons knowledgeable about the culture regarding the appropriateness of the anticipated interventions, acquire information about specific coping strategies regarded as beneficial by the culture, and monitor for any negative or unexpected reactions from survivors and local staff during the implementation of interventions. Asking for feedback from staff regarding culturally acceptable behavior by the interventionist is also critically important to the success of an intervention (e.g., the use of nonverbal gestures, facial expressions, or direct discussion of the traumatic event).

For those unfamiliar with working through translators, it is helpful to speak slowly, pause frequently, and avoid colloquialisms, metaphors, and jargon. When possible, it is preferable to allow local, newly trained personnel to implement the interventions under the supervision of, or together with, the interventionist than to have the interventionist do so solely via a translator. If working in international settings where few speak English, and there are few translators available, it is important to choose interventions that are activity- rather than language-based. For example, in the Sri Lanka relief effort, some activities were too difficult to translate to a large audience to be implemented effectively. However, activity-based interventions were consistently understood by and effective for both children and local staff seeking to learn new intervention tools. When possible, have materials translated prior to arrival. To assist in selecting useful interventions, a summary of evidence-informed techniques that have been used in disasters in the Americas, Europe, and Asia are described in the pages that follow.

EVIDENCE-INFORMED PLAY INTERVENTIONS FOR DISASTER MENTAL HEALTH

When selecting interventions, the interventionist should consider a variety of factors, including (1) disaster-related variables (proximity to the disaster, exposure, length of time since the disaster, amount of devastation, loss of life), (2) the level of immediate physical needs of the child and family, (3) the sociopolitical and religious contexts of the region, including culture and language, (4) the existing mental health infrastructure and access to ongoing psychological and/or medical intervention, (5) the developmental level of the child, (6) the availability of caretakers to participate in interventions, (7) the child's coping resources and level of adaptive functioning, and (8) contextual issues (e.g., intervention space, materials available, skill of the interventionists, whether translators must be used or not) (Shelby & Felix, 2005; Vernberg, 2002). An assessment of these contextual factors will influence the choice and scope of the intervention. Even the most empirically valid intervention may not work as planned in the wrong culture, setting, or context or through translation. Flexibility and adaptation to local styles of coping is essential.

The interventions below directly focus on enhancing or providing coping skills, sometimes in relation to specific characteristics of traumatic stress. There are several important reasons for this focus, including the ideas that clinical levels of posttraumatic stress among children vary widely across disastrous events and that resilience in coping is often common among survivors (Norris et al., 2001). Second, the limited time and access to direct mental health services for survivors in many third-world countries need to be considered. Lengthy and less-focused treatment approaches may be viewed as unhelpful given time and resource limitations or may not be provided in sufficient dosage to show an effect. For example, nondirective or child-centered treatment approaches may require several sessions before the child shows symptom reduction or coping skills gains compared to the shorter period of time that targeted approaches take. Third, user-friendly global interventions (e.g., coping skills training and activities) that can be taught to local healers and caregivers—as opposed to more sophisticated interventions that target symptoms—can strengthen natural supports for recovery. Investing training resources in the existing local networks rather than primarily with survivors develops an infrastructure for continued intervention provision beyond the relief mission. Caregivers and local leaders will be there long after relief operations end, thus building their capacity to respond to the mental health needs of their community is more likely to have a lasting benefit. In addition, they are experts on their own culture and community and thus can adapt the interventions to best fit the needs of children within their culture.

Assessment of Coping Strategies

Before beginning an intervention, it is important to assess the child's coping strengths and psychosocial needs. Information about children's coping abilities is usually best gathered through a multisource approach in which both the adult caregivers and child provide reports. Although a question-and-answer technique may be sufficient for adults, an interventionist may be much more likely to obtain accurate information from a child by engaging him or her with a more experiential activity to assess coping behavior. Interventionists in Sri Lanka used a depiction of a banana tree in which healthy and ripe bananas are labeled with adaptive coping strategies (e.g., thinking thoughts that make me feel better, talking to someone I trust), while rotten bananas on the ground are labeled with maladaptive coping mechanisms (e.g., blaming self, focusing on how awful things are). Some labels are left blank for children to name the coping strategies that they have been using. Children are told that some bananas make them feel better when eaten, while others are likely to make them feel worse. Children are then asked to identify which of the bananas they are consuming, allowing the interventionist to tailor the intervention activities to each child's specific coping needs.

Enhancing Coping Skills

Enhancing and reinforcing the child's ability to cope effectively is a cornerstone of crisis and acute intervention. Effective goals for coping enhancement interventions should include improving the child's ability to (1) carry out developmentally appropriate activities of daily living, (2) reduce negative or fearful thoughts, and (3) seek out and receive social support (Watson & Shalev, 2005). Several play-based activities that promote adaptive coping among young survivors are described below.

Puppetry can be an effective tool for helping children build and enhance coping skills. Using puppets, the interventionists portray a story of a young character who has experienced an unnamed traumatic event.

Reactions to the trauma are described and normalized (e.g., the children are scared, some of them are hurt, and the main character is afraid that he or she will be alone). Soon, grown-up characters come to take the child character(s) to a safe place. The main character is given food and reassurances of safety, and his or her fears are addressed. The emphasis should be placed on characters' development of coping skills, including seeking social support when needed, returning to normal routines, using positive self-talk, and engaging in self-soothing activities. When using this intervention with young children, they may practice coping along with the character. For example, when the character learns a deep breathing exercise, the interventionist can have the audience breathe along with him or her. Extensions of the puppet show might demonstrate the character experiencing trauma reminders. Perhaps something makes a loud noise similar to what was heard during the disaster. The character and the children might then practice positive self-talk together.

In another activity, "Go Fishing for Coping Skills," the interventionist prepares paper cards similar to those used in the classic game of Go Fish. In the coping version, instead of matching colors, the children will match skills (e.g., players ask whether their playmates have a "play or do something fun" card). Both adaptive (e.g., deep breathing, talking to a friend, planning a pleasurable activity, positive imagery) and maladaptive (e.g., hitting, hiding, engaging in destructive activities, focusing on how bad things seem) coping skills are pictured and written on each "fish." Adaptive skills have matches, but maladaptive skills do not and must therefore be discarded. When a child selects a coping skill, the interventionist asks him or her, "Will that make you feel better or worse?" With each adaptive coping strategy that is selected, the child is encouraged to describe how that coping strategy can be individualized for him or her and successfully implemented.

Correcting Cognitive Distortions and Misattributions

Young children are susceptible to misunderstandings about the nature and causes of traumatic events (Shelby, 2000); therefore, interventions designed to correct cognitive distortions are commonly needed after disasters. An informational puppet show can be effective in providing corrective information, normalizing responses, and universalizing children's reactions regarding the disaster. After information has been collected regarding the child's misconceptions, these distortions are incorporated into the puppet show. In the dramatization, for example, one puppet is an older, wise character, while the rest are children who, like those in the audience, have many questions. The child puppets then ask each other—without answering—their many questions, including those with cognitive distortions and misattributions. Finally, one of the young puppets suggests that they take their questions to the wise elder. The elder should be sure to explain that it is normal to have questions and that most children have similar ones. Examples of questions that some puppets can ask include "Will I ever be able to sleep at night again?" or "Will things ever be back to normal?" and "Is it my fault?" Finally, the elder puppet provides factual information and clarification of the puppets' questions. When the show is over, the children in the audience may be given the opportunity to play the role of one of the child puppets and ask questions of their own.

When tailoring the puppet show to address misattributions particular to a specific culture or subculture, the range of misattributions can vary widely. For example, in one village in Sri Lanka, many children believed the tsunami was caused by sea snakes who wanted to drink the coconut milk. The puppet show was altered to include questions about reptiles and tropical fruit.

Skills to Decrease Hyperarousal and Panic Symptoms

Relaxation skills training posttrauma is a widely advocated intervention (see La Greca & Prinstein, 2002 and Watson & Shalev, 2005 for reviews) that can empower survivors to manage panic and hyperarousal symptoms. One example is diaphragmatic breathing (belly breathing), which is a quick, simple intervention to counteract the onset of panic symptoms. This can be coupled with positive imagery, which involves having the survivor visualize scenes that elicit positive feelings or relaxation in him or her. The interventionist may lead the child in imagining him- or herself in a favorite place with time spent focusing on the images, smells, sounds, and other sensations related to it. Although this intervention is best suited for children in middle childhood and older, younger children with symptoms of hyperarousal (e.g., frequent crying or anger spells) can be helped to relax with adult-delivered soothing sessions (Shelby & Felix, 2005; Shelby, 2000), which may be scheduled several times throughout the day. During this special time, the adult engages in all of the child's favorite relaxing activities (e.g., rocking, singing, dimming the lights, bathing, storytelling, giving young children something to suck). Massage might also be included in the soothing session if the young child enjoys the activity (Field, Seligman, Scafidi, & Schanberg, 1996) given its myriad benefits to anxious and depressed children. To make the soothing sessions more effective, it is important for the caregiver first to identify, based on each child's individual needs, environments and soothing activities suitable for the young survivor.

Another method of intervention involves creating an individualized soothing menu that incorporates all of the senses and cues children to use their relaxation skills. In this activity, children can create a menu of images, smells, touches, tastes, and sounds that make them feel calm, relaxed, and happy. For example, the interventionist can lead the child to identify three things she can visualize that will help her relax or feel positive, then three things she can imagine smelling that make her feel calm and happy, and so on until an individualized menu of soothing activities that incorporate all five senses is developed. When possible, the identified items should involve both something imagined (e.g., a long-wanted pet, or a food item not readily available) and something real (e.g., looking at something blue, smelling mother's scarf, or touching a soft item of clothing) to provide dual avenues of coping tools.

Managing Intrusive Reexperiencing

Flashbacks, nightmares, repetitive trauma-related play, and other forms of intrusive reexperiencing have long been thought to result from physiological attempts to organize and integrate the trauma experience (Horowitz, 1976). Providing concrete coping skills for these symptoms can empower survivors in situations in which they are reexperiencing the traumatic event. Physical activities may be particularly well suited for young survivors because they can more readily engage in play and movement than in more verbal methods of intervention. One coping activity involves having the child actively take control of his or her intrusive memories. A metaphor of a television show, a radio station, or a tape/CD player is used with the child. Care is taken to ensure that the metaphor is appropriate for the child's economic, cultural, and social context: in cultures without televisions, a radio may be more familiar. The interventionist describes how it is to be watching or listening to a show only to have it interrupted with static, a broken tape, or the emergency broadcasting network. Many children have a similar experience allowing them to relate to the frustration of an interrupted program. For example, when asked what they can do when a favorite radio show is interrupted by static, most children can articulate or agree that changing the channel would allow them to feel better. So the interventionist helps the survivor think of ways to "change the channel" when the intrusive memory occurs. To facilitate this activity, the interventionist and child might draw the television or radio and attach various positive images to the drawing to replace unwanted images.

Identifying and Building Social Support

Following a trauma, early social support facilitates recovery from traumatic stress (Watson & Shalev, 2005). In fact, a child's ability to seek out and receive social support is among the greatest indicators of effective recovery (Norris et al., 2001; Watson & Shalev, 2005). Social support of all types helps children by reducing the risk of depression and anxiety (Ostrander, Weinfurt, & Nay, 1998; White, Bruce, Farrell, & Kliewer, 1998), improving social skills (Demaray & Elliott, 2001; Malecki & Elliott, 1999), and enhancing academic performance (Richman, Rosenfeld, & Bowen, 1998). When entire communities are affected, such as in large-scale disasters, less social support may be available to help with the recovery process because all community members are coping with loss and destruction (Silverman & La Greca, 2002). Particularly following massive disasters, it is vital to enhance a child's ability to identify multiple sources from which to obtain various kinds of support (e.g., emotional, instrumental, informational; Tardy, 1985). The interventionist should take steps to ensure that children and their families know about available resources to meet their social support needs (e.g., "Who do you go to if you feel sad or scared? When you need a hug, something to eat, someone to talk to, someone to play with, someone to help with homework, etc.?"). If a child cannot identify anyone, or if members of his or her usual support system have not survived, the interventionist should take steps to identify alternative individuals who are available to the child for social support (Saltzman, Layne, & Pynoos, 2003). These individuals might include older children, shelter workers, teachers, or clergy. The child may then role-play with the interventionist how to solicit social support from the identified persons. In Sri Lanka, one popular activity designed to help young survivors identify sources of social support involved having them write the names of potential sources of social support on wooden beads, string them, and wear them as social support necklaces. In a similar activity, children traced their hands on paper and wrote the names or drew the faces of people on each finger to whom they could turn for support.

Restoring Developmentally Appropriate Activities

Following a significant trauma, it is common for children to regress developmentally from previously mastered skills (NCCTS, 2005). Therefore, it is important for children to regain developmentally appropriate opportunities so that they can return to the adaptive behaviors and activities typical for their age and developmental level. Activities designed to identify and return to normal daily routines are helpful to children. Even if schools or places of worship have been destroyed, an interventionist should seek to promote a return to the daily structure that existed before the disaster (Vernberg, 2002). This includes restoring to the extent possible getting ready for the day, playtime, study time, or family time. It is also helpful to assist children and caregivers in planning pleasurable activities so that they can feel positive anticipation for future events. In Sri Lanka, children were yearning to play soccer, dance, sing, and play with balloons or bubbles, despite their dire circumstances. Their play brought smiles not only to the faces of the children, but also to the adult survivors.

Maintaining Hope for the Future

In our experiences in many parts of the world, one of the most powerful early intervention tools to promote resilience and healthy recovery is helping survivors regain and hold positive images about their future and that of their community. Being surrounded daily by the devastation following a disaster, compounded by the possibility of slow or delayed reconstruction efforts, can take a toll on a survivor's emotional and psychological well-being. Therefore, engaging children in role-play activities of the rebuilding effort can not only improve their sense of mastery over their environment, but also help them create and hold specific, hopeful images of the future. The interventionist leads this activity by gathering groups of children and stating, "Something bad has happened to your village (town, school, etc.)." He or she proceeds, "Well, today you have the power to do something about it. Today, we can pretend to rebuild your village." As the interventionists encourage them, the children typically express enthusiasm, and "rebuilding" efforts begin. Adults can lead them to gather resources from their natural environment to use to role-play the rebuilding effort. In posttsunami Sri Lanka, children excitedly rebuilt their "homes" with strong, protective stone walls. They created schools, temples, and community gardens with paths connecting homes to community buildings. They created wells and water purification systems for their villages and included tsunami warning systems. The children smiled and took great pride in showing their rebuilt homes with beautiful gardens to the interventionists and other adults. Adults from the entire village gathered to watch the children rebuild. Many seemed to take pride in the children's play construction activities. Following the completion of the village, pictures of the children with their village were taken and left with them as reminders of their rebuilding efforts.

Parental/Caregiver Involvement in Child Recovery

One of the greatest indicators for children's posttraumatic recovery is caregiver involvement (Cohen & Mannarino, 1996, 1997, 1998; Norris et al., 2001). It is crucial for the therapist to seek to engage parents or caregivers in intervention efforts (Norris et al., 2001). A primary focus should be to educate parents about stress reactions. Adults may not realize the level to which children are distressed and underestimate their problems (Silverman & La Greca, 2002). Children may also shield their parents from information that may be distressing to the parents (Yule & Williams, 1990).

A primary goal of parental/caretaker intervention is to help parents or caretakers promote recovery in their child(ren). Psychoeducation with the parent/caregiver includes normalization about responses to traumatic events. An emphasis should be placed on refraining from shaming or punishing a child for having posttraumatic symptoms. For example, some parents need to be reminded that loss of a previously acquired skill (e.g., enuresis, clinginess, or crying) is common following disasters and that normal functioning usually returns (NCCTS, 2005).

Enhancing parents' ability to address their children's stress reactions can also be a helpful way of alerting them to issues of which they might not have previously been aware. Parents may be interested in learning about soothing techniques, including addressing their children's nightmares or flashbacks, and may benefit from tips on how to discuss the event with their children. Here, an emphasis should be placed upon actions that parents or others are taking to increase safety, including being prepared in the case of a similar emergency (La Greca & Prinstein, 2002; Shelby, 2000). Helping a parent offer realistic reassurances (e.g., "I will do everything I can to keep you safe," or "We will build a much stronger house than we had before") of safety to a child can help the child regain a sense of safety.

When possible, an interventionist should engage parents in interventions and games that will be played with the children. In fact, all of the activities described above can be modified to include parents or caregivers. Although attaining parental participation may be difficult, particularly in places where adults do not typically play with children, it is critical to the child's posttraumatic adjustment and recovery to involve the caretaker as much as possible (e.g., Norris et al., 2001). Providing psycho-educational information to parents in naturally occurring settings, such as while they are standing in line to receive humanitarian assistance, can help to involve parents who might otherwise be disinterested or avoid psychosocial interventions. Also, providing media interviews (particularly radio), disseminating informational literature, and directly offering assistance to parents for their own material needs are all possible methods of informing caregivers.

INTERVENTIONISTS

Although often overlooked, the interventionist may well be the most important part of the relief effort. Below, several aspects of the interventionist's experience are discussed. Skills, training, and responsibilities of the interventionist are explored, with recommendations for training disaster mental health workers, then factors related to the interventionist's health and emotional resiliency are discussed. Practical tips for success in the field are described, and a discussion of job-related stress and reentry into the interventionist's normal routine closes the chapter.

Skills, Training, and Responsibilities of the Interventionist

To maximize the likelihood of a positive intervention effect, the interventionist is ideally a highly trained mental health professional with training and experience in evidence-based trauma interventions. The ideal interventionist keeps abreast of the latest findings in the disaster, trauma, and child mental health fields given the large responsibility of training other professionals who often have less access to contemporary research findings. Thus, the interventionist must be knowledgeable about the most empirically and ethically sound intervention tools available, coupled with clinical experience and sound judgment. Under ideal circumstances, the interventionist is licensed in a mental health field (and thus, does not require on-site supervision) and able to demonstrate knowledge of a variety of individual and group activities that seek to achieve the goals of the mission. This includes an ability to deliver services with an understanding of both potential benefits and iatrogenic effects (Weine et al., 2002). A full grasp of the principles of cultural sensitivity is crucial (Watson &

Shalev, 2005), as international disaster relief contains issues and experiences not normally encountered in common clinical settings. Finally, the interventionist or the sponsor organization must ensure that adequate follow-up with host-country interventionists or survivors takes place. A host of psychological issues arise during the recovery period, and those who introduce interventions to survivors also have a responsibility to maintain relations with the appropriate agencies to ensure that the interventions are being used appropriately and effectively (Weine et al., 2002). In addition to the training typically required as part of the interventionist's discipline, care should be taken to adequately prepare interventionists to perform interventions in the unique setting of disaster relief work. The training should include (1) evidence-based or evidence-informed interventions, (2) the role of the interventionist (e.g., play activities versus crisis intervention versus psychotherapy), (3) methods to adapt and modify interventions to meet special circumstances (e.g., large groups, timid children, little access to caretakers), and (4) chain of supervisory command.

Health and Emotional Resiliency

An international volunteer who works in primitive conditions should be of good physical health and strong emotional resiliency. Field conditions are usually severe. The stress on the body can begin with long flights, lengthy land travel, or primitive sea travel necessary to reach remote areas of need. Work in developing countries may take place over a variety of terrains, including places inaccessible by roads. Moreover, the volunteer should possess an accurate ability to assess his or her physical and mental health status. Therapists with limited mobility or physical fitness should accurately describe their limitations to the humanitarian aid organization prior to departure to be sure that their circumstances will not hinder their work or the work of the team. On several relief missions, the authors have encountered well-intentioned volunteers who had not accurately predicted the dire physical conditions, climate, or grueling work circumstances of the mission. Occasionally, a volunteer's health was jeopardized. More typically, the relief team or organization was frustrated by the mismatch between the volunteer and the demands of the work.

It is also important to research and receive appropriate vaccinations and prophylactic measures before volunteering (see the Centers for Disease Control and Prevention website, www.cdc.gov). Wearing protective clothing, using insect repellent, and knowing about water safety are all important considerations for international disaster relief work. Similarly, knowledge of local foods can help those with special dietary needs anticipate what conditions they will face.

Interventionists should also consider that some accepted forms of behavior or physical presentation in Western countries may not be acceptable. Smoking is a cultural taboo in some countries, especially for women, and care should be taken to minimize withdrawal symptoms while on assignment if this is a concern. Similarly, some forms of body art (e.g., piercings, tattoos) may not be acceptable in the host country. Though individuality may be celebrated in the United States, it is best to conform to local customs when possible for the sake of the work.

Practical Tips

When working with populations that are unfamiliar to the interventionist, it is important to monitor the use of self in the environment. For example, an interventionist with an interpersonal style that is gregarious and flamboyant may not be received well in some cultures, whereas one with an interpersonal style more subdued and timid may not be received well in another culture. It is important to be mindful of the fact that survivors may be confused or put off by behaviors that are uncharacteristic of their behavioral customs. Assessing and matching levels of emotionality, articulation, and opinion sharing is an important disaster mental health skill. Equally important is the selection of toys and activities; one must ensure that they are positive, or at least benign, to the host region. The dress or shapeliness of some dolls, for example, may be too provocative in some cultures. Sports equipment, especially balls used in the host country's most popular sport (e.g., soccer, baseball, or basketball), is always popular. At times, toys may be altogether unobtainable. If this is the case, the interventionist should be creative, making use of items found in nature. Some interventions may not work as planned; therefore, it is important for an interventionist to be prepared to modify an intervention with little notice. New information about a religious belief may be uncovered that makes it inappropriate for interventionists to employ the intervention in the way planned (e.g., decrease fears of ghosts when ghosts serve an important cultural function). Likewise, it helps to integrate local behavioral norms and practices when possible and to resist adhering rigidly to any intervention that does not appear to be working.

Nontrainable Factors

There are a number of personality characteristics that an interventionist should possess in order to contribute most effectively to disaster relief, especially when working on a team. Among these, flexibility and ingenuity are essential. Disaster work, by its nature, tends to be chaotic, especially in developing nations. In disaster relief work, parameters and mission objectives change constantly as new information becomes available to relief organizations. Therefore, the interventionist may be called upon to perform unanticipated tasks with little notice. Whereas a less flexible interventionist may feel frustrated, angry, or overwhelmed, the flexible interventionist anticipates such conditions and quickly incorporates the new information into intervention plans. It may be necessary to alter planned interventions to be more appropriate for a wider audience than initially realized. For example, in Sri Lanka, two groups of interventionists were deployed, each to a different region. In both cases, the number of children present in the mass care settings had been grossly underestimated. The first group of interventionists quickly and effectively converted their prearranged activities to puppet shows, large-group games, and activity stations while retaining the original objectives of the techniques, whereas the second group of therapists abandoned the prearranged interventions altogether without attempting to adapt them for their large group. The first group received accolades from the host agency and provided evidence-informed interventions to the survivors. The second group was less creative in adapting the interventions to the large group and instead opted to spend time in unstructured play activities with the children, who haphazardly received interventions related to the tsunami. In contrast to the first group, this group was described by the host organization as having little structure and providing less benefit to the children.

As can be seen from the example, international interventionists are called upon to adjust quickly to changing needs, resources, or instructions. Likewise, it is important that the interventionist understand the importance of following the established chain of command within the relief organization he or she is serving. Many mental health professionals are accustomed to being leaders and having professional independence; however, due to safety concerns and the rapidity of altered plans, protocols, local circumstances, and resources, it is imperative that interventionists follow the directives of their superiors in the organization.

Although it is not often discussed, it is necessary to emphasize the importance of self-awareness and group cohesion with members of a relief mission. Interventionists should be encouraged to be aware of and engage in discussion with team members regarding their interactions and functioning within the group. The intensity and nature of the work can promote a deep sense of personal fulfillment and growth. Under ideal circumstances, relief workers gain an enriched understanding of themselves as they work alongside and elicit feedback from their fellow team members.

Compassion Fatigue and Reentry

Therapists who are more susceptible to vicarious stress should be warned that disaster tends to be a trigger that may bring the interventionist's own reactions to the surface. Graphic scenes and stories are often described, which can lead the interventionist to experience profound sadness upon exposure to the harsh reality of the survivors. Emotional fatigue can set in quickly when so much is asked of someone in such a concentrated manner. The interventionist may find it difficult to focus on the successes of the mission in the face of massive devastation. Taking time for physical and emotional self-care (Weine et al., 2002), as well as holding debriefing experiences with other members of the relief effort can be important to sustain even experienced relief workers. On the other hand, many workers report their disaster relief experiences as some of the most precious of their lives. When the interventionist is appropriately prepared, the privilege of bearing witness to the suffering and recovery of others can be deeply moving.

Volunteers can also experience stress upon reentry to their home country. Often, more time and mental energy is spent on preparing for the relief operation than on preparing for the reentry process. It is common for relief workers to experience the routine of their normal lives as mundane in contrast to the intensity of the work they performed in the field. Following our relief trip to Sri Lanka, many of the mental health volunteers reported irritability, difficulty concentrating, increased emotionality, and feeling as if their heart was still in Sri Lanka. Volunteers, as is common for many relief workers, questioned the strength and longevity of their impact in the face of such massive devastation. As time passed, reactions shifted toward focusing on the value of the work that was done. Some volunteers found value in continuing to assist with the ongoing relief efforts, such as giving presentations on needs and recruiting donations, others returned to Sri Lanka, and yet others used their experiences to cultivate their clinical interests and skills. Thus, the affect of the work continues to manifest.

CONCLUSION

Disaster relief work is certainly challenging, but it can also be an incredibly rewarding experience for volunteers. Many developing countries are not able to provide this type of specialized service to their young survivors, making foreign mental health specialists a welcomed and extremely appreciated resource. Effectively contributing to the psychosocial well-being of children in the aftermath of a disaster not only assists on the individual level, but can help the rehabilitation efforts of entire communities. Just as it is necessary to have skilled laborers for the reconstruction effort, it may be considered equally imperative to have capable interventionists with adequate preparation, motivation, and strength of character to aid emotional recovery. When implemented effectively, this type of service has the potential to leave a lasting effect on the children who receive it and can do the same for the individuals who provide it.

ACKNOWLEDGMENTS

We would like to thank Operation USA, a nongovernmental organization committed to providing needed relief services around the world, for sponsoring our psychosocial rehabilitation efforts in Sri Lanka. Their commitment, guidance, and vision helped make this volunteer trip a success.

REFERENCES

Cohen, J. A., & Mannarino, A. P. (1996). A treatment outcome study for sexually abused preschool children: Initial findings. *Journal of the American Academy of Child and Adolescent Psychiatry, 35*, 42–50.

Cohen, J. A., & Mannarino, A. P. (1997). A treatment study for sexually abused preschool children: Outcome during a 1-year follow-up. *Journal of the American Academy of Child and Adolescent Psychiatry, 36*, 1228–1235.

Cohen, J. A., & Mannarino, A. P. (1998). Interventions for sexually abused children: Initial treatment outcome findings. *Child Maltreatment, 3*, 17–26.

Demaray, M. K., & Elliott, S. N. (2001). Perceived social support by children with characteristics of attention-deficit/hyperactivity disorder. *School Psychology Quarterly, 16*, 68–90.

Field, T., Seligman, S., Scafidi, F., & Schanberg, S. (1996). Alleviating posttraumatic stress in children following Hurricane Andrew. *Journal of Applied Developmental Psychology, 17*, 37–50.

Horowitz, M. J. (1976). *Stress response syndromes*. New York: Aronson.

Jacobs, G. A. (1995). The development of a national plan for disaster mental health. *Professional Psychology: Research and Practice, 26,* 543–549.

La Greca, A., & Prinstein, M. J. (2002). Hurricanes and earthquakes. In A. M. La Greca, W. K. Silverman, E. M. Vernberg, & M. C. Roberts (Eds.), *Helping children cope with disasters and terrorism* (pp. 55–72). Washington, DC: American Psychological Association.

Lindemann, E. (1944). Symptomatology and management of acute grief. *American Journal of Psychiatry, 101,* 141–148.

Malecki, C. K., & Elliott, S. N. (1999). Adolescents' ratings of perceived social support and its importance: Validation of the Student Social Support Scale. *Psychology in the Schools, 36,* 473–483.

National Center for Child Traumatic Stress (NCCTS). (2005). Psychological impact of the tsunami across the Indian rim. Retrieved January 21, 2005, from www.NCTSNet.org

Norris, F. H., Byrne, C. M., Diaz, E., & Kaniasty, K. (2001). 50,000 disaster victims speak: An empirical review of the empirical literature, 1981–2001. Retrieved April 5, 2005, from www.istss.org/terrorism/victims_speak.htm

Ostrander, R., Weinfurt, K. P., & Nay, W. R. (1998). The role of age, family support, and negative cognitions in the prediction of depressive symptoms. *School Psychology Review, 27,* 121–137.

Reyes, G., & Elhai, J. D. (2004). Psychosocial interventions in the early phases of disasters. *Psychotherapy: Theory, Research, Practice, Training, 41,* 399–411.

Richman, J. M., Rosenfeld, L. B., & Bowen, G. L. (1998). Social support for adolescents at risk of school failure. *Social Work, 43,* 309–323.

Saltzman, W. R., Layne, C. M., & Pynoos, R. S. (2003). *Trauma/grief-focused group psychotherapy manual for adolescents.* Unpublished treatment manual, University of California, Los Angeles.

Shelby, J. S. (2000). Brief therapy with traumatized children: A developmental perspective. In H. Kaduson & C. Schaefer (Eds.), *Short-term play interventions* (pp. 69–104). New York: Guilford Press.

Shelby, J. S., & Felix, E. D. (2005). Posttraumatic play therapy: The need for an integrated model of directive and non-directive approaches. In L. Reddy & C. Schaefer (Eds.), *Empirically based play interventions for children* (pp. 79–104). Washington, DC: American Psychological Association Press.

Silverman, W. K., & La Greca, A. M. (2002). Children experiencing disasters: Definitions, reactions, and predictors of outcomes. In A. M. La Greca, W. K. Silverman, E. M. Vernberg, & M. C. Roberts (Eds.), *Helping children cope with disasters and terrorism* (pp. 11–33). Washington, DC: American Psychological Association.

Tardy, C. (1985). Social support measurement. *American Journal of Community Psychology, 13,* 187–202.

Vernberg, E. M. (2002). Intervention approaches following disasters. In A. M. La Greca, W. K. Silverman, E. M. Vernberg, & M. C. Roberts (Eds.), *Helping children cope with disasters and terrorism* (pp. 55–72). Washington, DC: American Psychological Association.

Watson, P. J., & Shalev, A. Y. (2005). Assessment and treatment of adult acute responses to traumatic stress following mass traumatic events. *CNS Spectrums, 10*(2), 123–131.

Weine, S., Danieli, Y., Silove, D., Van Ommeren, M., Fairbank, J. A., & Saul, J. (2002). Guidelines for international training in mental health and psychosocial interventions for trauma exposed populations in clinical and community settings. *Psychiatry, 65,* 156–164.

White, K. S., Bruce, S. E., Farrell, A. D., & Kliewer, W. (1998). Impact of exposure to community violence on anxiety: A longitudinal study of family social support as a protective factor for urban children. *Journal of Child and Family Studies, 7,* 187–203.

Yule, W., & Williams, R. M. (1990). Post-traumatic stress reactions in children. *Journal of Traumatic Stress, 3,* 279–295.

Index

"n" following a page number indicates a note.